T0182120

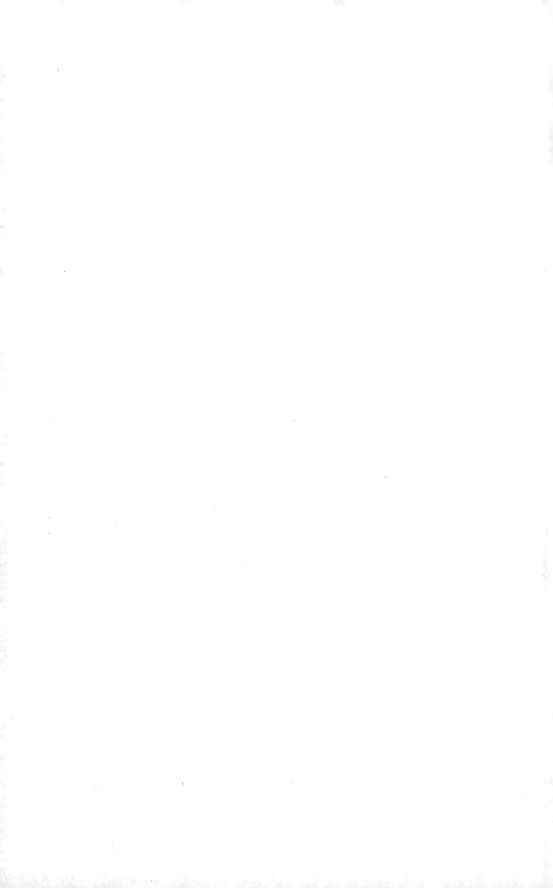

Multivariate Analysis of Ecological Data with ade4

Jean Thioulouse • Stéphane Dray
Anne-Béatrice Dufour • Aurélie Siberchicot
Thibaut Jombart • Sandrine Pavoine

Multivariate Analysis of Ecological Data with ade4

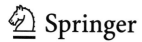 Springer

Jean Thioulouse
Laboratoire de Biométrie
et Biologie Evolutive
CNRS UMR 5558 – Université de Lyon
Villeurbanne, France

Stéphane Dray
Laboratoire de Biométrie
et Biologie Evolutive
CNRS UMR 5558 – Université de Lyon
Villeurbanne, France

Anne-Béatrice Dufour
Laboratoire de Biométrie
et Biologie Evolutive
CNRS UMR 5558 – Université de Lyon
Villeurbanne, France

Aurélie Siberchicot
Laboratoire de Biométrie
et Biologie Evolutive
CNRS UMR 5558 – Université de Lyon
Villeurbanne, France

Thibaut Jombart
Department of Infectious
Disease Epidemiology
London School of Hygiene
and Tropical Medicine
London, UK

Sandrine Pavoine
Centre d'Ecologie et des Sciences
de la Conservation (CESCO)
Muséum national d'Histoire naturelle,
CNRS, Sorbonne Université
Paris, France

ISBN 978-1-4939-9402-1   ISBN 978-1-4939-8850-1   (eBook)
https://doi.org/10.1007/978-1-4939-8850-1

This Springer imprint is published by the registered company Springer Science+Business Media, LLC
part of Springer Nature.
The registered company address is: 233 Spring Street, New York, NY 10013, U.S.A.

Foreword

« Les programmes sont des objets scientifiques bizarres : les uns y cachent la compréhension mathématique des modèles qui les supportent, les autres en font des objets expérimentaux. Lieu par excellence d'échanges et de conflits, d'appropriation souhaitable ou abusive, produit sans auteur présumé pour les camelots de la démonstration (lesquels programment rarement) ou objet largement surestimé, sa valeur dépend du moment et de l'environnement. Il faut concilier deux logiques, celle de l'utilisateur et celle du statisticien. Notons à ce propos qu'on peut militer pour la libre circulation des programmes ou (exclusif) des données : il faut rassurer tout le monde. Image d'une méthode pour celui qui l'écrit, le programme change de nature pour celui qui l'emploie, image d'une problématique pour celui qui l'acquiert, les données changent de nature quand elles servent d'illustration. La libre circulation des données et des programmes est un facteur décisif du développement : une seule chose est inconcevable, c'est qu'il n'y ait qu'un seul point de vue sur ces objets. »

Daniel Chessel, 1992

Contents

Chapter 1
Introduction

Abstract This introductory chapter presents the intended readership of the book and a short history of the **ade4** software. It also describes the associated packages of the **ade4** family and how to install and use these packages with **R**. Lastly, we provide a short presentation of the types of ecological data sets found in real case studies.

1.1 Intended Readership

Multivariate data analysis methods are not restricted to any particular application field: they have been used in many scientific domains. However, because of the background of its authors, **ade4** has always been more particularly intended for biologists, especially in the field of Ecology. The subject area analysis of the list of scientific papers citing the three **ade4** references (Thioulouse et al. 1997; Dray and Dufour 2007; Thioulouse and Dray 2007) highlights this trend (Fig. 1.1, source: ISI Web of Knowledge).

Researchers and students in ecological fields are therefore potentially interested in using multivariate analysis methods, and this book was primarily written for them. Other areas with fewer citations include, for example, Tropical Medicine, Physics Particles and Fields, Spectroscopy, Sociology and Literature. Researchers in these areas can also be interested in this book, but the examples used throughout the text come from ecological case studies.

Multivariate data analysis methods are particularly useful to analyse large data sets, for example tens or hundreds of variables measured on hundreds or thousands of samples. The synthetic properties of these methods are really helpful in this case. When fewer parameters and/or samples are available, other methods should be considered. Today, molecular biology methods provide huge data sets belonging to almost any biology area, that can be analysed very effectively with multivariate analysis methods.

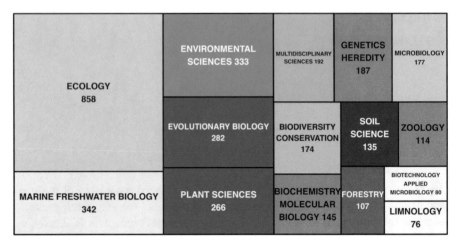

Fig. 1.1 Number of citations of the three **ade4** papers by ISI research area (top 15 research areas). The total number of citations reaches 2655 in March 2018. This figure is created with the **treemap** package (Tennekes 2017).

1.2 Evolutions of ade4

1.2.1 The ade4 Add-On Package for R

The current version of **ade4** is an add-on package for the **R** software. This has important consequences for the user: you need to install **R** on your computer and learn to handle it before you can start using **ade4**. But it also has many advantages: learning to deal with **R** will be valuable beyond the use of **ade4**, as all the common statistical computations needed by biologists can be performed with **R**.

There is also an easy-to-use Graphical User Interface (GUI) implemented in the **ade4TkGUI** add-on package (Thioulouse and Dray 2007, see Appendix B). This GUI can facilitate the transition from previous versions of **ade4** to the **R** package, or help beginners start to use **R** and **ade4**.

Another advantage is the fact that **R** is a multi-platform software. This means that it runs on Windows, Mac and many Unix-like platforms, with optimised performances. Multi-platform compatibility also includes datafile format. You can, for example, start computations on one computer (say a Windows PC) and save the results in the `.RData` file created at the end of the work session. You can then copy this `.RData` file to another computer (including a Mac or Linux PC) and continue computations without problem. The `.RData` file can even be stored on a network file server and used through the network on a Linux, Mac or Windows computer.

The first version of the **ade4** package was submitted to CRAN in late 2002. It has kept evolving since that time, many functions have been added and several "spin-off" packages have appeared. The current version of the **ade4** package is number 1.7–11. It comprises 225 functions and 108 data sets.

1.2.2 Previous Versions of ade4

Previous versions of **ade4** date back to the early 1980s. Their evolution was cyclic, with periods of intense development that were needed to catch up with the fast evolution of operating systems and computer hardware. These periods were followed by several years of distribution of a stable version, during which the evolution was limited to the addition of new statistical or graphical methods.

Everything started from a small set of programs written in BASIC on the Data General Nova 3 minicomputer of the Biometry Lab (Lyon 1 University, France). The first move occurred in 1985: a diagonalisation procedure in assembly language was written for the Eclipse S/140 that had replaced the Nova. This procedure allowed to compute the eigenvalues and eigenvectors of a matrix in a reasonable time, and this made possible using multivariate data analysis methods interactively on real-size ecological data sets.

In the late 1980s, the Eclipse was discontinued and we switched from Data General to the new Apple Macintosh microcomputer. We ported the programs to Microsoft QuickBasic, and added a HyperCard interface. The first version of this new setup was called ADECO and its distribution started in 1989.

ADECO developed into ADE-3.7 in 1994, but it was still written in QuickBasic, which had been abandoned by Microsoft at that time. So in the mid-1990s, we switched again and started a new version, called ADE-4, completely re-written in C. This allowed us to propose a multi-platform solution in 1995, using a HyperCard user interface on Macintosh, and WinPlus on Windows PC.

A few years later, we decided to start teaching S-Plus to Master's students. Courses began in 1999, but we eventually switched to **R** in 2001. After a few months of hesitation, we started working on the **R** version of the new **ade4** package in early 2002, and submitted ade4-1.0 to CRAN in December 2002. Since that date, **ade4** stands for "Analysis of Ecological Data: Exploratory and Euclidean Methods in Environmental Sciences".

All these developments, during almost 40 years, were the fruit of the work of many people. Only a few are cited here, please forgive inconsistencies, errors or omissions. The first Basic programs were written by (among others) Jean-Dominique Lebreton, Daniel Chessel and Jean Thioulouse. A little while later, the ADECO software benefited from the help of Sylvain Dolédec and Jean-Michel Olivier. During the 1980s and 1990s, many other people contributed to the work, including Yves Auda, Stéphane Champely, François Chevenet, James Devillers, Mohamed Hanafi, Yves Lasne, Monique Simier, Claire Boisson. The ADE-4 development was financially supported by several contracts with the French Ministry of Environnement and the National Center for Scientific Research (CNRS). Alain Pavé, Richard Tomassone, Christian Gautier, Claude Amoros, Bernhard Statzner and Bernard Hugueny helped keep the boat afloat.

The **R** add-on package (**ade4**) started a new area, with many new contributors, among them Stéphane Dray, Anne-Béatrice Dufour, Aurélie Siberchicot, Jean

Lobry, Sandrine Pavoine, Clément Callenge, Thibaut Jombart, Sébastien Ollier. The recent switch to GitHub introduced a new open development model (svn/git) and new contributors:

> https://github.com/sdray/ade4/graphs/contributors

1.3 Using ade4

1.3.1 Computer Hardware

Any microcomputer sold today is sufficient to perform most ecological data analysis tasks. Even small laptops and netbooks have enough computing power to do a Principal Component Analysis (PCA) on a large ecological data table. Only a few computing-intensive tasks like permutation tests on large tables can necessitate a more powerful desktop workstation with a faster CPU.

The size of the disk and of the main memory of mainstream microcomputers is more than enough for almost any data analysis problem. Even large DNA fingerprint, microarray or even metagenomic data table will easily fit. Data tables with thousands of rows and columns can be analysed without problem.

1.3.2 Installing R

The first step to start using **ade4** is to install **R**. The **R** project homepage is here:

> https://www.r-project.org/

and precompiled binary distributions are available for the main operating systems (Linux, Windows, Mac). A list of international mirrors can be used to choose the nearest source:

> https://cran.r-project.org/mirrors.html

Instructions on how to download, install and run **R** can be found on all the mirrors. It is advisable to use the most recent version of the **R** software. Use the `sessionInfo()` function to get information about the current version of **R** and of attached or loaded packages.

1.3.3 Installing ade4

After installing **R**, you need to install the **ade4** package. The easiest way to do this is to launch **R** and type the following command:

```
install.packages("ade4")
```

This is to be done only once. After package installation, you must load the package with the following command:

```
library(ade4)
```

This must be redone each time **R** is launched, but it can be automated by placing the `library` command in the `.Rprofile` file. See the Startup documentation in **R** for more information about this:

```
help("Startup")
```

This documentation page is very important and explains many things about the **R** startup mechanism.

The latest development versions of **ade4** are available on GitHub:

https://github.com/sdray/ade4

The development version of **ade4** can be easily installed using the functionality provided by the **devtools** package (Wickham et al. 2018):

```
library(devtools)
install_github("sdray/ade4")
```

1.3.4   Dependencies

Using advanced features of the **ade4** package can necessitate the use of other **R** packages (called *dependencies*). You can install all the dependencies (i.e., all the packages potentially needed by **ade4**) at once by using the following install command:

```
install.packages("ade4", dependencies = TRUE)
```

This will download many other packages and can take some time, depending on your internet connection speed.

1.3.5   Packages of the ade4 Family

Since the first release of **ade4** on CRAN, several associated packages have been developed. These packages improve or extend the original functionalities of **ade4**:

- **adegraphics**: An S4 Lattice-Based Package for the Representation of Multivariate Data
- **ade4TkGUI**: Tcl/Tk Graphical User Interface
- **adespatial**: Multivariate Multiscale Spatial Analysis
- **adephylo**: Exploratory Analyses for the Phylogenetic Comparative Method

- **adegenet**: Exploratory Analysis of Genetic and Genomic Data
- **adehabitat(HR/HS/LT/MA)**: Analysis of Habitat Selection by Animals
- **adiv**: Analysis of Diversity

Some chapters of this book also require the use of packages **adegraphics**, **ade4TkGUI, adespatial** and **adephylo**.

1.3.5.1 adegraphics

The **adegraphics** package (Siberchicot et al. 2017, see Chapter 4) offers a flexible framework to create and manage graphics. It is based on the **lattice** package (Sarkar 2008) and contains the definitions of graphical S4 classes and methods that were previously implemented in **ade4** as plain functions and S3 classes. A full chapter of this book is dedicated to this package (see Chap. 4).

adegraphics is available from CRAN mirrors, and it can be installed and loaded independently from **ade4**. **adegraphics** replaces some former implementations of graphical functions in **ade4**. If both packages should be used, always load **adegraphics** *after* **ade4** to make sure you are using the right version of the functions:

```
install.packages("adegraphics")
library(ade4)
library(adegraphics)
```

adegraphics is distributed with a tutorial vignette which can be accessed using:

```
vignette("adegraphics", package = "adegraphics")
```

The latest development versions of **adegraphics** are available on GitHub:

https://github.com/sdray/adegraphics

1.3.5.2 ade4TkGUI

The **ade4TkGUI** package (Thioulouse and Dray 2007, see Appendix B) provides a graphical user interface for **ade4**. It *depends on* **ade4** and **adegraphics**, which means that these two packages must be installed and that they are automatically loaded when **ade4TkGUI** is loaded. It is also available from CRAN mirrors, and you can install it just like you installed **ade4**:

```
install.packages("ade4TkGUI")
library(ade4TkGUI)
```

The latest development versions of **ade4TkGUI** are available on GitHub:

https://github.com/aursiber/ade4TkGUI

1.3.5.3 adespatial

adespatial (Dray et al. 2018, see Chapter 12) provides tools for the multiscale spatial analysis of multivariate data. Several methods are based on the use of a spatial weighting matrix and its eigenvector decomposition (Moran's Eigenvectors Maps, MEM).

    adespatial is available from CRAN mirrors:

```
install.packages("adespatial")
library(adespatial)
```

    adespatial is distributed with a tutorial vignette which can be accessed using:

```
vignette("tutorial", package = "adespatial")
```

    The latest development versions of **adespatial** are available on GitHub:

> https://github.com/sdray/adespatial

1.3.5.4 adephylo

adephylo (Jombart et al. 2010a, see Chapter 13) has been developed at the interface between packages for exploratory data analysis (**ade4**), phylogenetic reconstruction (**ape**, Paradis et al. 2004) and phylogenetic comparative methods (**phylobase**, R Hackathon et al. 2017). **adephylo** is available from CRAN mirrors:

```
install.packages("adephylo")
library(adephylo)
```

    adephylo replaces some former implementations of phylogenetic comparative methods in **ade4**, which are now deprecated.

    adephylo is distributed with a tutorial vignette which can be accessed using:

```
vignette("adephylo", package = "adephylo")
```

    The latest development versions of **adephylo** are available on GitHub:

> https://github.com/thibautjombart/adephylo

1.3.6 Version of the Packages Used in This Book

The versions of **R** and of the packages that were used to compile this book are given by the sessionInfo function:

```
sessionInfo()
```

```
R version 3.5.0 (2018-04-23)
Platform: x86_64-apple-darwin15.6.0 (64-bit)
Running under: macOS High Sierra 10.13.5
```

```
Matrix products: default
BLAS: /Library/Frameworks/R.framework/Versions/3.5/Resources/lib
    /libRblas.0.dylib
LAPACK: /Library/Frameworks/R.framework/Versions/3.5/Resources
    /lib/libRlapack.dylib

locale:
[1] fr_FR.UTF-8/fr_FR.UTF-8/fr_FR.UTF-8/C/fr_FR.UTF-8/fr_FR.UTF-8

attached base packages:
[1] stats       graphics  grDevices utils       datasets  methods
[7] base

other attached packages:
[1] adephylo_1.1-11    adespatial_0.2-0   adegraphics_1.0-10
[4] ade4_1.7-11        treemap_2.4-2

loaded via a namespace (and not attached):
 [1] Rcpp_0.12.17          ape_5.1              lattice_0.20-35
 [4] tidyr_0.8.1           deldir_0.1-15        gtools_3.5.0
 [7] prettyunits_1.0.2     assertthat_0.2.0     digest_0.6.15
[10] gridBase_0.4-7        mime_0.5             R6_2.2.2
[13] plyr_1.8.4            coda_0.19-1          httr_1.3.1
[16] ggplot2_2.2.1         pillar_1.2.3         rlang_0.2.1
[19] progress_1.1.2        lazyeval_0.2.1       spdep_0.7-7
[22] uuid_0.1-2            adegenet_2.1.1       data.table_1.11.4
[25] gdata_2.18.0          vegan_2.5-2          gmodels_2.16.2
[28] Matrix_1.2-14         RNeXML_2.1.1         splines_3.5.0
[31] stringr_1.3.1         igraph_1.2.1         munsell_0.4.3
[34] shiny_1.1.0           compiler_3.5.0       httpuv_1.4.3
[37] pkgconfig_2.0.1       mgcv_1.8-23          htmltools_0.3.6
[40] tidyselect_0.2.4      expm_0.999-2         tibble_1.4.2
[43] XML_3.98-1.11         permute_0.9-4        dplyr_0.7.5
[46] later_0.7.2           MASS_7.3-50          grid_3.5.0
[49] nlme_3.1-137          spData_0.2.8.3       xtable_1.8-2
[52] gtable_0.2.0          magrittr_1.5         scales_0.5.0
[55] KernSmooth_2.23-15    stringi_1.2.2        reshape2_1.4.3
[58] LearnBayes_2.15.1     promises_1.0.1       bindrcpp_0.2.2
[61] sp_1.3-1              phylobase_0.8.4      latticeExtra_0.6-28
[64] xml2_1.2.0            seqinr_3.4-5         boot_1.3-20
[67] RColorBrewer_1.1-2    tools_3.5.0          rncl_0.8.2
[70] glue_1.2.0            purrr_0.2.5          parallel_3.5.0
[73] colorspace_1.3-2      cluster_2.0.7-1      bindr_0.1.1
```

1.3.7 The adelist Forum

The **ade4** package homepage is here:

> http://pbil.univ-lyon1.fr/ade4/home.php?lang=eng

A public forum and mailing list can be found at this address:

> http://listes.univ-lyon1.fr/wws/info/adelist

This is the place where questions about all aspects of **ade4** and related packages should be asked. All the users of **ade4** should subscribe to this list, at least temporarily. To report problems or errors, you can use the GitHub functionality (e.g., https://github.com/sdray/ade4/issues for **ade4**). Do no forget to quote the result of the sessionInfo function.

1.3.8 Using the Help System

You are now ready to start using the **ade4** package. You can browse through the package documentation using the html interface (see the `help.start` functions). Like in any **R** package, all the functions and data sets have a documentation page, that can be accessed with the `help` command:

```
help("dudi.pca")
```

or

```
?dudi.pca
```

1.4 Interactive Code Snippets

The code snippets used throughout this book are available online. They can be run, modified and checked thanks to the shiny system at the following address:

> http://pbil.univ-lyon1.fr/ADE-4/book.php

1.5 Ecological Data Sets

The structure of ecological data sets can be very complex, but can generally be reduced to simpler forms, compatible with **R** data structures. Figures 1.2 and 1.3 show the main data structures used in ecological data analysis. These structures also correspond to particular data analysis methods in **ade4**.

The most frequent data structure is a rectangular table with samples (sites) as rows and variables as columns (Fig. 1.2A). This structure corresponds to quantitative environmental variable data tables (sites × variables, see Chap. 5), and also to floro-faunistic tables (sites × species, see Chap. 6). It perfectly fits the **R** data frame structure, and can be used directly in the **ade4** package for single-table multivariate analysis methods. The case of qualitative (or categorical) environmental variables also fits well **R** data frames, with columns class set to `factor`. Mixes of quantitative and qualitative variables can also be stored in data frames, since data frame columns can have mixed types.

Another common practice in Ecology is to consider distance matrices. These distances can be either directly measured by ecologists or derived from original raw data (see functions `dist.binary`, `dist.quant`, etc. in **ade4**). Distances are used to describe dissimilarities among individuals such as genetic, morphometric or geographic distances. The analysis of distance matrices (Fig. 1.2B) requires an adequate statistical treatment and some methods are implemented in **ade4** for that purpose (Sect. 6.5). In **R**, distance matrices are stored as objects of class `dist`.

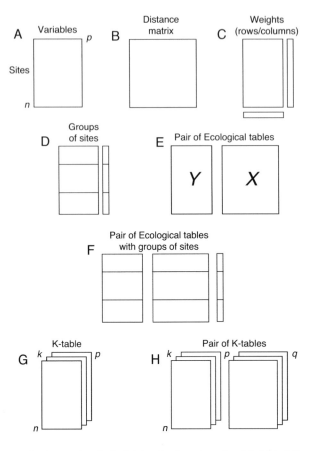

Fig. 1.2 Common structures of ecological data sets. A: rectangular data table (site × environmental variables or site × species), B: distance matrix, C: row and column weights, D: data table with groups of sites, E: pair of ecological tables (X = environmental variables, Y = species data), F: pair of ecological tables with groups of sites, G: *K*-table, H: pair of *K*-tables.

In **ade4**, all the multivariate analysis methods make use of row and column weights, and they are a very important part of the analysis itself. The row and column weights of a data table can be stored in numeric vectors (Fig. 1.2C). Weights are generally not defined by the user: they are associated to a particular analysis and are computed directly by **ade4** functions. For instance, in correspondence analysis (Sect. 6.2), rows and columns weights are derived from the row and column totals of the data set. However, in some cases, these weights can also be defined by the user as external constraints. For instance, in the case of differential sampling effort, row weights can be chosen proportional to sampling intensities so that highly sampled sites have more weight in the analysis.

In many cases, it is useful to define groups of samples to take into account different geographical locations, several types of habitats, or successive sampling dates

(Fig. 1.2D). More generally, groups of samples can correspond to the experimental design used to collect the data, and it is very important to be able to take this information into account in the statistical analysis of the data set. We shall see in Chap. 7 that several methods exist in the **ade4** package for this purpose. In **R**, a vector of class `factor` with a length equal to the number of rows of the data table (sites, or samples) can be used to define groups of rows in a data table.

When both the abundance of species and environmental variables are recorded at the same site, it is possible to study how the species respond to environmental gradients. This is the most classical problem of ecological data analysis (see Chap. 8) and requires to analyse simultaneously a pair of tables. The rows of the two tables must be identical, as they correspond to the same sampling sites. In **ade4**, one data frame is used to store the environmental variables and another to store the species data. These two data frames can be pre-processed by simple one-table analysis methods, and the resulting objects can then be passed to two-table coupling methods (Fig. 1.2E). If the rows of these two tables are also partitioned in groups, it is possible to study species-environment relationships in different conditions, treatments or areas (Fig. 1.2F).

When sampling is repeated over time, one gets a series of tables, called a K-table. In **ade4** this information is stored in a compact and easy-to-use data structure (a list of class `ktab`). This structure provides functions allowing a straightforward manipulation of individual tables and of the whole series (Fig. 1.2G). Many methods are available in **ade4** to analyse `ktab` *globally* (see Chap. 9) and study how the structure of ecological communities change in time. Pairs of `ktab` can be used to analyse the evolution of the relationships between species and environment (Fig. 1.2H, see Chap. 10).

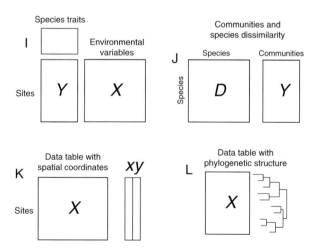

Fig. 1.3 Common structures of ecological data sets (continued). I: pair of ecological tables with species traits, J: dissimilarities between species and communities composition tables, K: rectangular data table (site × environmental variables or site × species) with geographical coordinates (xy), L: rectangular data table with phylogenetic information between rows.

To improve our understanding of the functioning of ecological systems, it is possible to integrate information on species. Species traits can be integrated to identify which characteristics of species drive their response to environmental conditions. Several methods focusing on this question are presented in this book (Fig. 1.3I, see Chap. 11). Species traits can also be used to define species dissimilarities that are then used to measure functional diversities within or among communities (Fig. 1.3J, see Chap. 14).

Lastly, it should be noticed that neither sites nor species can be considered as independent samples. Sites are usually georeferenced and thus have geographical attributes (Fig. 1.3K, see Chap. 12). On the other hand, species share some common evolutionary history that can be represented by a phylogenetic tree (Fig. 1.3L, see Chap. 13). The **adespatial** and **adephylo** packages provide tools to study spatial and phylogenetic autocorrelation, respectively, in order to understand how ecological properties are affected by spatial and phylogenetic relatedness.

Chapter 2
Useful R Functions and Data Structures

Abstract This chapter explains the basic **R** functions needed for data import and export operations, and for handling vectors, data tables and qualitative variables (factors). This introductory presentation is limited to a few key elements needed for *multivariate data analysis in Ecology* with the **ade4** package. It is not intended as a general introduction to **R**, and if needed, the reader should refer to a basic book on **R**. See, for example, here: https://cran.r-project.org/manuals.html or here: https://cran.r-project.org/other-docs.html.

2.1 Introduction

Data preparation and importation are one of the most time-consuming operations in the process of analysing ecological data with the **ade4** package in **R**. Raw data sets are often stored in spreadsheet documents, and there is a long way between these raw documents and the data table that can be used in a multivariate analysis. Both technical and theoretical considerations must be taken into account during these preparation steps.

Technical problems arise in the task of *cleaning up* the data, that is, for example, checking for special characters that could prevent normal reading of the raw file, checking for row and column names, verifying aberrant values, removing missing data, etc. Some of these steps must be taken in the spreadsheet software, and some should preferably be done in **R**.

More theoretical questions appear later, and they are related, for example, to which variables should be included or not in the data table, which type of data should be considered, which data analysis method should be used, etc. Most of these steps should be performed inside **R**, using its powerful data handling functions.

2.2   Basic Data Import and Export Functions

The basic functions for reading and writing data tables in **R** are `read.table` and `write.table`. The `data` function can be used to load a *predefined data set*, either from the base **R** distribution or from a contributed package like **ade4**.

2.2.1   read.table

The main data import function is `read.table`. This is the function to use when reading a text file (for example, a spreadsheet exported from Excel).

```
> read.table(file, header = FALSE, dec = ".")
```

The first argument (`file`) is the name of the file which the data are to be read from. The argument `header` is a logical value indicating whether the file contains the names of the variables as its first line. The `dec` argument can be used to set the decimal mark ("." by default). Many other arguments are described in the `read.table` documentation. Use `help("read.table")` in **R** to get access to this documentation.

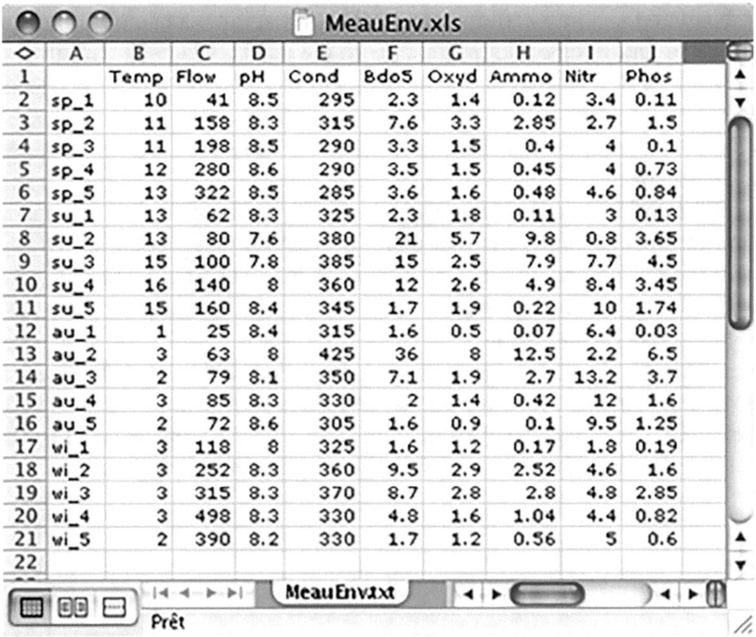

◇	A	B	C	D	E	F	G	H	I	J
1		Temp	Flow	pH	Cond	Bdo5	Oxyd	Ammo	Nitr	Phos
2	sp_1	10	41	8.5	295	2.3	1.4	0.12	3.4	0.11
3	sp_2	11	158	8.3	315	7.6	3.3	2.85	2.7	1.5
4	sp_3	11	198	8.5	290	3.3	1.5	0.4	4	0.1
5	sp_4	12	280	8.6	290	3.5	1.5	0.45	4	0.73
6	sp_5	13	322	8.5	285	3.6	1.6	0.48	4.6	0.84
7	su_1	13	62	8.3	325	2.3	1.8	0.11	3	0.13
8	su_2	13	80	7.6	380	21	5.7	9.8	0.8	3.65
9	su_3	15	100	7.8	385	15	2.5	7.9	7.7	4.5
10	su_4	16	140	8	360	12	2.6	4.9	8.4	3.45
11	su_5	15	160	8.4	345	1.7	1.9	0.22	10	1.74
12	au_1	1	25	8.4	315	1.6	0.5	0.07	6.4	0.03
13	au_2	3	63	8	425	36	8	12.5	2.2	6.5
14	au_3	2	79	8.1	350	7.1	1.9	2.7	13.2	3.7
15	au_4	3	85	8.3	330	2	1.4	0.42	12	1.6
16	au_5	2	72	8.6	305	1.6	0.9	0.1	9.5	1.25
17	wi_1	3	118	8	325	1.6	1.2	0.17	1.8	0.19
18	wi_2	3	252	8.3	360	9.5	2.9	2.52	4.6	1.6
19	wi_3	3	315	8.3	370	8.7	2.8	2.8	4.8	2.85
20	wi_4	3	498	8.3	330	4.8	1.6	1.04	4.4	0.82
21	wi_5	2	390	8.2	330	1.7	1.2	0.56	5	0.6
22										

(MeauEnv.xls — MeauEnv.txt — Prêt)

Fig. 2.1 Screenshot of an example Excel spreadsheet "MeauEnv.xls". The first row contains variable names, and the first column contains row names. The first cell (A,1) is left empty.

From the spreadsheet software (see Fig. 2.1), the data table should be saved to a text file using the "Save as…" command. It is then possible to read this text file using the `read.table` function in **R**, and to store the result in a data frame. In the following example, the text file "MeauEnv.txt" is read and the resulting data are stored in the `env` data frame.

```
env <- read.table(file = "MeauEnv.txt", header = TRUE)
```

Note that for **R**, row names *must* be unique. Failing to follow this rule will prevent reading of the file. It results in the error message "`duplicate 'row.names' are not allowed`".

Column names should not contain any special character, particularly spaces, as they would be interpreted by default as column separators. These names will be used by **ade4** graphical functions as labels on factor maps, so they should be kept short and informative. For example, do not use long species names that would clutter factor maps, but short species codes (like "irve" for *Iris versicolor*). Usually, rows correspond to items (individuals, samples, etc.) and columns correspond to descriptors (variables, species, etc.).

Depending on the spreadsheet software preferences and on the computer system settings, the decimal mark in the text file can be a dot "." or a comma "," (this is particularly the case in some European countries). It is necessary to check this point and to set the `dec` argument accordingly, or to change the decimal mark in the text file using a compatible text editor.

By default, `read.table` transforms all the character variables (variables containing character strings) into factors. However, quoted strings containing numerical values (for example, the quoted string "42") are transformed into numeric type. The `as.is` arguments can be used to prevent character variables form being treated as factors. And the `colClasses` argument allows to specify exactly how each variable should be interpreted.

Other useful functions for importing and exporting data can be found in some suitable packages. For instance, the **readODS** package (Schutten et al. 2016) is relevant to handle OpenDocument spreadsheets and the **xlsx** package (Dragulescu and Arendt 2018) to handle Excel files.

2.2.2 write.table

Writing **R** results to output text files can be done with the `write.table` function:

```
write.table(env, "EnvData.txt")
```

The `read.csv` and `write.csv` variants can also be used to ease compatibility problems with Excel or other spreadsheet software.

2.2.3   Data

The base **R** distribution, and also many contributed packages, contain predefined
data sets. They are often used in the **R** documentation system to illustrate particular
functions. These data sets can be loaded using the `data` function. Such data sets can
contain a list of elements: data tables, vectors and others. The `names` function can
be used to get the name of these elements, and the `class` function gives their type:

```
library(ade4)
data(meaudret)
names(meaudret)
```

```
[1] "env"        "design"     "spe"        "spe.names"
```

```
class(meaudret)
```

```
[1] "list"
```

```
class(meaudret$env)
```

```
[1] "data.frame"
```

2.3   Vectors

Vectors are the base elements of **R**. A vector is just a series of values, with a
given `length` and a type (called `mode`), for example `numeric`, `logical` or
`character`. Vectors can be handled as whole entities, but they can also be indexed
and sub-setted.

```
x <- 1:4
length(x)
```

```
[1] 4
```

```
x
```

```
[1] 1 2 3 4
```

Vectors of character strings are particularly useful. The `c` function can be used to
build vectors:

```
(x <- c("Eda", "Bsp", "Brh", "Bni"))
```

```
[1] "Eda" "Bsp" "Brh" "Bni"
```

The square bracket operator can be used to index a vector and select some of its elements:

```
x[1]
```

```
[1] "Eda"
```

A range of values can be specified with the colon notation:

```
x[1:3]
```

```
[1] "Eda" "Bsp" "Brh"
```

A negative index excludes the corresponding element (but positive and negative indices cannot be mixed):

```
x[-2]
```

```
[1] "Eda" "Brh" "Bni"
```

Indexing can also be made using logical constants or expressions:

```
x[c(TRUE, FALSE, TRUE, TRUE)]
```

```
[1] "Eda" "Brh" "Bni"
```

```
x[substr(x, 1, 1) == "B"]
```

```
[1] "Bsp" "Brh" "Bni"
```

Many other possibilities are available, but they are out of the scope of this book.

2.4 Data Frames

Ecological data sets used for multivariate analysis can be quite complex, but they must be organised in one or more rectangular data tables. The most common of these tables is the species table: its rows correspond to the sampling sites, and its columns correspond to animal or plant species. The values contained in the table can be, for example, the number of individuals of each species found at each site, or the presence/absence of the species, or any kind of abundance index. Another common type of table is the environmental variables table. It contains the values of some environmental variables (quantitative or categorical) measured in a set of sites. Here also, sites are in rows and variables in columns.

The most convenient data structure available in **R** for storing these tables is the data frame. A data frame is a table with unique row names and (preferably unique) column names. Columns correspond to variables and they can be of any type (numeric, character, factor), so it is easy to handle mixed type variables.

The first rows of a data frame can be displayed using the head function, and argument n gives the number of rows that should be displayed:

```
head(env, n = 4)
```

```
      Temp Flow  pH Cond Bdo5 Oxyd Ammo Nitr Phos
sp_1    10   41 8.5  295  2.3  1.4 0.12  3.4 0.11
sp_2    11  158 8.3  315  7.6  3.3 2.85  2.7 1.50
sp_3    11  198 8.5  290  3.3  1.5 0.40  4.0 0.10
sp_4    12  280 8.6  290  3.5  1.5 0.45  4.0 0.73
```

2.4.1 Dimensions

The dimension of a data frame is given by the dim function. For example, in the **ade4** package, the meaudret data set contains a data frame called env, that has 20 rows and 9 columns, corresponding to 9 physico-chemical variables measured in 20 sampling sites along a small French stream (Pegaz-Maucet 1980, see the meaudret help page).

```
env <- meaudret$env
dim(env)
```

```
[1] 20   9
```

```
head(env, n = 4)
```

```
      Temp Flow  pH Cond Bdo5 Oxyd Ammo Nitr Phos
sp_1    10   41 8.5  295  2.3  1.4 0.12  3.4 0.11
sp_2    11  158 8.3  315  7.6  3.3 2.85  2.7 1.50
sp_3    11  198 8.5  290  3.3  1.5 0.40  4.0 0.10
sp_4    12  280 8.6  290  3.5  1.5 0.45  4.0 0.73
```

The number of rows and columns are given by the nrow and ncol functions:

```
nrow(env)
```

```
[1] 20
```

```
ncol(env)
```

```
[1] 9
```

2.4.2 Row and Column Names

The names of variables can be accessed and modified with the names function:

```
names(env)
```

```
[1] "Temp" "Flow" "pH"    "Cond" "Bdo5" "Oxyd" "Ammo" "Nitr"
[9] "Phos"
```

```
names(env)[2] <- "Disch"          # Disch: Discharge = Flow
names(env)
```

```
[1] "Temp"  "Disch" "pH"      "Cond"  "Bdo5"  "Oxyd"  "Ammo"
[8] "Nitr"  "Phos"
```

The corresponding function for rows is the `row.names` function:

```
row.names(env)
```

```
[1]  "sp_1" "sp_2" "sp_3" "sp_4" "sp_5" "su_1" "su_2" "su_3"
[9]  "su_4" "su_5" "au_1" "au_2" "au_3" "au_4" "au_5" "wi_1"
[17] "wi_2" "wi_3" "wi_4" "wi_5"
```

2.4.3   Accessing Data Frame Elements

Data frames can be handled very easily in **R**, thanks to powerful functions and operators that can be used to select rows and columns and to perform many operations on them. The square bracket operator can be used to select rows and columns within a data frame. The element of a data frame located at row *i* and column *j* is obtained using the syntax `[i, j]`.

```
env[2, 2]
```

```
[1] 158
```

A range of elements can be selected using the colon operator. The syntax `i:j` represents elements *i* through *j*, and it can be used for both rows and columns. With the same example data frame, we get:

```
env[1:5, 3:6]
```

```
      pH Cond Bdo5 Oxyd
sp_1 8.5  295  2.3  1.4
sp_2 8.3  315  7.6  3.3
sp_3 8.5  290  3.3  1.5
sp_4 8.6  290  3.5  1.5
sp_5 8.5  285  3.6  1.6
```

If *i* or *j* are not specified, then all the elements are selected. For example, the syntax `[1:3, ]` selects all the columns of rows 1–3:

```
env[1:3, ]
```

```
     Temp Disch  pH Cond Bdo5 Oxyd Ammo Nitr Phos
sp_1   10    41 8.5  295  2.3  1.4 0.12  3.4 0.11
sp_2   11   158 8.3  315  7.6  3.3 2.85  2.7 1.50
sp_3   11   198 8.5  290  3.3  1.5 0.40  4.0 0.10
```

By default, if the selection has only one dimension, then the type of the object is set to vector:

```
env[1:5, 4]
```

```
[1] 295 315 290 290 285
```

In this case, the `drop` argument can be used to keep the result as a data frame, preserving row and column names:

```
env[1:5, 4, drop = FALSE]
```

```
      Cond
sp_1   295
sp_2   315
sp_3   290
sp_4   290
sp_5   285
```

Additionally, the $ syntax can be used to access the columns of a data frame.

```
env$Cond
```

```
 [1] 295 315 290 290 285 325 380 385 360 345 315 425 350 330
[15] 305 325 360 370 330 330
```

The attachment mechanism is also very handy to handle data frames. After a data frame has been *attached* to the current environment, its variables can be accessed directly (i.e., without having to type the name of the data frame).

```
attach(env)
Cond
```

```
 [1] 295 315 290 290 285 325 380 385 360 345 315 425 350 330
[15] 305 325 360 370 330 330
```

```
detach(env)
```

2.4.4   Row and Column Sums and Means

R provides two functions to compute automatically the row and column sums of a data frame. These functions are `rowSums` and `colSums` (note that similar functions `rowMeans` and `colMeans` also exist to compute row and column means). In the `meaudret` data set, the `spe` data frame contains the abundance of 13 *Ephemeroptera* species in 20 samples (20 rows and 13 columns). The sums by species and by site can be computed easily:

```
dim(meaudret$spe)
```

```
[1] 20 13
```

```
colSums(meaudret$spe)
```

```
Eda Bsp Brh Bni Bpu Cen Ecd Rhi Hla Hab Par Cae Eig
 20 104 163  11  35  37  26  41  80   5  35  10  28
```

```
rowSums(meaudret$spe)
```

```
sp_1 sp_2 sp_3 sp_4 sp_5 su_1 su_2 su_3 su_4 su_5 au_1 au_2
  48   12   17   18   24   44    9   16   32   33   53    1
au_3 au_4 au_5 wi_1 wi_2 wi_3 wi_4 wi_5
  26   47   58   45   22    5   32   53
```

2.4.5   Row and Column Selection

Rows and columns of a data frame can be selected based on any complex criteria.
For example, we can select the rows of a data frame for which the row sum is higher
than a given threshold. In the meaudret data set, we can select the samples for
which the total abundance in the spe data frame is higher than 10:

```
spe <- meaudret$spe
spe2 <- spe[rowSums(spe) > 10, ]
dim(spe2)
```

```
[1] 17 13
```

   rowSums(spe) computes the vector of row sums, and rowSums(spe) >10
is a vector of logical values (TRUE or FALSE) that is used to select the rows: TRUE
selects the corresponding row in spe while FALSE excludes it. Here, only three
samples had a row sum less than 10.

2.4.6   Changing Values

Modifying any particular value in a data frame can be done automatically. For
example, replacing negative values by zeroes can be done with a simple user-defined
function. First, we put three negative values in a copy of our example data frame:

```
envNeg <- env
envNeg[2, 2] <- envNeg[4, 2] <- envNeg[3, 4] <- -1
head(envNeg, n = 4)
```

```
     Temp Disch  pH Cond Bdo5 Oxyd Ammo Nitr Phos
sp_1   10    41 8.5  295  2.3  1.4 0.12  3.4 0.11
sp_2   11    -1 8.3  315  7.6  3.3 2.85  2.7 1.50
sp_3   11   198 8.5   -1  3.3  1.5 0.40  4.0 0.10
sp_4   12    -1 8.6  290  3.5  1.5 0.45  4.0 0.73
```

   Then, we define the function repNeg. This function does the job: it takes one
variable (x) and replaces all negative values by zeroes. The ifelse function makes
this step easy (see the ifelse help page if needed):

```
repNeg <- function(x) ifelse(x < 0, 0, x)
```

The repNeg function is then applied to all the variables of the envNeg data frame using the apply function (Sect. 2.4.9). The result is stored in the new envPos data frame.

```
envPos <- apply(envNeg, 2, repNeg)
head(envPos, n = 4)
```

```
     Temp Disch  pH Cond Bdo5 Oxyd Ammo Nitr Phos
sp_1   10    41 8.5  295  2.3  1.4 0.12  3.4 0.11
sp_2   11     0 8.3  315  7.6  3.3 2.85  2.7 1.50
sp_3   11   198 8.5    0  3.3  1.5 0.40  4.0 0.10
sp_4   12     0 8.6  290  3.5  1.5 0.45  4.0 0.73
```

2.4.7   Missing Values in Data Frames

Usual multivariate analysis methods cannot be used on data sets that contain missing values. This is true for most methods available in the **ade4** package, although a few ones do admit missing values. The presence of missing values in a data frame can be tested using the is.na function. is.na returns a data frame of logical values, equal to TRUE if the corresponding element in the original data frame is a missing value (noted NA in **R**). The any function can then be used to check all the values of the data frame for missing values.

First, we make a copy of our example data frame, and we check that it does not contain any missing value:

```
env2 <- env
any(is.na(env2))
```

```
[1] FALSE
```

Then we put three missing values in the copy, and check it again:

```
env2[2, 2] <- env2[4, 2] <- env2[3, 4] <- NA
any(is.na(env2))
```

```
[1] TRUE
```

```
head(env2, n = 4)
```

```
     Temp Disch  pH Cond Bdo5 Oxyd Ammo Nitr Phos
sp_1   10    41 8.5  295  2.3  1.4 0.12  3.4 0.11
sp_2   11    NA 8.3  315  7.6  3.3 2.85  2.7 1.50
sp_3   11   198 8.5   NA  3.3  1.5 0.40  4.0 0.10
sp_4   12    NA 8.6  290  3.5  1.5 0.45  4.0 0.73
```

It is now possible to remove the rows (or columns) containing missing values. The expression is.na(env2) returns a data frame of logical values: TRUE if the corresponding value in env2 is missing, and FALSE if it is not. rowSums computes the row sums of this logical data frame, taking 1 for TRUE and 0 for FALSE. This means that if there is no missing value on one row of env2, then the sum of the same row of is.na(env2) will be equal to 0.

```
env3 <- env2[rowSums(is.na(env2)) == 0, ]
dim(env3)
```

```
[1] 17   9
```

```
head(env3, n = 4)
```

```
     Temp Disch  pH Cond Bdo5 Oxyd Ammo Nitr Phos
sp_1   10    41 8.5  295  2.3  1.4 0.12  3.4 0.11
sp_5   13   322 8.5  285  3.6  1.6 0.48  4.6 0.84
su_1   13    62 8.3  325  2.3  1.8 0.11  3.0 0.13
su_2   13    80 7.6  380 21.0  5.7 9.80  0.8 3.65
```

Note that the na.omit and complete.cases functions provide other ways to remove the rows of a data frame that contain missing values. Removing the columns containing missing values is also very easy:

```
env4 <- env2[, colSums(is.na(env2)) == 0]
dim(env4)
```

```
[1] 20   7
```

```
head(env4, n = 4)
```

```
     Temp  pH Bdo5 Oxyd Ammo Nitr Phos
sp_1   10 8.5  2.3  1.4 0.12  3.4 0.11
sp_2   11 8.3  7.6  3.3 2.85  2.7 1.50
sp_3   11 8.5  3.3  1.5 0.40  4.0 0.10
sp_4   12 8.6  3.5  1.5 0.45  4.0 0.73
```

Missing values for a given variable can be replaced by the mean of this variable, computed without the missing values. Note that this is probably not the best solution and there are some other alternatives (see, e.g., Dray and Josse 2015). In **R**, this can be done using a simple user-defined function:

```
envMiss <- env
envMiss[2, 2] <- envMiss[4, 2] <- envMiss[3, 4] <- NA
head(envMiss, n = 4)
```

```
     Temp Disch  pH Cond Bdo5 Oxyd Ammo Nitr Phos
sp_1   10    41 8.5  295  2.3  1.4 0.12  3.4 0.11
sp_2   11    NA 8.3  315  7.6  3.3 2.85  2.7 1.50
sp_3   11   198 8.5   NA  3.3  1.5 0.40  4.0 0.10
sp_4   12    NA 8.6  290  3.5  1.5 0.45  4.0 0.73
```

```
repMean <- function(x) {
        ifelse(is.na(x), mean(x, na.rm = TRUE), x)
     }
envEst <- apply(envMiss, 2, repMean)
head(envEst, n = 4)
```

```
     Temp Disch  pH  Cond Bdo5 Oxyd Ammo Nitr Phos
sp_1   10  41.0 8.5 295.0  2.3  1.4 0.12  3.4 0.11
sp_2   11 166.7 8.3 315.0  7.6  3.3 2.85  2.7 1.50
sp_3   11 198.0 8.5 337.9  3.3  1.5 0.40  4.0 0.10
sp_4   12 166.7 8.6 290.0  3.5  1.5 0.45  4.0 0.73
```

The user-defined function repMean uses the built-in function ifelse to replace the missing values by the mean of the variable, computed without missing values (thanks to the na.rm = TRUE argument).

2.4.8 Data Transformation

Data transformation is a matter of a few lines of **R** code. Applying a function to a data frame applies it to all its element, so transforming all the variables of a data frame is quite straightforward:

```
envLog <- log(env + 1)
head(envLog, n = 4)
```

```
      Temp Disch   pH Cond Bdo5  Oxyd  Ammo Nitr   Phos
sp_1 2.40  3.74 2.25 5.69 1.19 0.875 0.113 1.48 0.1044
sp_2 2.48  5.07 2.23 5.76 2.15 1.459 1.348 1.31 0.9163
sp_3 2.48  5.29 2.25 5.67 1.46 0.916 0.336 1.61 0.0953
sp_4 2.56  5.64 2.26 5.67 1.50 0.916 0.372 1.61 0.5481
```

2.4.9 Apply

`apply` is a very useful **R** function that can be used to apply a function to the rows or to the columns of a data frame. For example, computing the standard deviation of all the variables in a data frame is easy:

```
apply(env, 2, sd)
```

```
Temp Disch    pH  Cond  Bdo5  Oxyd  Ammo  Nitr  Phos
 5.5 130.3   0.3  36.7   8.5   1.7   3.6   3.4   1.8
```

The first argument (`env`) is the data frame to which the function should be applied. The third one (`sd`) is the function itself, and the second argument is the margin to which the function should be applied: 1 means rows and 2 means columns. So computing the row sums of the `spe` data frame (Sect. 2.4.5) can be done like this:

```
apply(spe, 1, sum)
```

```
sp_1 sp_2 sp_3 sp_4 sp_5 su_1 su_2 su_3 su_4 su_5 au_1 au_2
  48   12   17   18   24   44    9   16   32   33   53    1
au_3 au_4 au_5 wi_1 wi_2 wi_3 wi_4 wi_5
  26   47   58   45   22    5   32   53
```

Note, however, that the `rowSums` function is much faster in this case. `apply` can be used not only with built-in **R** functions but also with any user-defined function (Sect. 2.4.6).

2.4.10 Summary

The `summary` function can be useful to check the type and numerical characteristics of the variables of a data frame. For quantitative variables, it gives the minimum, maximum, first and third quartiles, the median and the mean. For qualitative variables, it gives the frequency of each level:

```
summary(cbind(env[, 1:3], meaudret$design$season))
```

```
        Temp              Disch                pH
Min.    : 1.0    Min.    : 25.0    Min.      :7.60
1st Qu.: 3.0    1st Qu.: 77.2    1st Qu.:8.07
Median : 6.5    Median :129.0    Median :8.30
Mean    : 7.7    Mean    :171.9    Mean      :8.25
3rd Qu.:13.0    3rd Qu.:259.0    3rd Qu.:8.43
Max.    :16.0    Max.    :498.0    Max.      :8.60
meaudret$design$season
spring:5
summer:5
autumn:5
winter:5
```

The summary function is generic, and it is often used in the **ade4** package to print a summary of multivariate analyses outputs.

2.4.11 Other Functions

There are many other utility functions that can be used to handle data frames. Here are a few among the most useful ones (see the documentation of each function for more details on how to use them):

- subset returns subsets of vectors, matrices or data frames that meet some conditions,
- split/unsplit divides the data into groups defined by a factor,
- by splits a data frame and applies a function to the subsets,
- aggregate splits the data and computes summary statistics for each subset,
- with uses a data frame as an environment to simplify the use of variable names,
- merge merges two data frames by common columns or row names, and other "join" operations.

2.5 Factors

Qualitative variables are often useful in multivariate analysis of ecological data. For example, they can be used to define groups of samples. In **R**, qualitative variables are called *factors*. In the meaudret data set of the **ade4** package, the meaudret$design data frame contains a description of the experimental design. There are two factors: season and site. The first one is the sampling season, the second the site number.

```
meaudret$design$season
```

```
 [1] spring spring spring spring spring summer summer summer
 [9] summer summer autumn autumn autumn autumn autumn winter
[17] winter winter winter winter
Levels: spring summer autumn winter
```

```
meaudret$design$site
```

```
[1]  S1 S2 S3 S4 S5 S1 S2 S3 S4 S5 S1 S2 S3 S4 S5 S1 S2 S3
[19] S4 S5
Levels: S1 S2 S3 S4 S5
```

The `meaudret$design$season` factor has 20 elements that can take the values `spring`, `summer`, `autumn` and `winter`. These values are called *levels*, they are character strings that can be modified with the `levels` function. Here, this factor defines groups of samples that were taken during the four seasons. The first five samples were taken in spring, the five following ones during summer, and so on.

2.5.1 Using Factors

Factors are used in several multivariate analysis methods that need the definition of groups, like Discriminant Analysis. They are also very handy to perform selections in a data frame. For example, to select all the samples that were taken during spring, we can do:

```
season <- meaudret$design$season
env[season == "spring", ]
```

```
     Temp Disch  pH Cond Bdo5 Oxyd Ammo Nitr Phos
sp_1   10    41 8.5  295  2.3  1.4 0.12  3.4 0.11
sp_2   11   158 8.3  315  7.6  3.3 2.85  2.7 1.50
sp_3   11   198 8.5  290  3.3  1.5 0.40  4.0 0.10
sp_4   12   280 8.6  290  3.5  1.5 0.45  4.0 0.73
sp_5   13   322 8.5  285  3.6  1.6 0.48  4.6 0.84
```

A selection in a data frame using a factor can be combined with a selection on the values of a variable. For example, to select the samples taken in spring where the water temperature was at least 12 °C:

```
env[season == "spring" & env$Temp >= 12, ]
```

```
     Temp Disch  pH Cond Bdo5 Oxyd Ammo Nitr Phos
sp_4   12   280 8.6  290  3.5  1.5 0.45  4.0 0.73
sp_5   13   322 8.5  285  3.6  1.6 0.48  4.6 0.84
```

The levels of a factor, like data frame row and column names, are used by **ade4** graphical functions. They should therefore be kept short and easy to identify. Changing the levels of a factor can be done with the `levels` function. For example, we can replace the season names by a two-character code in the `season` factor:

```
levels(season)
```

```
[1] "spring" "summer" "autumn" "winter"
```

```
levels(season) <- c("sp", "su", "au", "wi")
season
```

```
[1]  sp sp sp sp sp su su su su su au au au au au wi wi wi
[19] wi wi
Levels: sp su au wi
```

The `summary` function, when applied to a factor, gives the frequency of each level:

```
summary(meaudret$design)
```

```
      season    site
  spring:5     S1:4
  summer:5     S2:4
  autumn:5     S3:4
  winter:5     S4:4
               S5:4
```

The `table` function computes the contingency table of the counts for each combination of several factor levels:

```
table(meaudret$design)
```

```
            site
season   S1 S2 S3 S4 S5
  spring  1  1  1  1  1
  summer  1  1  1  1  1
  autumn  1  1  1  1  1
  winter  1  1  1  1  1
```

2.5.2 Generating Factors

Several **R** functions allow to generate automatically factors with the needed structure. The `rep` function repeats its first argument several times. The `as.factor`
function transforms the resulting series of character strings into a factor. For
example, the `season` and `site` factors of the `meaudret` data set can be
generated like this:

```
as.factor(rep(c("spring", "summer", "autumn", "winter"),
      each = 5))
```

```
[1]  spring spring spring spring spring summer summer summer
[9]  summer summer autumn autumn autumn autumn autumn winter
[17] winter winter winter winter
Levels: autumn spring summer winter
```

```
as.factor(rep(c("S1", "S2", "S3", "S4", "S5"), times = 4))
```

```
[1]  S1 S2 S3 S4 S5 S1 S2 S3 S4 S5 S1 S2 S3 S4 S5 S1 S2 S3
[19] S4 S5
Levels: S1 S2 S3 S4 S5
```

Note that by default, the levels are sorted in alphabetical order (autumn, spring,
summer, winter).

Another way to get the same result is to use the `gl` function. Here levels are
sorted in the same order as the user defines.

```
gl(4, 5, labels = c("spring", "summer", "autumn", "winter"))
```

```
 [1] spring spring spring spring spring summer summer summer
 [9] summer summer autumn autumn autumn autumn autumn winter
[17] winter winter winter winter
Levels: spring summer autumn winter
```

```
gl(5, 1, 20, labels = c("S1", "S2", "S3", "S4", "S5"))
```

```
 [1] S1 S2 S3 S4 S5 S1 S2 S3 S4 S5 S1 S2 S3 S4 S5 S1 S2 S3
[19] S4 S5
Levels: S1 S2 S3 S4 S5
```

2.5.3 Re-ordering Levels

The `reorder` function can be used to reorder the levels of a factor. In the
`meaudret` data set, the seasons are in chronological order. The boxplot of
ammonium concentration during the four seasons gives the result displayed in the
left panel of Fig. 2.2. The seasons can be reordered to have increasing seasonal
mean ammonium concentration (middle panel), or to have a different chronological
display starting in winter (right panel).

The `relevel` function also reorders factor levels, but only one level needs to be
specified. This level is set as being the first one, and the others are just moved down.

```
par(mfrow = c(1, 3), mar = c(3, 3, 0, 0))
boxplot(env$Ammo ~ season)
legend("topleft", "Original", cex = 1.5)
incrAmmo <- reorder(season, env$Ammo, mean)
boxplot(env$Ammo ~ incrAmmo)
legend("topleft", "Increasing ammo.", cex = 1.5)
chron <- reorder(season, rep(c(2, 3, 4, 1), each = 5))
boxplot(env$Ammo ~ chron)
legend("topleft", "Chronological", cex = 1.5)
```

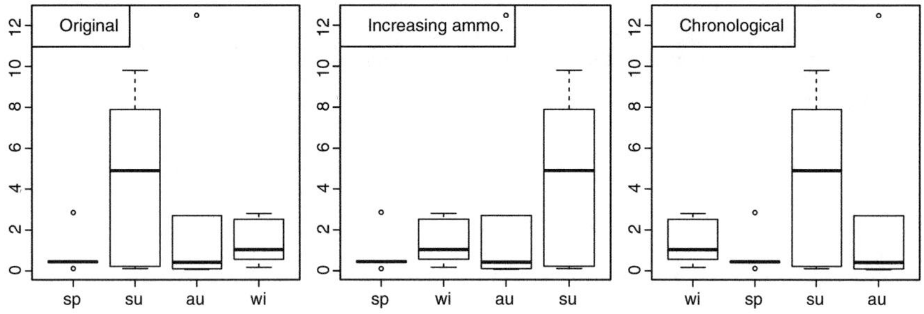

Fig. 2.2 Using the `reorder` function.

Chapter 3
The `dudi` Class

Abstract This chapter explains the structure of the `dudi` (S3) class, which is the core of the **ade4** package. All the multivariate data analysis methods available in **ade4** can be described in the framework of the duality diagram and an object of class `dudi` is a translation of this mathematical structure in **R**. In this chapter, we explain what is an object of class `dudi` and which functions are used to generate and handle it. We detail all its elements, how to use it to analyse data tables, and how to export its elements to use them outside **R**.

3.1 Introduction

`dudi` stands for "**du**ality **di**agram". The `dudi` class has been detailed in the paper dedicated to the **ade4** package (Dray and Dufour 2007). We give here a short summary of the structure of this class. Basic mathematical definitions and properties are given in Boxes 3.1 and 3.2. Readers interested in more details about the duality diagram should refer to Escoufier (1987) and Holmes (2006). The duality diagram can be seen as a picture of the mathematical objects used in the theoretical description of a multivariate analysis. This unifying framework has several objectives, like facilitating the comparisons of different multivariate methods, making easier to remember the characteristics of particular methods, finding out the operator needed to complete a given analysis, identifying the different outputs (row scores and variable loadings), the maximised criteria, how to compute them and how they are related.

© Springer Science+Business Media, LLC, part of Springer Nature 2018 29
J. Thioulouse et al., *Multivariate Analysis of Ecological Data with ade4*,
https://doi.org/10.1007/978-1-4939-8850-1_3

3.2   Principles of Multivariate Analysis

Multivariate analysis provides techniques to identify the main structures of large data sets. It produces graphical outputs that summarise the information of a large number of variables by a smaller number of dimensions. Basically, multivariate methods consist in geometric operations (orthogonal rotation and projection, see Appendix A) and associated computations are achieved by matrix diagonalisation.

The principles can be illustrated by a simple example where a data table contains the measurements of two variables (x1 and x2) for 30 individuals. Data can be represented on a standard scatterplot. On this plot, each observation is a point in a 2D plane and each dimension (axis) corresponds to a variable (Fig. 3.1A). Coordinates of individuals in this system of axes are simply given by the observed values. It is clear that both variables do not vary independently, they share a common information. Multivariate methods seek for a new system of axes that optimise the representation of the data by focusing on the common variation between the two original variables. Individuals are then projected on these new axes. The new set of orthogonal axes highlights the common variation by maximising the variance (or inertia) of the projections (Fig. 3.1B). Lastly, the new system of axes is used to represent the individuals. This new representation corresponds to a rotation of the original scatterplot. The rotation is also applied to represent the original variables in this new system of axes (Fig. 3.1C, x1 and x2 arrows). Dimension reduction can then be applied by selecting not all but only a few axes to represent the individuals and variables. In this 2D example, the coordinates on the first principal axis can be kept to summarise the information given by the two variables on a single dimension.

Computations associated to these geometric operations are achieved through the diagonalisation of the covariance matrix, with the `eigen` **R** base function. The coordinates of principal axes are given by the eigenvectors and associated eigenvalues are equal to the variance of the projections (or projected inertia). Coordinates of the individuals in the new system of axes are then obtained by matrix multiplication (see Box 3.2).

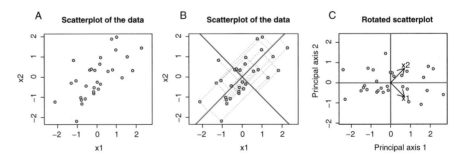

Fig. 3.1 A simple example with 2 variables and 30 individuals. Data can be represented on a standard scatterplot (A). A new system of axes can be defined to optimise the representation of the variation shared by the two variables and individuals are projected on these axes (B). An orthogonal rotation is performed to represent the individuals and the variables in the new system of axes (C).

Note that a symmetric viewpoint can be considered where variables are represented in a space where each axis corresponds to an individual (see Box 3.1). These two viewpoints are intimately related and the name *duality diagram* originates from these links. Details are given in Boxes 3.1, 3.2 and 3.3.

Box 3.1 The Duality Diagram: Basic Mathematical Definitions
Let $\mathbf{X}$ be a data table, with n rows (samples) and p columns (variables). This table can be seen as a cloud of n points in $\mathbb{R}^p$, or symmetrically as a cloud of p points in $\mathbb{R}^n$:

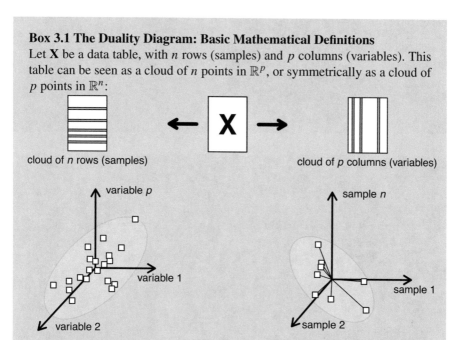

Multivariate analysis aims to summarise these two representations to identify (1) the main similarities between the samples and/or (2) the principal relationships between the variables. To deal with these two objectives, $\mathbf{Q}$, a $p \times p$ positive symmetric matrix and $\mathbf{D}$, an $n \times n$ positive symmetric matrix are defined. $\mathbf{Q}$ is a metric used as an inner product in $\mathbb{R}^p$ allowing to measure distances between the n samples. $\mathbf{D}$ is a metric used as an inner product in $\mathbb{R}^n$ allowing to measure the links between the p variables. These three matrices define a statistical triplet $(\mathbf{X}, \mathbf{Q}, \mathbf{D})$ which can be represented as a *duality diagram*:

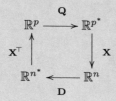

(continued)

Box 3.1 (continued)

$\mathbf{X}^\top$ denotes the transpose of $\mathbf{X}$ and the operators to navigate between spaces ($\mathbb{R}^n$, $\mathbb{R}^p$) and their duals ($\mathbb{R}^{n^*}$, $\mathbb{R}^{p^*}$) are obtained by turning around the diagram. For instance, in $\mathbb{R}^p$, the diagonalisation of $\mathbf{X}^\top\mathbf{DXQ}$ provides a low-dimensional space where the representation of samples is as close as possible to the observed one. Symmetrically, in $\mathbb{R}^n$, a small dimension space where the representation of variables is as close as possible to the original one is obtained by the diagonalisation of $\mathbf{XQX}^\top\mathbf{D}$. These two different diagonalisations are intimately linked and are the core of the duality diagram framework.

Box 3.2 The Duality Diagram: Mathematical Properties

$\mathbf{X}^\top\mathbf{DXQ}$ and $\mathbf{XQX}^\top\mathbf{D}$ are the *Escoufier operators* (Escoufier 1987). They share the same r non-null eigenvalues ($\lambda_1, \lambda_2, \ldots, \lambda_r$) stored in decreasing order in the $\mathbf{\Lambda}$ diagonal matrix. r is the rank of the diagram. The matrices $\mathbf{A}$ and $\mathbf{B}$ contain the associated eigenvectors as columns (i.e., $\mathbf{A} = [\mathbf{a}_1|\mathbf{a}_2|\ldots|\mathbf{a}_r]$ and $\mathbf{B} = [\mathbf{b}_1|\mathbf{b}_2|\ldots|\mathbf{b}_r]$) and satisfy the following conditions:

$$\mathbf{X}^\top\mathbf{DXQA} = \mathbf{A}\mathbf{\Lambda} \text{ with } \mathbf{A}^\top\mathbf{QA} = \mathbf{I}_r$$

and

$$\mathbf{XQX}^\top\mathbf{DB} = \mathbf{B}\mathbf{\Lambda} \text{ with } \mathbf{B}^\top\mathbf{DB} = \mathbf{I}_r$$

The columns of $\mathbf{A}$ are the *principal axes* (Pearson 1901) and those of $\mathbf{B}$ are the *principal components* (Hotelling 1933). The columns of $\mathbf{A}$ are usually known as the vectors of *loadings*. Note also that we adopt Hotelling's notation, while several authors consider $\mathbf{XQA}$ as the principal components (e.g., Jolliffe 2002).

The two diagonalisations are closely related and the two systems of axes are linked by the following transition formulas:

$$\mathbf{B} = \mathbf{XQA}\mathbf{\Lambda}^{-\frac{1}{2}} \text{ and } \mathbf{A} = \mathbf{X}^\top\mathbf{DB}\mathbf{\Lambda}^{-\frac{1}{2}}$$

Two other equivalent diagonalisations can be considered:

$$\mathbf{QX}^\top\mathbf{DXA}^* = \mathbf{A}^*\mathbf{\Lambda} \text{ with } \mathbf{A}^{*\top}\mathbf{Q}^{-1}\mathbf{A}^* = \mathbf{I}_r$$

and

$$\mathbf{DXQX}^\top\mathbf{B}^* = \mathbf{B}^*\mathbf{\Lambda} \text{ with } \mathbf{B}^{*\top}\mathbf{D}^{-1}\mathbf{B}^* = \mathbf{I}_r$$

(continued)

> **Box 3.2** (continued)
> The columns of $\mathbf{A}^*$ are the *principal factors* and those of $\mathbf{B}^*$ are the *principal cofactors*. We have also the following relationships:
>
> $$\mathbf{A}^* = \mathbf{QA} \text{ and } \mathbf{B}^* = \mathbf{DB}$$
>
> There are some important properties associated to the analysis of a duality diagram:
>
> **Property 3.1** *The vectors* $\mathbf{a}_1, \mathbf{a}_2, \ldots, \mathbf{a}_r$ *successively maximise, under the* $\mathbf{Q}$-*orthogonality constraint, the quadratic forms* $\|\mathbf{XQa}_i\|_{\mathbf{D}}^2 = \lambda_i$.
>
> **Property 3.2** *The vectors* $\mathbf{b}_1, \mathbf{b}_2, \ldots, \mathbf{b}_r$ *successively maximise, under the* $\mathbf{D}$-*orthogonality constraint, the quadratic forms* $\|\mathbf{X}^{\mathsf{T}}\mathbf{Db}_i\|_{\mathbf{Q}}^2 = \lambda_i$.
>
> **Property 3.3** *The pairs of vectors* $(\mathbf{a}_1, \mathbf{b}_1), \cdots, (\mathbf{a}_r, \mathbf{b}_r)$ *successively maximise, under the* $\mathbf{Q}$- *and* $\mathbf{D}$-*orthogonality constraints, the inner products* $\langle \mathbf{XQa}_i | \mathbf{b_i} \rangle_{\mathbf{D}} = \langle \mathbf{X}^{\mathsf{T}}\mathbf{Db}_i | \mathbf{a_i} \rangle_{\mathbf{Q}} = \sqrt{\lambda_i}$.
>
> In the following, we simplify the writing of these properties by considering $\mathbf{a}_i = \mathbf{a}$, $\mathbf{b}_i = \mathbf{b}$ and $\lambda_i = \lambda$. The row scores ($\mathbf{L}$), projection of the rows of $\mathbf{X}$ onto the principal axes, and the column scores ($\mathbf{C}$), projection of the columns of $\mathbf{X}$ onto the principal components, are given by:
>
> $$\mathbf{L} = \mathbf{XQA} \text{ and } \mathbf{C} = \mathbf{X}^{\mathsf{T}}\mathbf{DB}$$

3.3 Structure

An object of class `dudi` is a list that contains both input and output data. The input data are the elements of the statistical triplet, i.e., the data table (stored as a `data.frame`) and the weights for the rows and the columns which are stored as vectors.

The output data are the results of the analysis of this triplet. The eigenvalues, eigenvectors (principal components and principal axes) and row and column scores are stored directly in the `dudi` object.

The `dudi` class has several subclasses, corresponding to different types of analyses. Additionally, other classes exist in **ade4**, which are not subclasses of `dudi`. A summary of the `dudi` class hierarchy is displayed in Table 3.1.

Objects of class `dudi` are created by multivariate analysis functions in **ade4**. These functions belong to several categories, which are broadly:

- one-table analysis methods (e.g., Principal Component Analysis, Chessel et al. 2004),

Table 3.1 The dudi class hierarchy and corresponding analysis names.

Class	Subclass	Sub-subclass	Analysis name
dudi	pca		Principal Component Analysis
dudi	pco		Principal Coordinate Analysis
dudi	coa		Correspondence Analysis
dudi	coa	foucart	Foucart Analysis
dudi	coa	witwit	Internal Correspondence Analysis
dudi	acm		Multiple Correspondence Analysis
dudi	dec		Decentred Correspondence Analysis
dudi	fca		Fuzzy Correspondence Analysis
dudi	mix		Mixed type Analysis
dudi	nsc		Non-Symmetric Correspondence Analysis
dudi	between		Between-Class Analysis
dudi	within		Within-Class Analysis
dudi	coinertia		Coinertia Analysis
dudi	betcoi		Between-Class Coinertia Analysis
dudi	witcoi		Within-Class Coinertia Analysis
dudi	niche		Niche (OMI) Analysis
dudi	rlq		RLQ Analysis
dudi	pcaiv		PCA on Instrumental Variables
dudi	pcaivortho		Orthogonal PCAIV
dudi	pta		Partial Triadic Analysis

- one table with groups of items (e.g., Between-Class Analysis, Chessel et al. 2004),
- two-table coupling methods (e.g., Coinertia Analysis, Dray et al. 2007),
- *K*-table methods (e.g., Partial Triadic Analysis, Dray et al. 2007).

Functions of the first category have a name that begins with dudi (like dudi.pca for Principal Component Analysis) and they return an object of class dudi. This object is a list, and its elements can vary according to the function that created it. But there is a series of eleven basic elements that are always available. The first three of these constant elements are:

- tab
- cw
- lw

These three elements are used to create the dudi object so they are always present. tab is a data frame that contains the data (**X** in Box 3.1), and cw and lw are vectors containing the column and row weights (leading to **Q** and **D** matrices in Box 3.1). Three other elements are added after the main computations have been performed:

- eig
- rank
- nf

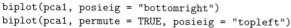

```
biplot(pca1, posieig = "bottomright")
biplot(pca1, permute = TRUE, posieig = "topleft")
```

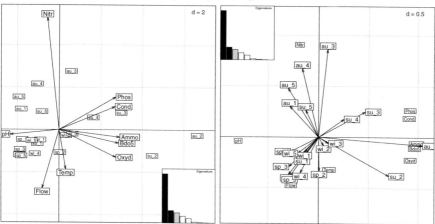

Fig. 3.2 PCA (distance) biplot. The left figure is a superimposition of three plots based on `pca1$c1` (arrows = variable loadings), `pca1$li` (labels = samples) and `pca1$eig` (eigenvalues screeplot, bottom-right corner). Comparison of the two figures shows the effect of the `permute` argument: the left figure is the usual "distance biplot" and the right is the "correlation biplot" obtained with the `permute = TRUE` option.

`eig` is a vector containing the eigenvalues ($\mathbf{\Lambda}$ in Box 3.2), `rank` is the rank of the matrix that has been diagonalised (r in Box 3.2), and `nf` is the number of axes (factors) that are kept to represent the results.

In the next step, five elements supplement the `dudi` object. The `call` element contains the function call (i.e., the command line that was typed by the user to run the analysis). It can be useful to redo the analysis if needed. The `c1` element contains the principal axes ($\mathbf{A}$ in Box 3.2) whereas `li` contains the row scores (i.e., projections of the individuals on the principal axes, $\mathbf{L}$ in Box 3.2). On the other hand, `l1` contains the principal components ($\mathbf{B}$ in Box 3.2) whereas `co` contains the column scores (i.e., projections of the variables on the principal components, $\mathbf{C}$ in Box 3.2).

These different elements can be used to draw factor maps where variables and/or individuals are represented (see Fig. 3.2 for an example).

In the following example, the `dudi.pca` function is used to do a Principal Component Analysis (PCA) of the data frame `env` (see Chap. 2). This provides the `pca1` object:

```
library(ade4)
library(adegraphics)
data(meaudret)
env <- meaudret$env
pca1 <- dudi.pca(env, scannf = FALSE, nf = 3)
```

`pca1` is an object of the class `dudi`, and of the subclass `pca`. We can check that this is indeed a list, and that the length of this list is equal to 13 (it has 13 elements).

```
class(pca1)
```

```
[1] "pca"   "dudi"
```

```
is.list(pca1)
```

```
[1] TRUE
```

```
length(pca1)
```

```
[1] 13
```

```
names(pca1)
```

```
[1] "tab"   "cw"    "lw"    "eig"   "rank" "nf"    "c1"    "li"
[9] "co"    "l1"    "call" "cent" "norm"
```

Two elements have been added to the eleven ones that make the basic dudi class: cent and norm. These elements are specific to objects created by dudi.pca and indicate if and how the initial variables have been centred and standardised.

3.4   Functions

Many other user-level functions create dudi objects. These are typically functions that are used to do multivariate analyses. As explained in the previous section, these functions belong to several categories. Table 3.2 shows a list of multivariate data analysis functions that create dudi objects, and Table 3.3 shows a list of multivariate data analysis functions that create objects similar but not strictly equivalent to a dudi object.

All these functions take several input arguments that can vary according to the type of analysis. The user should refer to each function help page to get information about the list of arguments and their default values. The str function can be used to obtain the list of arguments of a function.

```
str(dudi.pca)
```

```
function (df, row.w = rep(1, nrow(df))/nrow(df), col.w = rep(1,
    ncol(df)), center = TRUE, scale = TRUE, scannf = TRUE,
    nf = 2)
```

Some of these arguments are common to many functions, so we shall detail them here:

- df: data frame containing the data table
- row.w: vector of row weights (default varies according to the type of analysis)
- col.w: vector of column weights (default varies according to the type of analysis)

Table 3.2 Multivariate data analysis functions that create `dudi` objects.

Function name	Analysis name
dudi.pca	Principal Component Analysis
dudi.pco	Principal Coordinate Analysis
dudi.coa	Correspondence Analysis
dudi.acm	Multiple Correspondence Analysis
dudi.dec	Decentred Correspondence Analysis
dudi.fca	Fuzzy Correspondence Analysis
dudi.fpca	Fuzzy PCA
dudi.mix	Mixed type Analysis
dudi.hillsmith	Hill and Smith Analysis
dudi.nsc	Non-Symmetric Correspondence Analysis
bca	Between-Class Analysis
wca	Within-Class Analysis
withinpca	Normed Within-Class PCA
witwit.coa	Internal Correspondence Analysis
coinertia	Coinertia Analysis
bca.coinertia	Between-Class Coinertia Analysis
wca.coinertia	Within-Class Coinertia Analysis
niche	Niche (OMI) Analysis
rlq	RLQ Analysis
bca.rlq	Between-Class RLQ Analysis
wca.rlq	Within-Class RLQ Analysis
pcaiv	PCA on Instrumental Variables
pcaivortho	Orthogonal PCAIV
pta	Partial Triadic Analysis
costatis	Coinertia Analysis and STATIS
statico	STATIS and Coinertia Analysis
foucart	Foucart Analysis

- `scannf`: logical, toggles screeplot display and asking the user about the number of axes that should be kept and used in row scores and variable loadings computations
- `nf`: if `scannf` is FALSE, number of kept axes (defaults to `nf = 2`)
- `dudi`: duality diagram (created using one of the `dudi.*` functions)

High-level functions using `dudi` objects for multivariate data analysis will be detailed in the following chapters.

Table 3.3 Multivariate data analysis functions that create other types of objects.

Function name	Analysis name
amova	Analysis of Molecular Variance
discrimin	Discriminant Analysis
discrimin.coa	Discriminant Correspondence Analysis
procuste	Procrustes Analysis
dpcoa	Double Principal Coordinate Analysis
bwca.dpcoa	Between and Within-Class DPCoA
statis	STATIS Analysis
sepan	*K*-table Separate Analyses
mfa	Multiple Factor Analysis
mcoa	Multiple Coinertia Analysis
mdpcoa	Multiple DPCoA
nipals	NIPALS Analysis
multispati	Spatial Data Analysis
mbpcaiv	Multiblock PCA with Instrumental Variables
mbpls	Multiblock Partial Least Squares

3.5　Elements of dudi Objects

We have seen in the previous section the basic elements of a dudi object. Here, we shall detail them and see how to use them on a simple example.

The pca1 object created in the previous section is a PCA on correlation matrix (or "standardised PCA"). It is a dudi object, so a list, and this list contains thirteen elements. The first eleven elements are the basic elements of any dudi object. They were provided by the as.dudi function which creates the dudi object. The last two elements (cent and norm) were added to the pca1 object at the end of the dudi.pca function.

3.5.1　*pca1$tab*

The first element of pca1 is pca1$tab. This is a data frame, containing the data table (samples in rows, variables in columns), but the variables have been centred and standardised: the mean has been subtracted from raw values and they have been divided by the standard deviation. We can check this on the first values of the data frame, using the scale function:

```
pca1$tab[1:3, 1:6]
```

```
       Temp    Flow      pH     Cond      Bdo5     Oxyd
sp_1 0.4270 -1.0310  0.9695 -1.1332  -0.60553 -0.5350
sp_2 0.6127 -0.1095  0.1939 -0.5736   0.03061  0.5821
sp_3 0.6127  0.2056  0.9695 -1.2731  -0.48550 -0.4762
```

```
scale(env)[1:3, 1:6]
```

```
      Temp    Flow      pH    Cond     Bdo5     Oxyd
sp_1 0.4162 -1.0049 0.9449 -1.1045 -0.59019 -0.5215
sp_2 0.5972 -0.1067 0.1890 -0.5591  0.02983  0.5673
sp_3 0.5972  0.2004 0.9449 -1.2409 -0.47321 -0.4642
```

The difference comes from the fact that the **R base** function scale uses the unbiased variance estimator (divided by $n-1$), while **ade4** uses the biased estimator (divided by n). Introducing the $n/(n-1)$ correction factor brings back things in order:

```
corfac <- sqrt(nrow(env) / (nrow(env) - 1))
scale(env)[1:3, 1:6] * corfac
```

```
      Temp    Flow      pH    Cond     Bdo5     Oxyd
sp_1 0.4270 -1.0310 0.9695 -1.1332 -0.60553 -0.5350
sp_2 0.6127 -0.1095 0.1939 -0.5736  0.03061  0.5821
sp_3 0.6127  0.2056 0.9695 -1.2731 -0.48550 -0.4762
```

An alternative is to use the scalewt function of **ade4** instead of scale:

```
scalewt(env)[1:3, 1:6]
```

```
      Temp    Flow      pH    Cond     Bdo5     Oxyd
sp_1 0.4270 -1.0310 0.9695 -1.1332 -0.60553 -0.5350
sp_2 0.6127 -0.1095 0.1939 -0.5736  0.03061  0.5821
sp_3 0.6127  0.2056 0.9695 -1.2731 -0.48550 -0.4762
```

3.5.2 pca1$cw and pca1$lw

The next two elements are pca1$cw and pca1$lw. They contain column and row weights. In the case of a plain PCA, the default values are equal to 1 for columns and $1/n$ for rows:

```
pca1$cw
```

```
[1] 1 1 1 1 1 1 1 1 1
```

```
pca1$lw[1:6]
```

```
[1] 0.05 0.05 0.05 0.05 0.05 0.05
```

```
1 / nrow(env)
```

```
[1] 0.05
```

3.5.3 *pca1\$eig, pca1\$rank and pca1\$nf*

After the dudi.pca function has finished computing eigenvalues and eigenvectors, the eigenvalues screeplot is displayed and the user is asked for the number of dimensions on which row scores and variable loadings should be computed. Three new elements are added to the pca1 object: pca1\$eig is a vector containing the eigenvalues, pca1\$rank is the rank of the correlation matrix, and pca1\$nf is the number of dimensions chosen to perform the analysis.

```
pca1$eig[1:6]
```

```
[1] 5.1747 1.3204 1.0934 0.7321 0.4902 0.1098
```

```
pca1$rank
```

```
[1] 9
```

```
pca1$nf
```

```
[1] 3
```

In a correlation matrix PCA, pca1\$rank should be equal to the number of variables, unless some of the variables are linearly dependent. This is the case, for example, if one of the variables is a linear combination (e.g., the sum) of some other variables.

The default value for nf is 2.

3.5.4 *pca1\$c1, pca1\$l1, pca1\$co and pca1\$li*

After the user has answered the question about the number of axes (or immediately if the scannf argument was set to FALSE), the dudi.pca function computes variable loadings and row scores and adds them to the pca1 object.

pca1\$c1 is a data frame containing the principal axes (i.e., variable loadings), its rows correspond to the variables (columns of the input data table), and its columns are the axes on which loadings are computed.

pca1\$l1 is a data frame containing the principal components, its rows correspond to the samples (rows of the input data table), and its columns are the axes on which components are computed.

```
pca1$c1[1:4, ]
```

```
              CS1       CS2       CS3
Temp     0.04634  -0.27926   0.80092
Flow    -0.11990  -0.41278  -0.55580
pH      -0.34881  -0.03483  -0.07268
Cond     0.39986   0.16240  -0.18562
```

```
pca1$l1[1:4, ]
```

```
            RS1      RS2     RS3
sp_1  -0.77208  -0.4034  1.0799
sp_2   0.01734  -0.9348  0.5774
sp_3  -0.81759  -0.8141  0.5853
sp_4  -0.83512  -1.0326  0.3415
```

By definition, the norm of these vectors is equal to 1:

```
sum(pca1$cw * pca1$c1$CS1 ^ 2)
```

```
[1] 1
```

```
sum(pca1$lw * pca1$l1$RS1 ^ 2)
```

```
[1] 1
```

pca1$co is a data frame containing column coordinates (or scores), its rows correspond to the variables (columns of the input data table), and its columns are the components on which scores are computed. The norm of these coordinates is equal to the square root of the corresponding eigenvalue.

```
pca1$co[1:4, ]
```

```
        Comp1     Comp2     Comp3
Temp   0.1054  -0.32090   0.8375
Flow  -0.2728  -0.47433  -0.5812
pH    -0.7935  -0.04002  -0.0760
Cond   0.9096   0.18661  -0.1941
```

```
sqrt(sum(pca1$cw * pca1$co$Comp1 ^ 2))
```

```
[1] 2.275
```

```
sqrt(pca1$eig[1])
```

```
[1] 2.275
```

pca1$li is a data frame containing row coordinates (or scores), its rows correspond to the samples (rows of the input data table), and its columns are the axes on which scores are computed. The norm of these coordinates is equal to the square root of the corresponding eigenvalue.

```
pca1$li[1:4, ]
```

```
          Axis1    Axis2   Axis3
sp_1  -1.75632  -0.4635  1.1292
sp_2   0.03944  -1.0741  0.6038
sp_3  -1.85987  -0.9355  0.6120
sp_4  -1.89974  -1.1865  0.3571
```

```
sqrt(sum(pca1$lw * pca1$li$Axis1 ^ 2))
```

```
[1] 2.275
```

3.5.5   `pca1$cent` and `pca1$norm`

After computations are over, the `dudi.pca` function adds two new elements to the `pca1` object: `cent` and `norm`. `cent` is a vector containing variable means, except in the case of a non-centred PCA where it is a vector of 0. We can check this on the first 6 variables:

```
pca1$cent[1:6]
```

```
   Temp     Flow       pH     Cond      Bdo5     Oxyd
  7.700  171.900    8.250  335.500     7.345    2.310
```

```
apply(env, 2, mean)[1:6]
```

```
   Temp     Flow       pH     Cond      Bdo5     Oxyd
  7.700  171.900    8.250  335.500     7.345    2.310
```

For a standardised PCA (PCA on correlation matrix), `norm` is the vector of variable standard deviations. Note that in **ade4**, the variance estimator that is used is never the unbiased estimator (divided by $n - 1$) but always the biased estimator (divided by n). This is different from the `var` and `sd` functions, which use the unbiased estimator:

```
pca1$norm[1:6]
```

```
   Temp      Flow       pH      Cond      Bdo5     Oxyd
 5.3861  126.9618   0.2579   35.7386    8.3316   1.7009
```

```
apply(env, 2, sd)[1:6]
```

```
   Temp      Flow       pH      Cond      Bdo5     Oxyd
 5.5260  130.2600   0.2646   36.6671    8.5480   1.7450
```

```
corfac <- sqrt((nrow(env) - 1) / nrow(env))
corfac * apply(env, 2, sd)[1:6]
```

```
   Temp      Flow       pH      Cond      Bdo5     Oxyd
 5.3861  126.9618   0.2579   35.7386    8.3316   1.7009
```

3.6   Using `dudi` Objects

Many functions in **ade4** allow to handle `dudi` objects. In this section, we describe some functions that create, manipulate, display or plot these objects. Note also that high-level multivariate analysis functions, like `bca` (Sect. 7.3), `coinertia` (Sect. 8.3) or `rlq` (Sect. 11.2) also use `dudi` objects as argument.

The `as.dudi` function creates a `dudi` object, starting from a data frame and row and column weights. It is called by high-level functions (`dudi.pca`, dudi.coa, etc.) and not directly by the user. The is.dudi function can test if an object is a dudi. The redo.dudi function redoes all the computations of a dudi, eventually changing the number of kept axes. The t.dudi method (t function) transposes a dudi, switching the roles of rows and columns.

Other useful functions are detailed in this section.

3.6.1 The print and summary Functions

The print function displays the main components of a dudi object. It prints the class hierarchy of the object, the command-line call, the number of axes kept in the analysis, the rank of the matrix that was diagonalised, and the list of eigenvalues. It then lists vectors and data frames making up the dudi, with their dimensions, mode and content. Depending on the type of dudi, it finally prints the name of additional elements, like cent and norm in the case of a PCA.

```
pca1             # equivalent to print(pca1)


Duality diagram
class: pca dudi
$call: dudi.pca(df = env, scannf = FALSE, nf = 3)

$nf: 3 axis-components saved
$rank: 9
eigen values: 5.175 1.32 1.093 0.7321 0.4902 ...
    vector length mode      content
1 $cw      9           numeric column weights
2 $lw     20           numeric row weights
3 $eig     9           numeric eigen values

    data.frame nrow ncol content
1 $tab           20    9     modified array
2 $li            20    3     row coordinates
3 $l1            20    3     row normed scores
4 $co             9    3     column coordinates
5 $c1             9    3     column normed scores
other elements: cent norm
```

The summary function displays a more useful numerical summary of a dudi object: the dudi class, the function call, the total inertia, the list of eigenvalues, and the simple and cumulative projected inertia on the first five axes.

```
summary(pca1)


Class: pca dudi
Call: dudi.pca(df = env, scannf = FALSE, nf = 3)

Total inertia: 9

Eigenvalues:
    Ax1      Ax2      Ax3      Ax4      Ax5
 5.1747   1.3204   1.0934   0.7321   0.4902

Projected inertia (%):
    Ax1      Ax2      Ax3      Ax4      Ax5
 57.497   14.671   12.149    8.135    5.447
```

```
Cumulative projected inertia (%):
    Ax1    Ax1:2    Ax1:3    Ax1:4    Ax1:5
  57.50    72.17    84.32    92.45    97.90

(Only 5 dimensions (out of 9) are shown)
```

3.6.2   The scatter and biplot Functions

The scatter function has a scatter.dudi method that draws the biplot of the dudi passed as argument. The same function is called by the biplot.dudi method, a function from the generic **R** biplot (Gabriel 1971). Figure 3.2 shows the output of this function. Scores and loadings are used to plot samples and variables on the same graph, with simple labels for samples and arrows for variables. Arrows are used to symbolise the fact that variables are seen as vectors. The permute argument of the scatter function is a logical value to switch between a *distance biplot* (permute = FALSE, the default) or a *correlation biplot* (permute = TRUE). The first biplot is a superimposition of pca1$li and pca1$c1 whereas the second represents pca1$co and pca1$l1. See Legendre and Legendre (1998, pp. 403–404) for more information about biplots. If permute is set to TRUE, then arrows are used for samples, and simple labels for variables.

By default, the screeplot of eigenvalues is inserted in the biplot, to show the importance of each principal component. On this screeplot, the principal components kept by the user are coloured in grey, and the two components selected to form the biplot (by default, the first and second ones) are in black.

3.6.3   The score Function

The score function is another generic graphical function of **ade4**. Depending on the class of its input argument, it provides a graph that underlines the canonical property of a multivariate analysis method. This graph is called the "canonical graph" of a dudi object.

For a simple PCA (pca and dudi classes), this graph is a collection of plots displaying the values of each variable against sample scores. The mathematical property underlined here is the fact that principal components maximise the sum of squared correlations with all the variables. In the case of normed PCA, the correlation between variables and the component is indicated in parentheses.

These correlations are strictly equal to the PCA score of variables:

```
round(pca1$co[, 1, drop = FALSE], 2)
```

```
      Comp1
Temp   0.11
Flow  -0.27
pH    -0.79
```

```
Cond   0.91
Bdo5   0.97
Oxyd   0.92
Ammo   0.98
Nitr  -0.19
Phos   0.92
```

By default, the scores on the first principal component are used (see Fig. 3.3), but any component can be selected thanks to the xax argument of the score function.

```
score(pca1, xax = 1, psub.cex = 1.5)
```

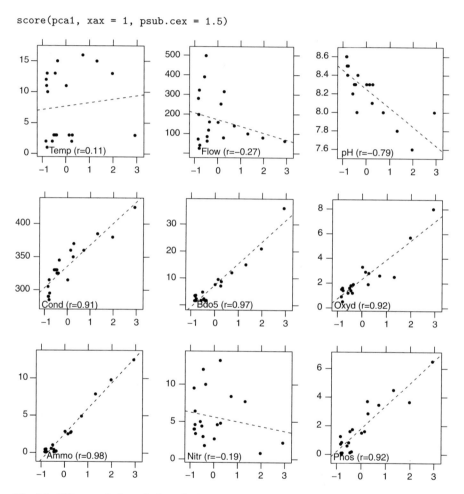

Fig. 3.3 PCA canonical graph. In each plot, the values of one variable are plotted against sample scores. This underlines one of the main properties of PCA, i.e., the fact that principal components maximise the sum of squared correlations with all the variables.

```
plot(pca1$li[, 1:2], type = "n", asp = 1)
text(pca1$li[, 1:2], label = row.names(env))
abline(h = 0, v = 0)
```

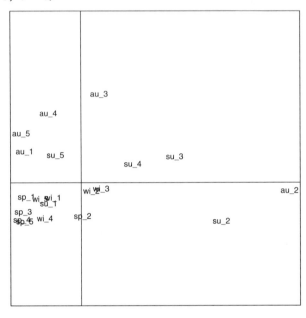

Fig. 3.4 PCA factor map plotted with the `plot` and `text` functions. Note that the limits of the graph are constrained by the `asp` argument so that the height/width ratio is equal to 1.

3.6.4   The s.label and plot Functions

Elements of a `dudi` object can also be used as arguments to **ade4** functions, or to general **R graphics** functions.

For example, row scores and variables loadings can be used as inputs to graphical functions. Usual **R** graphical functions like `plot` and `text` can draw the classical multivariate analysis graphs, called "factor maps" (Fig. 3.4).

The problem is that, by default, the height/width ratio of the graph is not equal to 1, which means that the real factor map can be distorted horizontally or vertically. The limits of the x-axis and the y-axis should therefore be passed as inputs to the `plot` function. The `asp` argument should also be modified to specify the aspect ratio of the graph. Figure 3.4 shows how to draw a factor map respecting the true height/width ratio using the `plot` function and the `asp` argument.

The simplest function to draw a factor map is the `s.label` function. It automatically draws factor maps with a height/width ratio equal to 1, even if the graphic window is not square (Fig. 3.5). The value `d = 2` in the upper right corner of the graph gives the scale: it is the size of the background grid.

```
ade4::s.label(pca1$li)
```

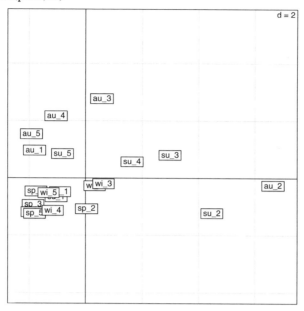

Fig. 3.5 PCA factor map plotted with the s.label function of the **adegraphics** package.

3.6.5 The *inertia* Function

The inertia function allows to compute inertia statistics described in Box 3.3.

Box 3.3 The Duality Diagram: Inertia Statistics

The total inertia associated to the triplet $(\mathbf{X}, \mathbf{Q}, \mathbf{D})$ represents the total variation contained in the data set. If we consider the clouds of points described in Box 3.1, the total inertia corresponds to a weighted sum of squared distances (using the appropriate metric) between the origin of the cloud and the points. For instance, for the cloud of p centred columns $\mathbf{x}_1, \mathbf{x}_2, \ldots, \mathbf{x}_p$ in $\mathbb{R}^n$, we have:

$$I_{(\mathbf{X},\mathbf{Q},\mathbf{D})} = \sum_{j=1}^{p} \omega_j \|\mathbf{x}_j\|_{\mathbf{D}}^2 = \mathrm{Trace}(\mathbf{X}^{\top}\mathbf{D}\mathbf{X}\mathbf{Q})$$

where $\mathbf{Q} = \mathrm{diag}(\omega_1, \ldots, \omega_p)$. As the clouds of columns and rows are linked, we have also:

(continued)

Box 3.3 (continued)

$$I_{(\mathbf{X},\mathbf{Q},\mathbf{D})} = \text{Trace}(\mathbf{X}^\top \mathbf{D}\mathbf{X}\mathbf{Q}) = \text{Trace}(\mathbf{X}\mathbf{Q}\mathbf{X}^\top \mathbf{D})$$

The analysis of a duality diagram finds two systems of orthogonal axes that decompose the total inertia (Box 3.2). For a given dimension, the projected inertia is maximised for the cloud of rows in $\mathbb{R}^p$ ($\|\mathbf{X}\mathbf{Q}\mathbf{a}\|_{\mathbf{D}}^2$) or column vectors in $\mathbb{R}^n$ ($\|\mathbf{X}^\top \mathbf{D}\mathbf{b}\|_{\mathbf{Q}}^2$) and is equal to λ (Properties 3.1 and 3.2 in Box 3.2). Hence the total inertia is decomposed in decreasing order and can be rewritten as:

$$I_{(\mathbf{X},\mathbf{Q},\mathbf{D})} = \text{Trace}(\mathbf{\Lambda}) = \sum_{i=1}^{r} \lambda_i$$

The inertia associated to each dimension can then be decomposed by points (i.e., rows or columns of $\mathbf{X}$). If we consider the cloud of variables, the *absolute contribution* $AC_i(j)$ measures the part of inertia of the i-th dimension explained by the j-th variable:

$$AC_i(j) = \frac{\omega_j \left(\mathbf{x}_j^\top \mathbf{D}\mathbf{b}_i\right)^2}{\lambda_i}$$

The *relative contribution* (also known as cos2) measures the part of inertia of the j-th variable explained by the i-th dimension:

$$RC_i(j) = \frac{(\mathbf{x}_j^\top \mathbf{D}\mathbf{b}_i)^2}{\|\mathbf{x}_j\|_{\mathbf{D}}^2}$$

Note that, we have:

$$\sum_{j=1}^{p} AC_i(j) = \sum_{i=1}^{r} RC_i(j) = 1$$

The previous definitions focused on contributions of variables but these statistics can also be computed for individuals (i.e., rows of $\mathbf{X}$).

By default, the function returns only the decomposition of the total inertia per axis:

```
inertia(pca1)
```

```
Inertia information:
Call: inertia.dudi(x = pca1)
```

```
Decomposition of total inertia:
      inertia     cum    cum(%)
Ax1  5.174737   5.175   57.50
Ax2  1.320419   6.495   72.17
Ax3  1.093376   7.589   84.32
Ax4  0.732113   8.321   92.45
Ax5  0.490214   8.811   97.90
Ax6  0.109835   8.921   99.12
Ax7  0.052960   8.974   99.71
Ax8  0.020031   8.994   99.93
Ax9  0.006316   9.000  100.00
```

Arguments `row.inertia` and `col.inertia` of the `inertia` function can be set to TRUE to compute relative and absolute contributions (Box 3.3) for samples or variables.

```
iner <- inertia(pca1, col.inertia = TRUE)
```

In this case, the function returns a list (class `inertia`) containing all the different inertia statistics. The main results can be obtained by applying the `summary` function:

```
summary(iner)
```

```
Total inertia: 9

Projected inertia (%):
   Ax1     Ax2     Ax3
 57.50   14.67   12.15

(Only 3 dimensions (out of 9) are shown)


Column absolute contributions (%):
      Axis1(%) Axis2(%) Axis3(%)
Ammo    18.73   0.2698  0.07917
Bdo5    18.00   0.8780  0.43463
Oxyd    16.39   3.7632  0.25313
Phos    16.37   5.2789  0.17503
Cond    15.99   2.6373  3.44540

Column relative contributions (%):
        Axis1    Axis2    Axis3
Ammo    96.95   0.3562 0.08657
Bdo5    93.16   1.1593 0.47521
Oxyd    84.80   4.9691 0.27677
Phos    84.71   6.9704 0.19138
Cond    82.74   3.4824 3.76711
```

The contributions are presented by decreasing order from the most important variable (sample respectively) to the least important on a defined axis. By default, sorting is done on the first axis of the analysis and only the five first variables are shown.

Inertia statistics can also be represented graphically. In this case, variables (or samples) are positioned by their coordinates and the size of the symbols or labels (using the `type` argument of the `plot` function) is proportional to their absolute or relative contributions (see the `plot.inertia` method, available in the **adegraphics** package, Fig. 3.6).

```
gcontabs <- plot(iner, contrib = "abs", plot = FALSE)
gcontrel <- plot(iner, contrib = "rel", plot = FALSE)
ADEgS(list(gcontabs, gcontrel))
```

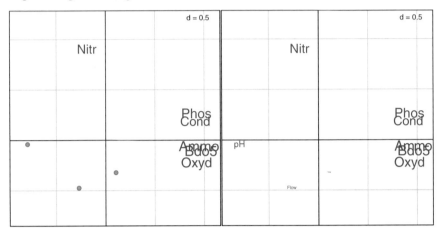

Fig. 3.6 The left plot shows the part of inertia of the first two axes explained by the variables: it shows how the axes can be interpreted. The right plot shows the part of inertia of variables explained by the first two axes: it shows whether variables are well described or not. These two plots are similar in PCA because all the variables (respectively samples) have the same weights.

```
screeplot(pca1, main = " ", xlab = " ")
```

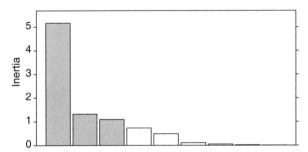

Fig. 3.7 Eigenvalues screeplot. Grey bars show the eigenvalues kept in the analysis (here, the first three ones). They correspond to the axes on which row and column coordinates have been computed.

3.6.6 Other Graphical Functions

There are many other graphical functions to draw multivariate analysis graphs. For example, the eigenvalues `pca1$eig` can be passed to the `barplot` function to draw the usual eigenvalues screeplot. The generic `screeplot` function also has a method for `dudi` objects (`screeplot.dudi`) that draws the eigenvalues

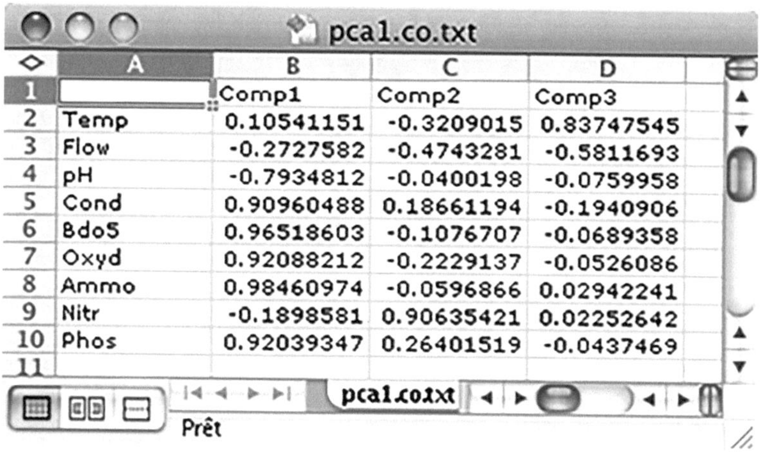
pca1.co.txt

	A	B	C	D
1		Comp1	Comp2	Comp3
2	Temp	0.10541151	-0.3209015	0.83747545
3	Flow	-0.2727582	-0.4743281	-0.5811693
4	pH	-0.7934812	-0.0400198	-0.0759958
5	Cond	0.90960488	0.18661194	-0.1940906
6	Bdo5	0.96518603	-0.1076707	-0.0689358
7	Oxyd	0.92088212	-0.2229137	-0.0526086
8	Ammo	0.98460974	-0.0596866	0.02942241
9	Nitr	-0.1898581	0.90635421	0.02252642
10	Phos	0.92039347	0.26401519	-0.0437469
11				

pca1.co.txt

Prêt

Fig. 3.8 Text file exported from **R** and imported in Excel.

screeplot (Fig. 3.7). This graph is the one displayed when the user is asked to choose the number of principal components that should be kept in the `dudi`, as this choice should be based on the shape of the decrease of eigenvalues.

The next chapter (Chap. 4) is dedicated to the **adegraphics** add-on package, and presents all the graphical functions that can be used with **ade4** multivariate data analysis outputs.

3.7 Exporting `dudi` Elements

Elements of `dudi` objects can be exported from **R** using the `write.table` function (see Sect. 2.2). This function creates text files that can be subsequently imported in a spreadsheet or drawing software. The argument `col.names = NA` should be used to include a null column name for the column containing row names.

```
write.table(pca1$co, file = "pca1.co.txt", col.names = NA)
```

In the spreadsheet software, during importation, the "delimited" type should be used with the delimiter set to the space character (Fig. 3.8).

Chapter 4
Multivariate Analysis Graphs

Abstract This chapter outlines the main characteristics of the **adegraphics** package. The structure of graphical objects, classes and associated methods are explained. Several examples show how user-level functions can be used to draw scientific graphs particularly adapted to multivariate data analysis. Automated collection of graphs, spatial representations, and the case of big data sets are detailed.

4.1 Introduction

Multivariate data analysis makes heavy use of graphical display. The first reason comes from the dimension reduction strategy of multivariate analysis. Indeed, this strategy leads to draw low-dimensional (1, 2 or 3) graphs, starting from multidimensional clouds of points (see Chap. 3). Another reason is that graphs can be seen as an interface between statistical data analysis theorems and biological interpretations (Thioulouse 1996). This point of view has been explained in the PhD thesis of Auda (1983) in the early 1980s, and we have continued in this way. The ideas expressed by Auda about graphs stemmed from the seminal work of Bertin (1967). They were implemented in a software called "Graphique" (in French), that was used for several years to drive a Tektronix pen plotter and several video CRT consoles.

These ideas were developed and adapted to multivariate data analysis in the ADECO and GraphMu software during the 1980s (Thioulouse 1989, 1990). They followed the evolution of the ADE-4 software (see Chap. 1) and were implemented in **R** in the **ade4** package in 2002. This implementation was based on plain **R** functions and it was intensively used during ten years. However, some capabilities of the previous version had been lost, and it was missing flexibility and extendability. A complete rewrite using the **lattice** package and S4 classes was undertaken in 2012 and the **adegraphics** package is the result of this effort (Siberchicot et al. 2017).

© Springer Science+Business Media, LLC, part of Springer Nature 2018
J. Thioulouse et al., *Multivariate Analysis of Ecological Data with ade4*,
https://doi.org/10.1007/978-1-4939-8850-1_4

4.2   Basics of adegraphics

In this new implementation, graphs are objects. They are created by a function, and saved into an **R** object that can later be displayed, modified or copied. The **adegraphics** package is based on S4 classes and on the **lattice** package developed by Sarkar (2008). The class architecture description is given in Box 4.1.

adegraphics is exclusively a graphical package, with no statistical or computational functions. It is a complete reimplementation of the graphical functions of **ade4**. Developing a new package for graphics instead of implementing these functions in **ade4** avoids to break other packages or code that used **ade4** graphical functions. However, users are encouraged to prefer the new graphical functionalities provided by **adegraphics** as the graphical functions of **ade4** will be maintained but not developed in the future.

Whereas the underlying implementation of **adegraphics** is completely new, we tried to keep the name and the basic syntax of **ade4** graphical functions. Simple **R** code written to draw graphs with **ade4** should therefore be re-usable, or easily re-written for **adegraphics**. Here we give a summary of the main features of **adegraphics** but a more detailed description can be found in Siberchicot et al. (2017).

4.2.1   *ADEg and ADEgS Objects*

Two types of graphical objects are defined in the **adegraphics** package:

- ADEg: elementary graph, with only one data source and one representation method
- ADEgS: a collection (list) of ADEg, ADEgS and trellis objects. Elements of this collection may result from several data sources and they can be handled individually, juxtaposed or superimposed.

ADEg objects are created with simple functions that keep the same name and the same basic parameters as previous **ade4** graphical functions. This makes the transition from **ade4** to **adegraphics** easier.

An ADEgS is a list of various graphical objects, with position information.

Box 4.1 Class Structure and User-Level Functions
The basic object of **adegraphics** is an ADEg graph. An ADEgS is simply a list of ADEg, with position and superposition information. A solid arrow represents an inheritance relation between two classes: the ADEg.S2 class inherits from the ADEg class. This inheritance mechanism was implemented

(continued)

Box 4.1 (continued)

to factorise some of the most common behaviours. For example, limits and background grid calculations in the ADEg.S2 class are identical in all the S2.class methods. These computations are all performed by a common method (prepare) in the ADEg.S2 class.

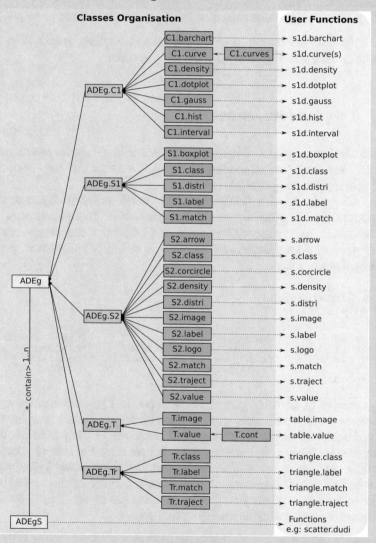

An elementary graph (ADEg object) belongs to one of the five categories:

- ADEg.C1: bidimensional graphs for one numeric score
- ADEg.S1: unidimensional graphs for one numeric score
- ADEg.S2: bidimensional graphs for x and y coordinates
- ADEg.T: table representation of distance matrix, contingency table or simple matrix or data frame
- ADEg.Tr: triangular representation for x, y and z coordinates

ADEg classes implement several methods for handling graphs, like plot, update, zoom, superpose, add, and the + operator.

4.2.2 Graphical Parameters

The most important graphical parameters defined in **adegraphics** can be modified directly. They can be set either globally for all subsequent drawings or during the creation of a particular graphical object.

The adegpar function (analogous to the par base function) can be used to get and set the value of all adegraphics parameters. These parameters consist of sublists that deal with specific elements of a graph and have easy to remember names: ppoints for point parameters, plabels for label parameters, psub for subtitle parameters, etc.

```
library(ade4)
library(adegraphics)
names(adegpar())
```

```
 [1] "p1d"        "parrows"    "paxes"      "pbackground"
 [5] "pellipses"  "pgrid"      "plabels"    "plegend"
 [9] "plines"     "pnb"        "porigin"    "ppalette"
[13] "ppoints"    "ppolygons"  "pSp"        "psub"
[17] "ptable"
```

A summary of available parameters is shown in Fig. 4.1. Columns represent the different sublists and rows give the name of the parameters available in each sublist. Parameters consist of dot-separated keys. The first key indicates the first sublist whereas the last key corresponds to the parameter. For example, parameters plabels.col and plabels.cex control the graphical aspect (colour and size) of the text of labels. Parameter plabels.cex is made of the parameter cex applied to the sublist plabels. These parameters can be set globally (i.e., for all subsequent drawings) with the adegpar function:

```
adegpar(plabels.col = "blue", plabels.cex = 1.5)
```

Here, the label character size is set to 1.5 and its colour to "blue". As both parameters applied to the plabels sublist, another syntax can be used to avoid repetitions:

```
adegpar(plabels = list(col = "blue", cex = 1.5))
```

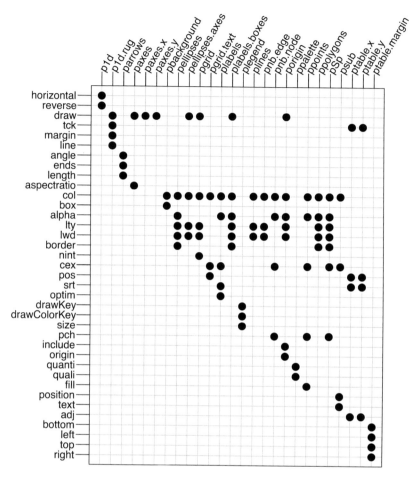

Fig. 4.1 Parameters that can be set with the `adegpar` function.

Another strategy is to set the parameters only for a particular graphical object during its creation:

```
xy <- cbind.data.frame(rnorm(10), rnorm(10))
s.label(xy, plabels = list(col = "blue", cex = 1.5))
```

Here parameters are passed using the "dots" (...) argument of the function `s.label` but all parameters do not apply to all functions. Figure 4.2 shows which parameters can be used in which function. The top axis shows the subset of parameters available through the `adegpar` function. The left axis lists the user functions in which these parameters can be set. A black point at position (i, j) means that a change in the sublist of parameter j will affect the display of the graphical object created by function i.

For example, all graphs can have a background grid (which gives the scale of the graph), but only a few graphs use polygons. So the parameters sublist `pgrid` can be used in all functions, whereas `ppolygons` is used in only six functions.

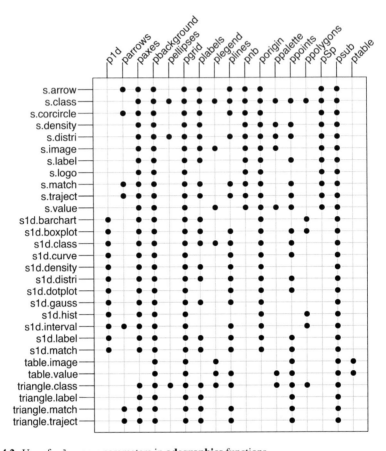

Fig. 4.2 Use of `adegpar` parameters in **adegraphics** functions.

Details about these parameters can be found in the help of the `adegpar` function (`?adegpar`).

All graphical functions of **adegraphics** have a "dots" (…) argument. Through this argument, it is possible to pass three type of parameters:

1. **adegraphics** parameters (see `adegpar` function)
2. **lattice** parameters
3. other graphical parameters, e.g.:

   - `xlim`, `ylim`: x and y bounds of the graph
   - `main`, `sub`: main title and subtitle
   - `xlab`, `ylab`: labels for x-axis and y-axis
   - `scales`: this is the `scales` parameter of the `xyplot` function of **lattice** to determine how x-axis and y-axis are drawn
   - `Sp`, `sp.layout`: objects from the **sp** package to display spatial objects
   - `nbobject`: objects of class nb to display neighbour graphs

The graphical display can be changed by passing these parameters as a "dots" argument to the graphical functions. It is also possible to modify some of the parameters globally, using the adegpar function for **adegraphics** parameters or the function trellis.par.set for specific **lattice** parameters.

4.2.3 Main Functions and Methods

All the graphical functions of **ade4** have been rewritten in **adegraphics**, and their capabilities have been largely improved. Tables 4.1, 4.2 and 4.3 give the list of the main functions that create ADEg or ADEgS objects.

A user function must be called to create an ADEg (or ADEgS) object (see first column of Tables 4.1, 4.2 and 4.3). This function sorts the parameters, creates the object and eventually plots the object (if argument plot = TRUE). This object will be returned as a temporary copy (using invisible), and stored if assigned in the command line. If it is stored, it can be modified later as needed.

After creation, various methods can be applied to the object to modify it and get the desired graphical representation:

- update: modifies the ADEg object after its creation. Most parameters passed through the "dots" argument (...) of the function can be changed using the update method.
- zoom: zooms in or out the display, changing the graphical boundaries
- +, add.ADEg, superpose: superposes an ADEg object on another one (previous plotted for add.ADEg, any ADEg object for +, and ADEg, ADEgS or trellis objects for superpose)

Table 4.1 One-dimensional graphical functions in **adegraphics** that return ADEg.C1 and ADEg.S1 objects.

Function	Object class	Type of representation
s1d.barchart	C1.barchart	1-D plot of a numeric score by bars
s1d.curve	C1.curve	1-D plot of a numeric score linked by a curve
s1d.curves	C1.curves	1-D plot of a numeric scores linked by curves
s1d.density	C1.density	1-D plot of a numeric score by density curves
s1d.dotplot	C1.dotplot	1-D plot of a numeric score by dots
s1d.gauss	C1.gauss	1-D plot of a numeric score by Gaussian curves
s1d.hist	C1.hist	1-D plot of a numeric score by histogram
s1d.interval	C1.interval	1-D plot of the interval between two numeric scores
s1d.boxplot	S1.boxplot	1-D box plot of a numeric score eventually partitioned in classes
s1d.class	S1.class	1-D plot of a numeric score partitioned in classes
s1d.distri	S1.distri	1-D plot of a numeric score by means/standard deviations computed using an external table of weights
s1d.label	S1.label	1-D plot of a numeric score with labels
s1d.match	S1.match	1-D plot of the matching between two numeric scores

Table 4.2 Bi-dimensional graphical functions in **adegraphics** that return ADEg.S2.

Function	Object class	Type of representation
s.arrow	S2.arrow	2-D scatter plot with arrows
s.class	S2.class	2-D scatter plot with a partition in classes
s.corcircle	S2.corcircle	Correlation circle
s.density	S2.density	2-D scatter plot with kernel density estimation
s.distri	S2.distri	2-D scatter plot with means/standard deviations computed using an external table of weights
s.image	S2.image	2-D scatter plot with loess estimation of an additional numeric score
s.label	S2.label	2-D scatter plot with labels
s.logo	S2.logo	2-D scatter plot with logos (pixmap objects)
s.match	S2.match	2-D scatter plot of the matching between two sets of coordinates
s.Spatial	S2.label	Mapping of a Spatial* object
s.traject	S2.traject	2-D scatter plot with trajectories
s.value	S2.value	2-D scatter plot with proportional symbols

Table 4.3 Other main graphical functions in **adegraphics**.

Function	Object class	Type of representation
table.image	T.image	Heat map-like representation with coloured cells
table.value	T.value or T.cont	Heat map-like representation with proportional symbols
triangle.class	Tr.class	Ternary plot with a partition in classes
triangle.label	Tr.label	Ternary plot with labels
triangle.match	Tr.match	Ternary plot of the matching between two sets of coordinates
triangle.traject	Tr.match	Ternary plot with trajectories
ADEgS	ADEgS	Association of multiple plots

- insert: inserts an ADEg or ADEgS object in an existing one or in the current device
- cbindADEg, rbindADEg: combines several graphs (ADEg, ADEgS or trellis) by columns or rows
- plot, print, show: displays ADEg or ADEgS objects

4.2.4   (Big) Data Storage

If the storeData argument of a graphical function is TRUE (the default value), the data used to draw the graphical object is stored inside the object itself. This is handy to redraw and update the object, but for large data sets it can be very memory consuming, particularly when many graphs pile up in the **R** global environment. To avoid this problem, storeData can be set to FALSE, and in this case only *the name* of the data objects (or function call) and their positions inside the **R** environments are stored. The drawback of setting `storeData` to `FALSE` is that, if the data object is no more available (e.g., if it has been deleted), the graph cannot be redrawn. A simulated data set is used to illustrate this possibility:

```
set.seed(15)
xy <- matrix(rnorm(1e+05), ncol = 2)
xy2 <- matrix(rnorm(1e+05, mean = 2), ncol = 2)
xy <- rbind(xy, xy2)
```

The resulting `xy` matrix has 100,000 rows originating from a mixture of two normal distributions and the function `s.label` is used to represent the data-points:

```
sl1 <- s.label(xy, plot = FALSE)
sl2 <- s.label(xy, storeData = FALSE, plot = FALSE)
print(object.size(sl1), units = "auto")
```

```
1.6 Mb
```

```
print(object.size(sl2), units = "auto")
```

```
92.7 Kb
```

The effect of setting `storeData = FALSE` is clear as the size of the ADEg object is drastically reduced. Note that by default, the `s.label` function remove labels when there are more than 1000 points (Fig. 4.3, left) but it remains hard to observe correctly the points distribution. The use of alpha transparency can help for this purpose (Fig. 4.3, centre).

```
sl3 <- s.label(xy, storeData = FALSE, plot = FALSE,
       points.alpha = 0.01)
```

The **adegraphics** package proposes also alternative graphical representations that are more suitable to observe structures in large data sets, but also to speed up the drawing of plots. For instance, the `s.density` function allows to draw density plots. Figure 4.3 (right) shows that the representation can be improved with specific parameters, like `contour` to add contour lines. `ppalette.quanti` is an `adegpar` parameter defining the colours of the density surface.

```
sd1 <- s.density(xy, nr = 0, threshold = 0.001, contour = TRUE,
       region = TRUE, ppalette.quanti =
       colorRampPalette(c(rgb(0, 0, 1, 0.05), rgb(0.5, 0, 0.5,
       0.9)), alpha = TRUE), plot = FALSE)
```

4.3 Simple Examples

We demonstrate **adegraphics** capabilities using data from the **Guerry** package (Friendly and Dray 2014) that contains data sets and maps of France in 1830. These data were analysed by Dray and Jombart (2011) to illustrate how to consider spatial information in classical multivariate methods. Although Guerry data are outside the ecological framework, they are suitable to illustrate graphical representations of multivariate and spatial data analysis.

```
ADEgS(list(sl2, sl3, sd1))
```

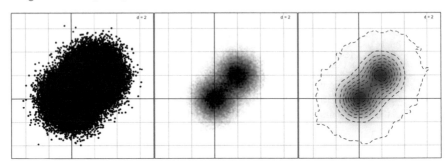

Fig. 4.3 Representing 100,000 individuals by points (left, sl2 object), transparent points (centre, sl3 object) and density surface (right, sd1 object). Only the representation on the right allows to visualise that data originate from a mixture of two normal distributions with different means.

```
library(Guerry)
library(sp)
data(gfrance85)
xy <- coordinates(gfrance85)
dep.names <- data.frame(gfrance85)[, 6]
region.names <- data.frame(gfrance85)[, 5]
df <- data.frame(gfrance85)[, 7:12]
names(df)
```

```
[1] "Crime_pers" "Crime_prop" "Literacy"    "Donations"
[5] "Infants"    "Suicides"
```

gfrance85 contains a map of France and associated data with 85 rows (departments) and 26 columns (variables). It is stored as a SpatialPolygonsDataFrame (class implemented in the **sp** package, Bivand et al. 2013; Pebesma and Bivand 2005). The map contains the department boundaries (administrative division of France) in 1830 and the region to which they belong (five regions: South, North, East, West, Centre). The data contains Guerry's 1833 data on moral statistics in France.

Six quantitative variables (numbered from 7 to 12) are kept and saved in the df data frame. Several variables are expressed as "Population per ..." to get a positive correlation with moral value (e.g., "Population per illegitimate birth" instead of "Illegitimate birth per 1000 people").

- Crime_pers: Population per Crime against persons
- Crime_prop: Population per Crime against property
- Literacy: Percent Read and Write, percent of literate military conscripts
- Donations: Donations to the poor
- Infants: Population per illegitimate birth
- Suicides: Population per suicide

A standardised PCA (see Sect. 5.2) is applied to the table of quantitative variables. The factor map of departments is then built with the s.label function and stored in the object g.lab.pca (Fig. 4.4, left):

```
pca.guerry <- dudi.pca(df, scannf = FALSE, nf = 3)
g.lab.pca <- g.lab.pca.u <- s.label(pca.guerry$li, labels =
    dep.names, plot = FALSE)
```

```
ADEgS(list(g.lab.pca, g.lab.pca.u))
```

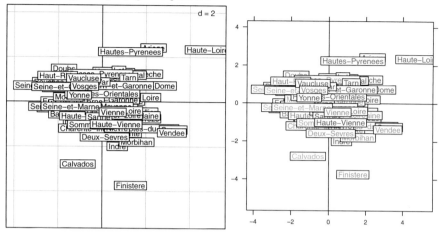

Fig. 4.4 Simple PCA factor map of the department scores (left, g.lab.pca) and use of the update function to change some graphical parameters (right, g.lab.pca.u).

This graph is then modified using the update function to draw x-axis and y-axis with scales, remove the background grid, and colour the labels of departments according to the region they belong to. Each of the five regions is given a colour (South = purple, North = green, East = blue, West = orange, Centre = red). These colours are created using the **RColorBrewer** package (Neuwirth 2014), and used to define a new palette for regions (col.region) and departments (col.dep).

```
library(RColorBrewer)
col.region <- brewer.pal(5, "Set1")
col.dep <- col.region[region.names]
g.lab.pca.u <- update(g.lab.pca.u, paxes.draw = TRUE,
        pgrid.draw = FALSE, plabels.col = col.dep, plot = FALSE)
```

Both graphics are then combined in a multiple graphical object using the ADEgS function (Fig. 4.4). The use of this function is detailed in Sect. 4.6.

To focus on differences among regions (North, South, Est, West, Centre), a Between-Class Analysis (BCA, bca function, see Chap. 7) is performed and results of the analysis are stored in bca.guerry.

```
bca.guerry <- bca(pca.guerry, fac = region.names, scannf = FALSE)
randtest(bca.guerry)$pvalue
```

```
[1] 0.001
```

The p-value of the permutation test of the BCA is extremely significant, meaning that there are strong differences in the "moral variables" measured in the departments belonging to the five regions. The scores of departments on BCA factor map are represented using the s.label function (Fig. 4.5, left):

```
g.lab.bca <- s.label(bca.guerry$ls, labels = dep.names,
        plabels.cex = 0.7, plot = FALSE)
```

```
ADEgS(list(g.lab.bca, g.lab.bca.o))
```

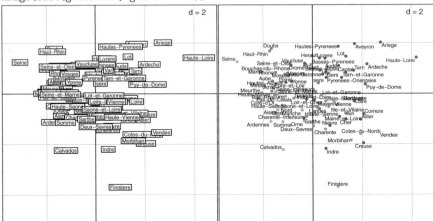

Fig. 4.5 Label positions can be optimised (right, g.lab.bca.o) using a simulated annealing algorithm based on the pointLabel function developed by Tom Short in the **maptools** package (Bivand and Lewin-Koh 2017). This algorithm tries to avoid overlapping and outside bounds labels.

Overlapping labels on these types of graphs is often a problem, and an optimisation function has been introduced in the **adegraphics** package to avoid this. This option is only available for s.label and triangle.label functions using the plabels.optim parameter:

```
g.lab.bca.o <- s.label(bca.guerry$ls, labels = dep.names,
        plabels = list(cex = 0.7, optim = TRUE), ppoints.col =
        col.dep, plot = FALSE)
```

Figure 4.5 shows the result of the simulated annealing algorithm used in this optimisation function. The graph on the left (g.lab.bca) is the standard graph, with several overlapping labels, while the graph on the right (g.lab.bca.o) shows how optimised label positions reduces overlapping. Clearly, this optimisation is really useful only when the number of labels on the factor map is high enough to cause overlaps but not too high, as overlaps cannot be avoided when hundreds of labels are present. In this case, an alternative is to draw labels only for individuals with the strongest contribution to inertia (see Sect. 3.6.5).

However, the representation of scores on the factorial map is not optimal. When spatial information is available, plotting geographical maps can be very useful to represent scores provided by multivariate methods and describe their spatial structure. In this context, the **adegraphics** package has greatly improved the possibilities of **ade4**. The next section shows how to do this, and how to handle spatial objects to draw nice geographical maps with **adegraphics**.

4.4 Spatial Representations

In **ade4**, background geographical maps could be plotted using custom `area` objects. In **adegraphics**, we decided to use **sp**, a package that provides classes and methods for spatial data (Bivand et al. 2013; Pebesma and Bivand 2005). Any kind of spatial object implemented in **sp** can be used as a background for ADEg objects using the `Sp` or `sp.layout` arguments.

We applied the `s.value` function to represent the first score of the BCA over the geographical map of France using a `SpatialPolygonsDataFrame` (`gfrance85` object) as background map (`Sp` parameter). The `s.value` function draws factor maps (or any kind of map) with symbols proportional to the value of a quantitative argument called `z`. Some graphical parameters are set globally using the `adegpar` function: `porigin.include`, `pgrid.draw` and `pbackground.box`. The value of these parameters will be applied to all graphical objects, unless stated otherwise during object creation. The new and old values of parameters are stored in `mappar` and `oldpar`, respectively, for further use.

```
oldpar <- adegpar()
mappar <- adegpar(porigin.include = FALSE, pgrid.draw = FALSE,
     pbackground.box = TRUE)
g1.map.bca <- s.value(xy, bca.guerry$ls[, 1], Sp = gfrance85,
     symbol = "circle", pSp.col = col.dep, psub.text = "BCA axis 1",
     psub.cex = 1.5)
```

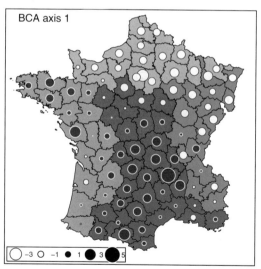

Fig. 4.6 Geographical map (`g1.map.bca`) of the first score of the BCA on the `Guerry` data. There is a clear division between the North-East of France (white circles, negative values) and the South-West/Centre (black circles, positive values).

The g1.map.bca object (Fig. 4.6) is created so that the size of symbols (black and white circles) is proportional to the department score on the first axis of the BCA (bca.guerry$ls[, 1]), and their location is given by the two-columns xy data frame (centres of the departments). Note that the pSp parameters can be used to customise the drawing of the map.

The spatial structure of the BCA score is obvious: there is a very clear division between the North-East of France and the South-West/Centre. BCA (and also PCA) is therefore able to extract spatial information from a data table, even though the spatial location of samples is not included explicitly in the analysis. Spatial methods like the multispati analysis (see Chap. 12) will optimise the mathematical properties of usual methods from this point of view.

4.5 Automatic Graph Collections

The **lattice** package introduced Trellis formulae, conditioning variables and panels to handle graph collections. Although **adegraphics** is based on **lattice**, it uses a different approach to graph collection. We detail here the three main alternatives to build automatically multiple graphics (ADEgS objects) with **adegraphics**.

4.5.1 Splitting Individuals with the facets Argument

The facets argument allows to split a graph according to the levels of a factor.

For instance, Fig. 4.7 shows how the BCA factor map can be split into five graphs (one for each region) using the facets argument of the s.label function and the region.names factor. This allows to facilitate the reading of the information compared to Fig. 4.5. Note that we reassigned old values of graphical parameters (stored in oldpar) using the adegpar functions.

4.5.2 Multiple Variables

Whereas the facets argument allows to produce multiple plots corresponding to groups of individuals, **adegraphics** offers also the possibility to build collection of graphics when a data frame with several variables is given as an argument to a function that usually requires a vector. For instance, the geographical maps of the first two BCA axes can be plotted using the s.value function using the same code than for Fig. 4.6 but using bca.guerry$ls instead of bca.guerry$ls[,1] as argument z. Figure 4.8 (g2.map.bca object) shows the results of this strategy.

Note that using both a facets argument and multiple variables is not allowed.

```
adegpar(oldpar)
s.label(bca.guerry$ls, labels = dep.names, plabels.optim = TRUE,
        facets = region.names)
```

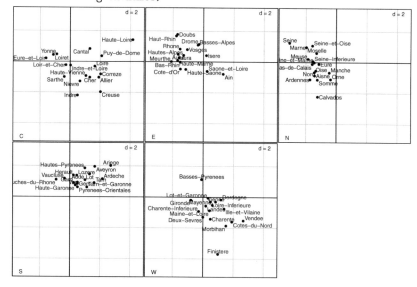

Fig. 4.7 The factor map of the BCA is split by region, using the `facets` argument of the `s.label` function. Note that the same limits on x and y axes are used to allow comparison among graphs.

4.5.3 Outputs of Multivariate Methods

All functions formerly available in **ade4** to display the outputs of multivariate analyses have been reimplemented in **adegraphics**. These new functions are generally (S3) instances of the generic `plot` function for high-level analyses (`plot.coinertia`, `plot.rlq`, etc.) and return an `ADEgS` object. For instance, the main results of BCA are returned by the `plot.between` function (Fig. 4.9).

The `bca.plot` object is made of six subgraphs and can be manipulated as a standard list:

```
length(bca.plot)
```

```
[1] 6
```

```
names(bca.plot)
```

```
[1] "loadings" "col"       "eig"       "row"       "Xax"
[6] "class"
```

Each subgraph is an element of this list and can be extracted using the names of elements (for the $ operator) or their index in the list (for [[ ]]).

```
adegpar(mappar)
g2.map.bca <- s.value(xy, bca.guerry$ls, Sp = gfrance85,
      symbol = "circle", pSp.col = col.dep, psub.cex = 1.5)
```

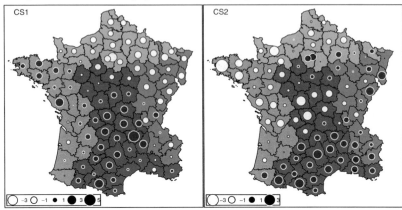

Fig. 4.8 The geographical maps (g2.map.bca object) of the first two BCA axes produced using the data frame bca.guerry$ls as argument.

```
identical(bca.plot[[2]], bca.plot$col)
```

```
[1] TRUE
```

The ADEgS object stored in bca.plot can be customised using graphical parameters to produce publication-ready figures. The **adegraphics** package also provides the possibility to create an ADEgS object from several simple graphs. This strategy is illustrated in the next section.

4.6   Step-by-Step Creation of an ADEgS

The ADEgS function can simply create an ADEgS object, taking as parameter a list of *n* graphical objects (ADEg, ADEgS or trellis) and some information about their respective positions. The position of the subgraphs can be defined using a positions matrix (positions argument, *n* rows and four columns) to define the drawing area (position of the bottom-left and top-right corners) for the *n* graphs. An alternative is the layout argument (see the layout function of the **graphics** package). If positions and layout are both omitted (as in Figs. 4.4 and 4.5), the positions matrix is computed automatically as a function of *n*.

A square matrix (add argument, *n* × *n*) handles superpositions: graphs *i* and *j* are superposed if $add[i, j] = 1$. The order of graphs in the list is important: the position of the first element in the list is defined by the first row of the positions matrix. In Figs. 4.4 and 4.5, the add matrix is equal to its default value, i.e., is null (no superposition).

```
adegpar(oldpar)
bca.plot <- plot(bca.guerry, row.col = TRUE)
```

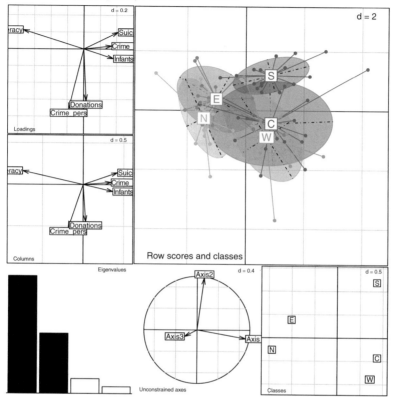

Fig. 4.9 Main outputs of BCA produced by the `plot` method. The returned object `bca.plot` is an ADEgS.

The creation of `ADEgS` objects is very flexible and is a real advantage when dealing with multiple graphs. In this section, we show how to create `ADEgS` objects to summarise the outputs of a multivariate analysis (BCA) on one or two axes.

4.6.1   Graphical Representations of One Axis

To interpret BCA axes, the score of variables on the first BCA axis is represented by a barchart (`g.barch` in Fig. 4.10). This one is negatively correlated to `Literacy` and positively correlated to variables `Crime_prop`, `Infants`, `Suicides`. Remember, however, that these last three variables are measured as "Population per ...". This means that high positive values correspond to low rates of suicides, crimes against property, and illegitimate births.

```
g.barch <- s1d.barchart(bca.guerry$co[, 1], xlim = c(-1.2, 1.2),
        labels = row.names(bca.guerry$co), plabels.cex = 1.5,
        p1d.horizontal = TRUE)
```

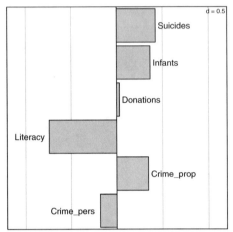

Fig. 4.10 Barchart of variable scores on the first BCA axis (g.barch object). The axis is negatively correlated to Literacy and positively correlated to variables Crime_prop, Infants, Suicides.

The screeplot of BCA eigenvalues is saved in g.eig (C1.barchart object) but not displayed here.

```
g.eig <- s1d.barchart(bca.guerry$eig, p1d.horizontal = FALSE,
        pgrid.draw = FALSE, plot = FALSE)
```

To customise the next graphs, some graphical parameters for one-dimensional representations are set, using the adegpar function and the p1d parameter list:

```
adegpar(p1d = list(horizontal = FALSE, rug.tck = 1,
        margin = 0.07), porigin.lwd = 0.5, ppoints.cex = 0.8)
```

Two one-dimension graphs are built (g.1lab.bca and g.1class.bca) but not displayed here, using s1d.label and s1d.class functions.

g.1lab.bca is an S1.label object and displays the department scores along the first BCA axis, with associated labels. Labels are department names, with a colour corresponding to the region to which they belong to.

```
g.1lab.bca <- s1d.label(bca.guerry$ls[, 1], label = dep.names,
        plabels.col = col.dep, ppoints.col = col.dep,
        plines.col = col.dep, plabels.box.draw = FALSE,
        plabels.cex = 1.6, plot = FALSE)
```

g.1class.bca is an S1.class object and displays the department scores by rugs grouped by region. The argument poslab is set to regular, which means that the region labels will be evenly spaced. The graphical display is reversed (with p1d.reverse = TRUE) to join the two representations side by side (Fig. 4.11).

```
g.1class.bca <- s1d.class(bca.guerry$ls[, 1], fac = region.names,
        poslab = "regular", col = col.region, p1d.reverse = TRUE,
        p1d.rug.margin = 0.1, plabels.cex = 2, plot = FALSE)
```

```
mat.lay <- matrix(c(1, 2, 3, 1, 2, 4, 1, 2, 5), nrow = 3, byrow = TRUE)
g.multi1.bca <- ADEgS(list(g.1class.bca, g.1lab.bca, g1.map.bca, g.barch,
      g.eig), layout = list(mat = mat.lay))
```

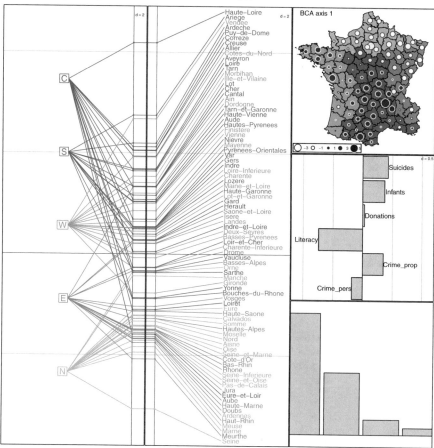

Fig. 4.11 Synthetic graph (`g.multi1.bca`) of the results on the first BCA axis. Two groups of departments can be distinguished: North–East (mostly negative scores) and West–South–Centre (mostly positive scores). The `g.1lab.bca` graph gives useful information on the position of each department individually. For example, Seine and Haute-Loire appear as outliers on each sides of the axis.

At the end, an ADEgS multiple graph object (`g.multi1.bca`) is created as a list containing the five previous graphical objects. The positions of subgraphs are defined in the matrix `mat.lay` used as `layout` information. The final figure (Fig. 4.11) contains the two one-dimensional graphs of the first BCA axis score, the map of this score on the France background, the barchart of the variable scores, and the screeplot of eigenvalues.

4.6.2   Graphical Representations of Two Axes

Here we show how the results of BCA can be represented for the first two axes of
BCA. The final figure will contain graphs to represent:

- the correlation circle of variables, to understand the meaning of the two axes,
- the BCA factor map, with department labels grouped by region,
- the geographical maps of the two BCA axes, to show the spatial structure of these
  axes,
- the screeplot of eigenvalues, to evaluate the importance of each dimension.

The correlation circle between observed variables and BCA axes is stored in a
g.cor object (Fig. 4.12). As seen previously, the first axis is negatively correlated
to Literacy and positively correlated to variables Crime_prop, Infants,
Suicides. On the second axis, a high positive score means low values of
donations and a high rate of crime against persons.

The BCA factor map is stored in g.class.bca (S2.class object). It
represents the five regions with convex hulls containing 70% of the departments
of each region (chullSize = 0.7).

Then an S2.label object, named g.lab.bca, is created with the department
names. The position of labels is optimised to avoid superpositions (plabels =
list(optim = TRUE)).

```
g.cor <- s.corcircle(cor(pca.guerry$tab, bca.guerry$ls),
        porigin.include = TRUE, pbackground.box = FALSE,
        plabels.cex = 1.2)
```

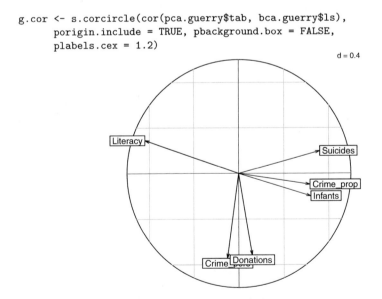

Fig. 4.12 Correlation circle between observed variables and BCA axis (g.cor object). The first
axis is negatively correlated to Literacy and positively correlated to variables Crime_prop,
Infants, Suicides. On the second axis, a high positive score means low values of donations
and a high rate of crime against persons.

```
g.class.bca <- s.class(bca.guerry$ls, region.names,
      ellipseSize = 0, starSize = 0.5, chullSize = 0.7,
      ppoints.cex = 0, col = col.region, plabels.cex = 0,
      pgrid.text.pos = "bottomright", plot = FALSE)
g.lab.bca <- s.label(bca.guerry$ls, as.character(dep.names),
      ppoints.col = col.dep, plabels = list(optim = TRUE,
          cex = 1, col = col.dep), plot = FALSE)
g.bca.dep <- g.class.bca + g.lab.bca
g.bca.dep <- insert(g.eig, posi = "topleft", ratio = 0.2)
```

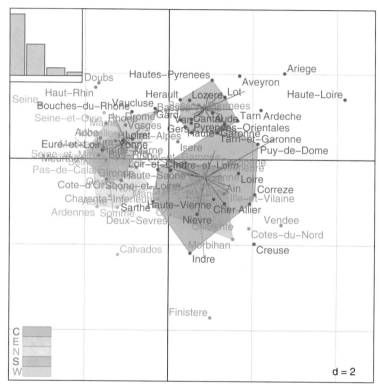

Fig. 4.13 Superposition of the two ADEg objects `g.class.bca` and `g.lab.bca`, with eigenvalues screeplot inserted as an ADEg object.

These last two graphs are superposed using the **adegraphics** + operator and the result is stored in a new ADEgS object named `g.bca.dep`.

The screeplot of eigenvalues of the BCA previously created is added to `g.bca.dep` with the `insert` function (Fig. 4.13).

On the first axis, North and East regions are characterised by a high level of literacy, together with high rates of suicides, crimes against properties, and illegitimate births. They are opposed to South, Centre and West on these variables. On the second axis, South is opposed to the four other regions and shows low levels of donations to the poors and high levels of crimes against persons. Globally, Centre and West seem comparable, and North and East too.

The maps of department scores on the two BCA axes have been stored in g2.map.bca object (Fig. 4.8).

Lastly a new ADEgS object (g.multi2.bca) is created with the ADEgS function (Fig. 4.14). The list of graphs of this object contains four elements:

- an ADEgS object, g.bca.dep (containing itself three ADEg, see Fig. 4.13),

```
positions <- rbind(c(0, 0, 0.8, 0.8), c(0.6, 0.6, 1, 1),
     c(0.6, 0.1, 1, 0.5), c(0.2, 0.6, 0.6, 1))
g.multi2.bca <- ADEgS(
     list(g.bca.dep, g2.map.bca[[1]], g2.map.bca[[2]], g.cor),
     positions = positions)
```

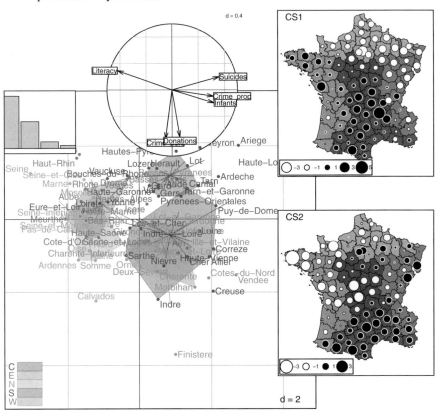

Fig. 4.14 This figure (g.multi2.bca) sums up the analysis on the selected subset of Guerry's data. On the first axis, North and East regions are characterised by a high level of literacy, together with high rates of suicides, crimes against properties, and illegitimate births. They are opposed to South, Centre and West on these variables. On the second axis, South is opposed to the four other regions and shows low levels of donations to the poors and high levels of crimes against persons. Globally, Centre and West seem comparable, and North and East too.

- two ADEg objects of class S2.value, g2.map.bca[[1]] and g2.map.bca[[2]],
- an S2.corcircle object, g.cor.

The position of each object is given in a positions matrix with four columns (x0, y0, x1, y1) giving the coordinates of the bottom-left and top-right corners of each graph.

g.multi2.bca is an object of formal class ADEgS, and it is possible to explore its contents. Its slots can be listed with the slotNames function:

```
slotNames(g.multi2.bca)

[1] "ADEglist"  "positions" "add"        "Call"


names(g.multi2.bca)

[1] "g1" "g2" "g3" "g4"
```

The Call slot contains the command line that was used to create the ADEgS object (g.multi2.bca@Call). The first slot (ADEglist) is the list of graphs, and the names function can be used to get their names. It is possible to select a subset of graphs in this list and to display them, for example using the [operator to select the first two subgraphs of the g.multi2.bca object:

```
g.multi2.bca[c(1, 2)]
```

4.7 Conclusion

The **adegraphics** package makes easier the manipulation of complex graphical displays obtained from multivariate analysis methods. Basic functions can be used to draw usual multivariate graphs (factor maps), but also special types of graphs, like one-dimensional graphs to study scores individually, or spatial representations (with the help of the **sp** package). Thanks to the **lattice** package, **adegraphics** also brings easy ways to use colours and transparency in multivariate analysis graphs.

Graphs are now objects that can be handled easily. Most of the parameters of a graph can be changed after its creation, allowing to precisely set all the characteristics of the final figure. These parameters can be set globally, for all the graphs subsequently drawn, or locally, for just one particular graph.

Many high-level functions are based on these new functions. They allow to draw synthetic displays of complex multivariate methods (e.g., plot.coinertia, plot.rlq, plot.pcaiv, etc.). Many examples of use of these high-level functions are shown in the next chapters of this book.

Another very important improvement is the automatic management of collections of graphs. Using the new graphical functions of **adegraphics**, it is easy to draw automatically all the graphs corresponding to the different columns (variables) of a data table, or all the graphs corresponding to any subsets of rows (individuals/samples) defined by a factor. This is very useful in multivariate analysis in general, and even more in the case of the analysis of three-way tables (see Chaps. 9 and 10). Additionally, all the graphs of a collection can be easily arranged, juxtaposed or superposed to make the final figure more easily understandable.

Chapter 5
Description of Environmental Variables Structures

Abstract This chapter is organised in three parts, corresponding to three data analysis methods: standardised PCA for quantitative variables, Multiple Correspondence Analysis (MCA) for qualitative variables (`factors` in **R**), and the Hill and Smith Analysis for tables containing a mix of qualitative and quantitative variables.

5.1 Introduction

Several simple data analysis methods can be used to describe the structure of environmental variables tables. Simple here means that these methods are adapted to the analysis of only one data table. If *more information* is available, for example information on the structure of the table (e.g., groups of rows or of columns), or if information is contained in *more than one* data table, then other methods should be used. According to the type of measured variables (quantitative, qualitative or both), different methods can be considered.

These different approaches will be illustrated using the `doubs` data set, from **ade4** (see Verneaux 1973, and `help("doubs", package = "ade4")`). The `doubs$env` data frame contains eleven environmental variables measured at 30 sites along the Doubs river in the Jura region (France). The `doubs$fish` data frame contains the abundances of 27 fish species that were found in the same sites. The `doubs$xy` data frame contains the spatial coordinates of the 30 sites (two columns, *x* and *y*).

```
library(ade4)
library(adegraphics)
data(doubs)
names(doubs)
```

```
[1] "env"     "fish"    "xy"      "species"
```

```
names(doubs$env)
```

```
[1] "dfs" "alt" "slo" "flo" "pH"  "har" "pho" "nit" "amm"
[10] "oxy" "bdo"
```

© Springer Science+Business Media, LLC, part of Springer Nature 2018
J. Thioulouse et al., *Multivariate Analysis of Ecological Data with ade4*,
https://doi.org/10.1007/978-1-4939-8850-1_5

The eleven variables are:

1. dfs: distance from the source (km * 10)
2. alt: altitude (m)
3. slo: log(x + 1) where x is the slope (per mil * 100)
4. flo: minimum average stream flow (m^3/s * 100)
5. pH (* 10)
6. har: total hardness of water (mg/l of Calcium)
7. pho: phosphates (mg/l * 100)
8. nit: nitrates (mg/l * 100)
9. amm: ammonia nitrogen (mg/l * 100)
10. oxy: dissolved oxygen (mg/l * 10)
11. bdo: biological demand for oxygen (mg/l * 10)

This environmental table can be represented graphically using the table.value or table.image function of the **adegraphics** package. Here, a colour palette function mypal is defined and the raw data are then represented using the table.image function. As the ranges of variation of the environmental variables are quite different, we scaled the data to allow a common and meaningful graphical representation (Fig. 5.1):

```
env <- doubs$env
apply(env, 2, range)
```

```
      dfs alt   slo   flo pH har pho nit amm oxy bdo
[1,]    3 172 1.099    84 77  40   1  15   0  41  13
[2,] 4530 934 6.176  6900 86 110 422 620 180 124 167
```

As the spatial coordinates are also available, sites can be plotted in the geographical space. The s.label function can be used to draw the position of sites, with the site number as label (Fig. 5.2).

To facilitate the interpretation of environmental data, information of Figs. 5.1 and 5.2 can be combined by creating thematic maps for all variables. To achieve this, we use the s.value function, with multivariate data in the z argument. It automatically loops over the variables and produces 11 geographical maps presented in Fig. 5.3. By default, this function plots squares which size is proportional to a set of values. The colour of the squares gives the sign of the value (white for negative values, black for positive). Here, we modify the method, symbol and ppalette.quanti parameters to obtain figures with coloured circles.

The maps presented in Fig. 5.3 highlight that some environmental variables have similar spatial distributions (e.g., distance from the source (dfs) and stream flow (flo)). The objective of multivariate methods is to provide a summary of this environmental table by identifying the main patterns of variation and which variables are involved in these structures.

```
table.value(scale(env), symbol = "circle")
```

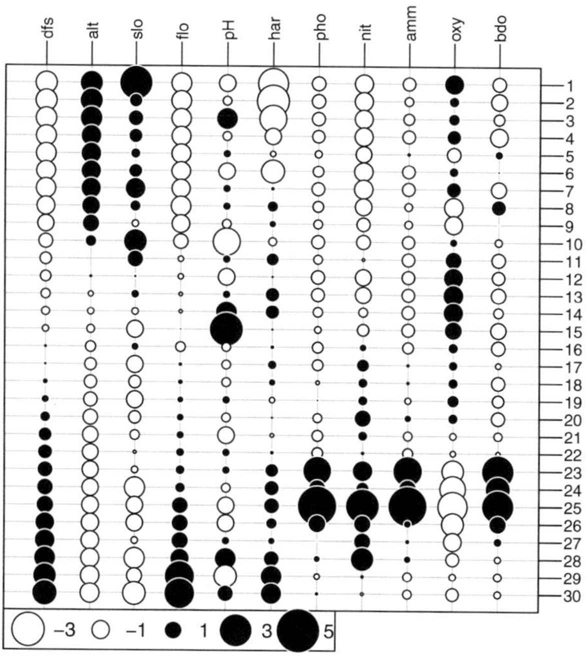

Fig. 5.1 Graphical representation of the environmental raw data table (sites as rows, variables as columns). Data are scaled.

5.2 Standardised Principal Component Analysis (PCA)

Principal Component Analysis (Pearson 1901; Hotelling 1933) is the most simple and the basis of all multivariate analysis methods. It allows to summarise the structure of a table containing quantitative variables. Many theoretical models lead to the same computations, but the duality diagram (Escoufier 1987) and the geometric model (LeRoux and Rouanet 2004) are the ones used in the **ade4** package.

Basic mathematical definitions are recalled in Box 5.1. In the **ade4** package, the dudi.pca function is used to compute a PCA. All the outputs of this function are grouped in a dudi object (subclass pca), and Box 5.2 recalls the corresponding output elements.

Two types of PCA are generally distinguished: *covariance matrix PCA* and *correlation matrix PCA*. They can be considered as the same method, applied after a different treatment of the data table: centring (subtracting the mean of each variable) for covariance matrix PCA and standardisation (subtracting the mean and dividing by the standard deviation) for correlation matrix PCA.

In the case of the env data table, the choice between covariance or correlation matrix PCA is easy: variables are not expressed in the same units and have

```
xy <- doubs$xy
sll <- s.label(xy, ppoints.cex = 0, plot = FALSE)
st1 <- s.traject(xy, ppoints.cex = 0, plabels.cex = 0, plot = FALSE)
s1 <- superpose(st1, sll, plot = TRUE)
```

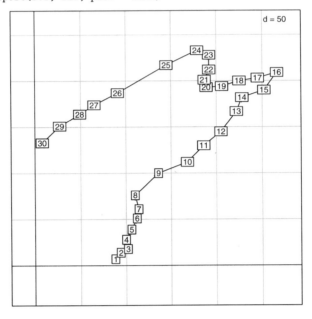

Fig. 5.2 Position of the 30 sampling sites along the Doubs river.

very different variances, ranging from 1 to more than 3.10^6. Here, differences in variances are meaningless and should not be considered in the analysis. Using a correlation matrix PCA is therefore necessary to remove these differences.

When all the variables are measured in the same units (homogeneous tables), both types of PCA can be applied. PCA on covariance matrix would give more importance to variables with high variance as they contribute more to the total inertia and thus will have more weight in the definition of axes. On the other hand, PCA on correlation matrix will give an equal importance to all the variables so that only the redundance (i.e., correlations) among variables drives the definition of axes. To choose between the two possibilities, users must decide if the differences between variances are (or not) a useful information that should be taken into account in the analysis. For example, in toxicity tables, all the values are LD50 (lethal dose 50, i.e., the concentration that kills 50% of organisms), and the columns correspond to different chemical compounds instead of different variables. Using a correlation matrix PCA on these tables will probably remove important information about the difference in toxicity between chemical compounds or between the diversity of species. In these cases, a covariance matrix PCA (argument `scale` set to `FALSE`) is preferable (see also Chap. 6).

```
mypal <- colorRampPalette(c("#EDF8FB", "#006D2C"))
s.value(xy, doubs$env, pgrid.draw = FALSE, porigin.draw = FALSE,
    plegend.drawKey = FALSE, psub.cex = 2, method = "color",
    symbol = "circle", ppalette.quanti = mypal, ppoints.cex = 0.5)
```

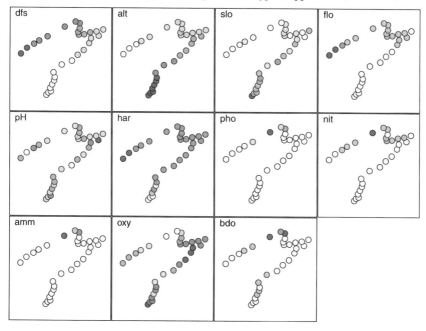

Fig. 5.3 Collection of 11 geographical maps of the doubs data set environmental variables. High values are in dark green, low values in light green.

Box 5.1 PCA: Basic Mathematical Definitions

Let $\mathbf{X}$ be a table of centred quantitative variables, with n rows (samples) and p columns (variables). Let $\mathbf{D} = \frac{1}{n}\mathbf{I}_n$ and $\mathbf{Q} = \mathbf{I}_p$ be the diagonal matrices of uniform row weights. The duality diagram of the PCA of $\mathbf{X}$ is:

$$
\begin{array}{ccc}
 & \mathbf{I}_p & \\
\mathbb{R}^p & \longrightarrow & \mathbb{R}^{p^*} \\
\mathbf{X}^{\top} \uparrow & & \downarrow \mathbf{X} \\
\mathbb{R}^{n^*} & \longleftarrow & \mathbb{R}^n \\
 & \frac{1}{n}\mathbf{I}_n &
\end{array}
$$

The corresponding PCA statistical triplet is $\left(\mathbf{X}, \mathbf{I}_p, \frac{1}{n}\mathbf{I}_n\right)$ and the total inertia of this statistical triplet is:

(continued)

Box 5.1 (continued)

$$I_{\left(\mathbf{X},\mathbf{I}_p,\frac{1}{n}\mathbf{I}_n\right)} = \text{Trace}\left(\frac{1}{n}\mathbf{X}^\top\mathbf{X}\right) = \sum_{j=1}^{p} \text{var}(\mathbf{x}_j)$$

According to Property 3.1 (Box 3.2) and Appendix A.3, PCA searches for a principal axis **a** maximising:

$$\left\|\mathbf{X}\mathbf{I}_p\mathbf{a}\right\|^2_{\frac{1}{n}\mathbf{I}_n} = \text{var}(\mathbf{X}\mathbf{a})$$

In $\mathbb{R}^n$, using Property 3.2 (Box 3.2) and Appendix A.5, it can be demonstrated that PCA searches for a principal component **b** maximising:

$$\left\|\mathbf{X}^\top\frac{1}{n}\mathbf{I}_n\mathbf{b}\right\|^2_{\mathbf{I}_p} = \sum_{j=1}^{p} \text{cov}^2(\mathbf{x}_j, \mathbf{b})$$

As variables are just centred, then this PCA is called a *covariance matrix PCA* or a *centred PCA* and $I_{\left(\mathbf{X},\mathbf{I}_p,\frac{1}{n}\mathbf{I}_n\right)}$ is the sum of the variances. If variables are also scaled to unit variance (dividing them by their standard deviation), then it is called a *correlation matrix PCA* or a *normed PCA*, and the total inertia $I_{\left(\mathbf{X},\mathbf{I}_p,\frac{1}{n}\mathbf{I}_n\right)}$ is equal to the number of variables. In this case, PCA maximises the sum of squared correlations with variables:

$$\left\|\mathbf{X}^\top\frac{1}{n}\mathbf{I}_n\mathbf{b}\right\|^2_{\mathbf{I}_p} = \sum_{j=1}^{p} \text{cor}^2(\mathbf{x}_j, \mathbf{b})$$

Box 5.2 PCA: `dudi` Output Elements
In the **ade4** package, the results of a PCA are stored in an object of class `dudi`, subclass `pca`. This object is a list with 13 elements, including the usual elements of any `dudi`. In this list, elements of particular interest are:

- `$eig`: eigenvalues ($\mathbf{\Lambda}$)
- `$cw`: column weights ($\mathbf{Q} = \mathbf{I}_p$)
- `$lw`: row weights ($\mathbf{D} = \frac{1}{n}\mathbf{I}_n$)
- `$tab`: transformed data table ($\mathbf{X}$)

(continued)

> **Box 5.2** (continued)
> - $c1: principal axes or variable loadings (**A**)
> - $li: row scores (**L = XA**)
> - $l1: principal components (**B**)
> - $co: column scores (**C** $= \frac{1}{n}$**X$^\mathsf{T}$B**)
>
> The two pairs of coordinates, ($c1, $li) or ($l1, $co), can be superimposed to draw two types of biplot (respectively, *distance biplot* and *correlation biplot*). See Legendre and Legendre (1998, pp. 403–404) for details.
>
> In the first interpretation, PCA finds coefficients for variables ($c1) to compute a linear combination ($li) that provides an ordination of individuals with the greatest dispersion (maximum variance).
>
> In the second interpretation, PCA provides a linear combination ($l1) that maximise the correlations ($co) with all variables (or covariances for centred PCA). Hence, it is the best summary of the variables.

The PCA of the doubs$env table is computed with the dudi.pca function and stored in the pca1 object:

```
pca1 <- dudi.pca(env, scale = TRUE, scannf = FALSE, nf = 3)
```

The scale argument is set to TRUE (the default value), so the PCA will be computed on the standardised (centred and normed) data table. The result is therefore a correlation matrix PCA.

The scannf argument ("**scan** the **n**umber of **f**actors") is set to FALSE, which means that the number of axes should not be asked to the user, but arbitrarily set to three. This value (three) is given by the third argument, nf. If nf is not set explicitly, it defaults to two. When running in interactive mode, the scannf argument should not be used, and its default value (TRUE) will cause the function to ask the number of axes (principal components) interactively to the user. This is the number of axes that should be "kept" in output files, and on which loadings and scores will be computed.

Many methods have been invented to try to guess the number of principal components that should be kept after a PCA. In **ade4**, users are simply asked how many components they want. To help answer this question, dudi functions display a barplot of eigenvalues in decreasing order. The user should then try to find a discontinuity in the shape of the decrease, and choose to keep the axes corresponding to eigenvalues placed before (on the left of) this discontinuity. For example, in Fig. 5.4, the user should keep (from left to right) 2, 3 and 4 axes.

Of course these examples are quite caricatural, and in real situations, it can be much harder to choose an appropriate number of principal components. However the principle remains that the shape of the decrease of eigenvalues is a good indicator of the presence of structures in the data table. Trying to keep the axes that correspond

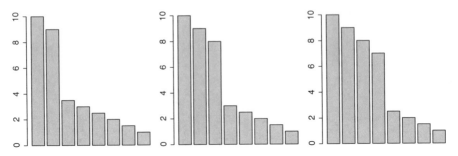

Fig. 5.4 Example eigenvalue barplots.

```
screeplot(pca1, main = " ", xlab = " ")
```

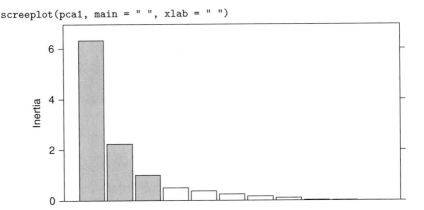

Fig. 5.5 Barplot of PCA eigenvalues for the Doubs environmental table.

to these potentially interesting structures is therefore a good and easy-to-use rule. As an alternative, the procedure developed by Dray (2008) is implemented in the `testdim` function that can be applied on correlation matrix PCA created by the `dudi.pca` function with `scale = TRUE`:

```
testdim(pca1)$nb.cor
```

```
[1] 2
```

Figure 5.5 shows the barplot of `pca1` eigenvalues. Two or three principal components can be kept (the `testdim` procedure says two).

The correlation circle (left) to represent variables and the factor map of sites (right) on the first two principal components are shown in Fig. 5.6.

This correlation circle (`sc1` object) shows two nearly orthogonal gradients: a geomorphological gradient opposing altitude and slope to hardness, distance from the source and stream flow, and a chemical gradient, opposing dissolved oxygen to phosphates, ammonium, and biological demand for oxygen. Oxygen concentration is higher upstream, and pollution is higher downstream, so these two gradients are not completely orthogonal. The first principal component is an upstream-downstream gradient, while the second component opposes geomorphology to chemical processes.

```
sc1 <- s.corcircle(pca1$co, plot = FALSE)
sl1 <- s.label(pca1$li, plabels.optim = TRUE,
      ppoints.cex = 0.5, plot = FALSE)
ADEgS(list(sc1, sl1))
```

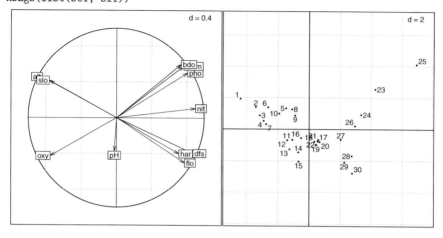

Fig. 5.6 Doubs environmental variables PCA factor maps. Left: correlation circle, right: factor map of sites.

The factor map on the right of Fig. 5.6 (sl1 object) shows that the sites are ordered along the first principal component, from site 1 (upstream, 300 m from the source) to site 30 (downstream, 453 km from the source). Departures from this geomorphology gradient are explained by the chemical gradient: sites with a high concentration of oxygen (1, 4, 7, 11, 12, 13, 14, 15) are in the lower-left part of the graph, and sites with a high concentration of ammonium, phosphates and a high BDO (23, 24, 25) are in the upper-right part of the graph.

The site coordinates can also be used to draw geographical maps of site scores, using the s.value function. Figure 5.7 shows the map of site scores on the first two principal components. The first principal component (left) is clearly an upstream-downstream gradient, with the exception of sites 23 to 25 (see site numbers in Fig. 5.2). The second principal component (right) cuts this gradient in four parts: the upper stream (sites 1 to 22) is divided in two, according to altitude and slope, and the lower stream (sites 23 to 30) is divided according to the pollution variables (ammonium, phosphates and BDO) which are higher in sites 23 to 26 and lower in sites 27 to 30.

The upstream-downstream gradients and the particular characteristics of highly polluted sites (sites 23 to 26) or of sites with high oxygen concentration (11 to 15) appear very clearly on these maps.

More generally, the geographical maps of site scores and their comparison with the collection of maps of standardised variables (Fig. 5.3) can be very useful to help interpret the outputs of a PCA. Drawing these maps is not possible when there are hundreds of variables (as it is the case for DNA fingerprints, for example), but then, particular variables of interest (e.g., variables with the most important relative contributions, see Box 3.3) can be chosen and mapped.

```
s.value(xy, pca1$li[, 1:2], pgrid.draw = FALSE, porigin.draw = FALSE,
    method = "size", symbol = "circle", col = mypal(2),
    ppoints.cex = 1)
```

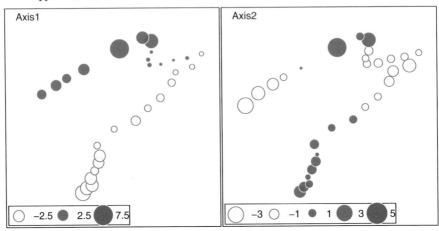

Fig. 5.7 Geographical maps of the first (left) and second (right) principal components of the PCA on the `doubs` data set environmental variables.

5.3   Multiple Correspondence Analysis (MCA)

Multiple Correspondence Analysis (MCA) is the basic method to analyse tables of qualitative variables (see synthesis by Tenenhaus and Young 1985) that are stored as `factors` in **R** (see Sect. 2.5). We illustrate MCA with the same data set as in Sect. 5.2 but we obtain qualitative variables by splitting the quantitative variables into categories. Four categories are defined automatically for each variable using the `cut` function. This function is applied to the environmental variables with `apply` (Sect. 2.4.9), and the resulting qualitative variables are stored in the `fenv` data frame.

```
fenv <- apply(env, 2, cut, breaks = 4, labels = 1:4)
fenv <- as.data.frame(fenv)
```

This transformation induces a loss of information as different values for a quantitative variable are regrouped into a single category of the recoded qualitative variable (Fig. 5.8). However, this approach can be useful when non-linear relationships occur between variables. In this case, PCA which is based on correlations, will only be able to extract linear relationships whereas MCA can identify non-linear trends by reordering the categories. When the relationships between variables are (at least approximately) linear, the results of both methods should be comparable.

MCA allows to identify associations between the categories (`levels`) of different qualitative variables (`factor`). Basic mathematical definitions are recalled in Box 5.3. The method is implemented in the `dudi.acm` function of the **ade4**

```
plot(env[, 1] ~ fenv[, 1], ylab = "Quantitative dfs",
     xlab = "Qualitative dfs")
```

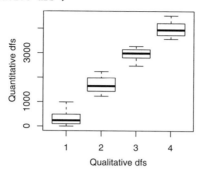

Fig. 5.8 Recoding of the quantitative variable `dfs` (distance from the source) in four categories.

package. All the outputs of this function are grouped in a `dudi` object (subclass `acm`), and Box 5.4 describes the main output elements. Here, we applied MCA on the data frame `fenv`.

Box 5.3 MCA: Basic Mathematical Definitions

Let $\mathbf{Z}$ be a table of qualitative variables, coded as integers, with n rows (samples) and v columns (variables). Let m_j be the number of categories of the j-th variable. The total number of categories for all variables is:

$$m = \sum_{j=1}^{v} m_j$$

The $n \times m$ disjunctive table $\mathbf{X}$ is associated to table $\mathbf{Z}$. It is made of the dummy variables that correspond to the categories of the qualitative variables of table $\mathbf{Z}$ (see Appendix A.7 for details).

The matrix $\mathbf{D} = \frac{1}{n}\mathbf{I}_n$ is the diagonal matrix of uniform row weights and $\mathbf{D}_m = \mathrm{diag}(\mathbf{X}^{\mathsf{T}}\mathbf{D}\mathbf{1}_n)$ is the $m \times m$ diagonal matrix of column weights. It contains the category frequencies computed as the sum of the weights of the individuals belonging to each category.

Let $\mathbf{Y} = \mathbf{X}\mathbf{D}_m^{-1} - \mathbf{1}_n\mathbf{1}_m^{\mathsf{T}}$ be the transformed and centred disjunctive table, where $\mathbf{1}_n$ is the $n \times 1$ vector of ones.

The duality diagram of the MCA of $\mathbf{Z}$ is defined by:

(continued)

Box 5.3 (continued)

$$
\begin{array}{ccc}
\mathbb{R}^m & \xrightarrow{\frac{1}{v}\mathbf{D}_m} & \mathbb{R}^{m^*} \\
\mathbf{Y}^{\top} \Big\uparrow & & \Big\downarrow \mathbf{Y} \\
\mathbb{R}^{n^*} & \xleftarrow{\frac{1}{n}\mathbf{I}_n} & \mathbb{R}^n
\end{array}
$$

The corresponding MCA statistical triplet is $\left(\mathbf{Y}, \frac{1}{v}\mathbf{D}_m, \frac{1}{n}\mathbf{I}_n\right)$.

According to Property 3.1 (Box 3.2) and Appendix A.3, PCA searches for a principal axis **a** maximising:

$$
\left\|\mathbf{Y}\frac{1}{v}\mathbf{D}_m\mathbf{a}\right\|^2_{\frac{1}{n}\mathbf{I}_n} = \left\|\frac{1}{v}\mathbf{X}\mathbf{a}\right\|^2_{\frac{1}{n}\mathbf{I}_n} = \mathrm{var}\left(\frac{1}{v}\mathbf{X}\mathbf{a}\right)
$$

In $\mathbb{R}^n$, using Property 3.2 (Box 3.2) and Appendix A.7, it can be demonstrated that MCA searches for a principal component **b** maximising:

$$
\left\|\mathbf{Y}^{\top}\frac{1}{n}\mathbf{I}_n\mathbf{b}\right\|^2_{\frac{1}{v}\mathbf{D}_m} = \left\|\frac{1}{n}\mathbf{D}_m^{-1}\mathbf{X}^{\top}\mathbf{b}\right\|^2_{\frac{1}{v}\mathbf{D}_m}
$$

The vector $\frac{1}{n}\mathbf{D}_m^{-1}\mathbf{X}^{\top}\mathbf{b}$ contains means of **b** per category so that:

$$
\left\|\mathbf{Y}^{\top}\frac{1}{n}\mathbf{I}_n\mathbf{b}\right\|^2_{\frac{1}{v}\mathbf{D}_m} = \frac{1}{v}\sum_{j=1}^{v}\eta^2(\mathbf{z}_j, \mathbf{b})
$$

This quantity is the mean of correlation ratios computed for all the variables.

Box 5.4 MCA: `dudi` Output Elements

In the **ade4** package, the results of an MCA are stored in an object of class `dudi`, subclass `acm`. This object is a list with 12 elements, including the usual elements of any `dudi`. In this list, elements of particular interest are:

- `$eig`: eigenvalues ($\mathbf{\Lambda}$)
- `$cw`: column (i.e., category) weights ($\frac{1}{v}\mathbf{D}_m$)

(continued)

Box 5.4 (continued)

- `$lw`: row weights ($\mathbf{D} = \frac{1}{n}\mathbf{I}_n$)
- `$tab`: transformed and centred disjunctive data table ($\mathbf{Y}$)
- `$c1`: category loadings ($\mathbf{A}$)
- `$li`: row scores ($\mathbf{L} = \frac{1}{v}\mathbf{X}\mathbf{A}$)
- `$l1`: principal components ($\mathbf{B}$)
- `$co`: column scores ($\mathbf{C} = \frac{1}{n}\mathbf{D}_m^{-1}\mathbf{X}^\top\mathbf{B}$)
- `$cr`: correlation ratios between qualitative variables and axes

Two types of interpretation can be defined. In the first one, MCA positions categories by a normed score `$c1`. A score for individuals (`$li`) is derived from this categories score: an individual is located at the mean of the score of the categories that it carries. This second score provides an ordination of individuals with the highest possible dispersion (maximum variance).

In the second type of interpretation, MCA finds normed coordinates for individuals (`$l1`) and positions categories at the mean of the individual scores that belong to them (`$co`). This maximises the mean of the variance of the categories for all variables. In other words, it maximises the mean of the correlation ratios.

The main difference between PCA and MCA is that the columns of the analysed table are the variables in PCA but the categories of qualitative variables in MCA:

```
ncol(pca1$tab)
```

```
[1] 11
```

```
ncol(acm1$tab)
```

```
[1] 44
```

The categories correspond to the different columns in the disjunctive table analysed by the MCA (see Box 5.3) and their order is not taken into account, just like different variables in a PCA. As a consequence, the number of eigenvalues is also increased (Fig. 5.9) in MCA. Another important difference is that MCA weights columns proportionally to the number of individuals belonging to the categories so that all variables have the same weights (as in PCA):

```
acm1$cw[1:4] == table(fenv$dfs)/nrow(fenv)/ncol(fenv)
```

```
   1    2    3    4
TRUE TRUE TRUE TRUE
```

```
as.numeric(by(acm1$cw, rep(1:ncol(fenv), each = 4), sum)) *
    ncol(fenv)
```

```
[1] 1 1 1 1 1 1 1 1 1 1 1
```

```
acm1 <- dudi.acm(fenv, scannf = FALSE)
screeplot(acm1, main = " ", xlab = " ")
```

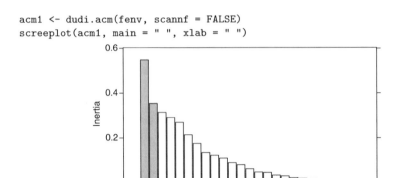

Fig. 5.9 Barplot of MCA eigenvalues for the Doubs environmental table.

```
sl1 <- s.label(acm1$co, ppoints.cex = 0.5, plabels.optim = TRUE,
      plot = FALSE)
sl2 <- s.label(acm1$li, ppoints.cex = 0.5, plabels.optim = TRUE,
      plot = FALSE)
ADEgS(list(sl1, sl2))
```

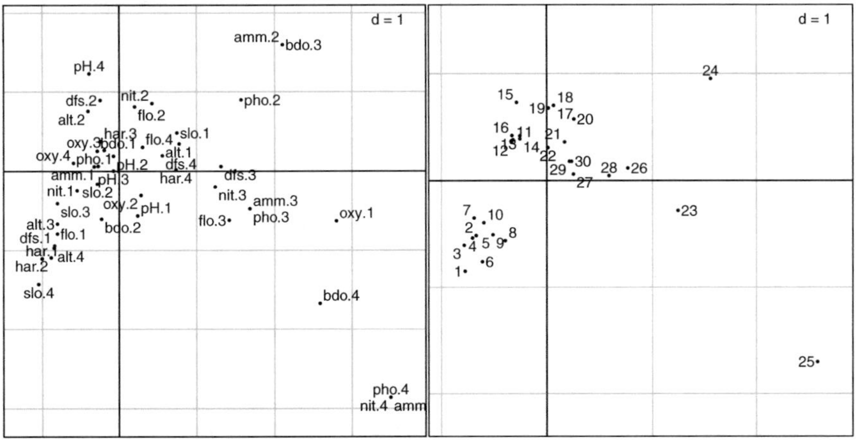

Fig. 5.10 Qualitative environmental variables MCA factor maps. Left: categories of qualitative variables, right: factor map of sites.

Figure 5.10 shows that, except for an inversion of the sign of the second axis, the factor map of sites is still very similar to the factor map obtained by the PCA (Fig. 5.6). The same typology of sampling sites along the stream is found: upper-stream sites (1 to 10) with high oxygen concentration and low ammonium and BDO are opposed to lower-stream sites (26 to 30), with sites 23 to 25 having an exceptionally high level of pollution.

The graph of categories (Fig. 5.10, left) is somewhat different because we now have one point for each category of each qualitative variable (44 categories as a whole) instead of 11 points only. The interpretation is however the same: categories corresponding to high levels of ammonium and BDO (amm.4, bdo.4) and to low levels of oxygen (oxy.1) are on the right of the graph, where highly polluted sites are found. Conversely, categories corresponding to high levels of oxygen (oxy.4), high values of slope (slo.4), low values of flow (flo.1) and hardness (hard.1, hard.2) are located on the left of the graph, where upper-stream sites are found.

MCA allows to carry out the interpretation of factors at the level of categories. This means that one can get a better (finer) explanation of the meaning of factors. In the **ade4** package, this property is used to draw particular graphs that show which individuals belong to each category. Two types of graphs can be drawn, using functions score (Fig. 5.11) and plot (Fig. 5.12).

The first type of graph (Fig. 5.11, using score function) shows the results of MCA for a given axis (specified by the xax argument which is equal to 1 by default). The normed coordinates of all the individuals (acm1$l1) are placed along the x-axis and the categories are displayed at the mean of the coordinates of their individuals. The vertical coordinate is given by the category score (acm1$co). It is then easy to interpret the meaning of the factor by looking at the positions of categories and individuals. For example, in Fig. 5.11, one can see that the categories

```
score(acm1, type = "points", col = TRUE, psub.cex = 1.5)
```

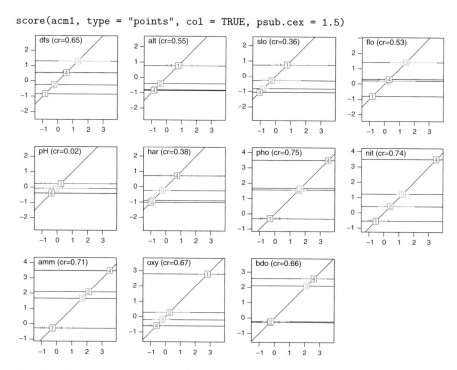

Fig. 5.11 The score graph of an MCA. Each elementary graph corresponds to one qualitative variable. The label of this variable is located in the top-left corner of the graph. In each graph, the horizontal lines correspond to the categories. See text for details.

```
plot(acm1, col = TRUE, psub.cex = 1.5)
```

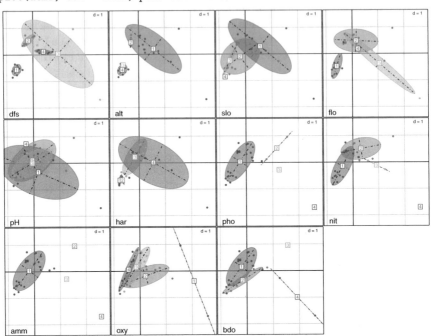

Fig. 5.12 The `plot` graph of an MCA. Like in Fig. 5.11, each elementary graph corresponds to one qualitative variable. The label of this variable is located in the bottom-left corner of the graph. In each graph, ellipses correspond to the categories of the qualitative variable. The coordinates of the individuals that belong to a category are represented by small dots, and category labels are placed at the centre of the ellipse. See text for details.

of variables hardness, phosphorus, nitrates, ammonium and BDO are ordered by increasing values along the first MCA factor. Conversely, the categories of variables altitude, slope, oxygen are ordered by decreasing values along the first MCA factor. On the vertical axis, the intervals between labels give information of the differences among categories (variance between categories). On the horizontal axis, the spacing among the tick marks allows to evaluate the homogeneity of individuals in a category (variance within categories). As the individual scores in MCA (`acm1$l1`) maximise the mean correlation ratio for all the qualitative variables, it is expected that the more vertical is the regression line for a qualitative variable, the higher is its correlation ratio value. Correlation ratios are stored in `acm1$cr`:

```
acm1$cr
```

```
        RS1      RS2
dfs 0.65017  0.54172
alt 0.54860  0.46824
slo 0.36286  0.18819
flo 0.52995  0.57221
pH  0.02396  0.15609
```

```
har 0.37616 0.26756
pho 0.75418 0.33689
nit 0.73984 0.53046
amm 0.71443 0.36912
oxy 0.67304 0.07847
bdo 0.65986 0.38953
```

The second type of graph is shown in Fig. 5.12. It can be drawn using the `plot` function. It is a bidimensional plot, with two MCA axes as abscissae and ordinates (specified by the `xax` and `yax` arguments). Each category of each variable is displayed by an ellipse. The position of the centre of the ellipse is given by the means of the coordinates of the individuals (`$li`) belonging to the category. The width and height of an ellipse are given by the variance of the coordinates of the individuals, and the covariance between the coordinates on the two axes gives the slope of the ellipse. The interpretation of this figure is the same as Fig. 5.10, but it is much more easy and detailed, as the categories of all the variables are not superimposed.

5.4   Hill and Smith Analysis (HSA)

Environmental data sets with exclusively qualitative variables are not very frequent. Some variables are easy to measure automatically on a continuous scale, while others are intrinsically qualitative. So the most frequent case is a table containing a mix of qualitative and quantitative variables. In this case, one can choose between two strategies: transforming quantitative variables to qualitative ones and using MCA, or considering qualitative variables as quantitative ones and using PCA.

The first strategy can be used when the number of quantitative variables is low. If this is not the case (most variables are quantitative with just a few qualitative ones), the loss of information may badly influence the results of the data analysis procedure. The second strategy can be used when qualitative variables are in fact ordered qualitative variables (e.g., categories *low*, *medium* and *high*). In this case, using PCA can be relevant (if linear trends are expected) but it is not a viable solution when qualitative variables contains categories that cannot be ordered (e.g., *blue*, *red* and *green*).

The Hill and Smith Analysis (HSA, Hill and Smith 1976) is a data analysis method that is able to deal directly with a data table containing a mix of quantitative and (ordered or unordered) qualitative variables. This method does not modify the original characteristics of the variables, avoiding the arbitrary choices of the two previous strategies. If all the variables are quantitative, then the results of HSA are identical to those of PCA. If all the variables are qualitative, then the results are identical to those of MCA. And if there is a mix of p quantitative variables and q qualitative variables, then the analysis is an optimal combination of the properties of the two analyses.

The row weights of this analysis are the same as the row weights of the PCA of the p quantitative variables, and are also equal to the row weights of the MCA

```
hs1 <- dudi.hillsmith(menv, scannf = FALSE)
scatter(hs1, posieig = "bottomleft")
```

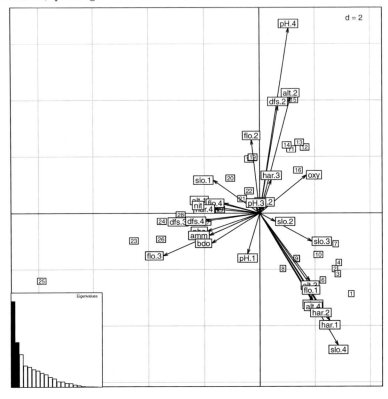

Fig. 5.13 The `scatter` graph of an Hill and Smith Analysis.

of the q qualitative variables. The column weights are different: for quantitative variables, column weights are equal to $1/(p + q)$, instead of 1 in a PCA. For qualitative variables, the weights are computed as in MCA (sum of the weights of the individuals belonging to each category, divided by q, see Box 5.3), except that it is divided here by the total number of variables $(p + q)$ instead of q. The total sum of column weights is therefore equal to 1, and qualitative and quantitative variables have the same weights.

To illustrate HSA, we consider the Doubs data where the first six variables are considered as qualitative and the last five as quantitative:

```
menv <- cbind(fenv[, 1:6], env[, 7:11])
```

The Hill and Smith Analysis is then computed on the resulting table using the `dudi.hillsmith` function of the **ade4** package. The `scatter` function can then be used to draw the biplot, where quantitative variables appear as simple labels, while qualitative ones appear with one label for each category.

`score(hs1, col = TRUE)`

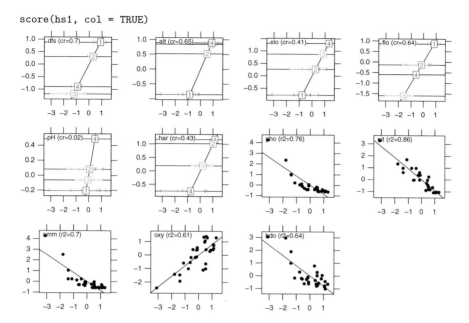

Fig. 5.14 The score graph of a Hill and Smith Analysis.

The `score` function can also be used to highlight the properties of the method (Fig. 5.14). HSA maximises the squared correlation for quantitative variables (i.e., the criteria of PCA) and the correlation ratio for qualitative variables (i.e., the criteria of MCA). As a consequence, Fig. 5.14 can be interpreted as Fig. 3.3 for quantitative variables and Fig. 5.11 for qualitative variables. These values are also stored in `hs1$cr`:

`hs1$cr`

```
          RS1        RS2
dfs  0.70222   0.840069
alt  0.65252   0.741726
slo  0.41026   0.157049
flo  0.63965   0.633381
pH   0.02332   0.225875
har  0.42895   0.320770
pho  0.75512   0.046149
nit  0.85903   0.008401
amm  0.70428   0.069365
oxy  0.61287   0.202631
bdo  0.63870   0.126527
```

The interpretation of Figs. 5.13 and 5.14 is identical to the interpretation of the PCA and MCA Figs. 5.6, 5.7, 5.10, 5.11 and 5.12: the first axis is an upstream-downstream gradient, while the second one opposes geomorphology to chemical processes. The data set under study is the same, with only quantitative to qualitative transformation for some variables and the three methods (PCA, MCA, HSA) give the same results, with the exception of possible axis inversions.

5.5   Other Simple Methods

The **ade4** package provides other methods for the analysis of an environmental table (see the first part of Table 3.2), but we are not going to detail them here. Here is the list of the functions and the corresponding methods (see the online documentation for more information on how to use them and examples of application):

- `dudi.fca`: Fuzzy Correspondence Analysis. Fuzzy variables are a generalisation of categorical variables, where items have a given probability of belonging to the categories of each fuzzy variable.
- `dudi.fpca`: Fuzzy PCA (see above)
- `dudi.mix`: Mixed type Analysis. This is an alternative to the `dudi.hillsmith` function.

Chapter 6
Description of Species Structures

Abstract Several simple data analysis methods can be used to analyse species data tables, i.e., tables having sites as rows and species as columns. Like in the previous chapter, simple means that these methods are adapted to the analysis of only one table. Three particular data analysis methods will be studied here: Correspondence Analysis (CA), centred Principal Component Analysis (cPCA), and Principal Coordinate Analysis (PCoA).

6.1 Introduction

Community ecology aims to study patterns and processes underlying the coexistence of individuals of different species (species assemblage). To achieve this goal, field works are performed to describe several sites by their species compositions (e.g., abundance, presence-absence). This information is stored as a sites × species table that can be graphically represented (Fig. 6.1). Following the continuum theory of Gleason (1926), a common approach (McIntosh 1978) consisted in rearranging the sequence of sites and species, both horizontally and vertically, to highlight the main organisation of ecological communities (Fig. 6.1). In the final arrangement, sites (respectively species) are ordered so that the position of a given site (respectively species) should reflect its similarity with others.

In the first works, the rearrangement is performed by hand (Curtis and McIntosh 1951) and the result is often subjective, depending on the experience of the ecologist. Hence, several methods have been proposed to perform an objective ordering of sites and species. Goodall (1954) proposed the generic term *ordination* to describe any techniques that allow to rearrange an ecological table. He suggested that this ordination can be performed on several dimensions and used Principal Component Analysis (PCA) to analyse a floristic data set. PCA has been widely used by ecologists but also strongly criticised due to its underlying assumption of linear species responses which is inadequate in the context of gradient analysis (Box 6.1, Swan 1970; Austin and Noy-Meir 1971; Beals 1973). Based on the principle of weighted averaging (Box 6.1), Correspondence Analysis (CA) considers unimodal species responses. This method developed by Benzécri (1969) has

© Springer Science+Business Media, LLC, part of Springer Nature 2018
J. Thioulouse et al., *Multivariate Analysis of Ecological Data with ade4*,
https://doi.org/10.1007/978-1-4939-8850-1_6

```
library(ade4)
library(adegraphics)
data(dunedata)
afc1 <- dudi.coa(dunedata$veg, scannf = FALSE)
g1 <- table.value(dunedata$veg, symbol = "circle", ppoints.cex = 0.5,
     plot = FALSE)
g2 <- table.value(dunedata$veg, coordsx = rank(afc1$co[,1]),
     coordsy = rank(afc1$li[,1]), symbol = "circle", ppoints.cex = 0.5, plot = FALSE)
cbindADEg(g1, g2, plot = TRUE)
```

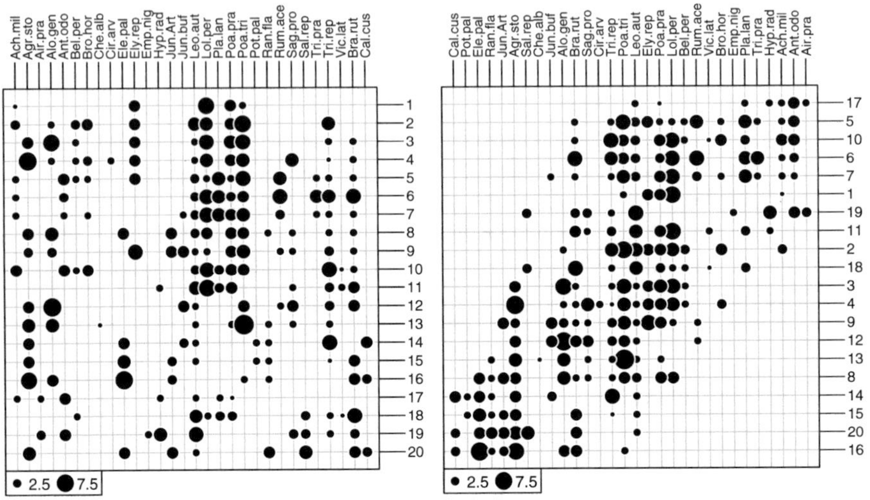

Fig. 6.1 Graphical representation of a floristic table (columns correspond to 30 species, rows to 20 sites). The size of symbols is proportional to species abundance. On the right, rows and columns are reordered using Correspondence Analysis (Sect. 6.2) to highlight the main structure. Data available in dunedata in **ade4**.

been popularised by Hill (1974, 1973) in Ecology using the iterative algorithm of *reciprocal averaging*. CA uses the χ^2 distance in a symmetric manner for sites and species. If the study mainly aims to characterise the variations of diversity among sites (i.e., β diversity), other types of distance can be envisaged. In this case, the analysis focuses on the similarities between sites (Box 3.1) and Principal Coordinate Analysis (PCoA) can be applied to summarise the information in few dimensions.

This chapter shows how the choice of a data analysis method should be driven by the type of data (count tables, presence-absence, abundance indices, etc.) but also by the objectives of the study. Indeed, each method has its own mathematical properties, and these properties relate to an underlying ecological model that must be adapted to the objectives of the study.

Box 6.1 Species Response Curve, Weighted Averaging and Ordination Methods

Usually, ecologists measure the abundances of m species and the values of p environmental variables in n sites. These data are stored in matrices

(continued)

Box 6.1 (continued)

Y and **X**, respectively. As both types of information are recorded for the same sites, it is possible to depict the abundance of a given species as a function of environmental gradient. Species distribution modelling aims to fit a statistical model to these data to describe species response curves and/or predict spatial distribution (Austin 2002). Principal Component Analysis (PCA) and related methods (e.g., Redundancy Analysis, RDA, Sect. 8.4.1) are based on correlations/covariances and thus assume implicitly linear species-environment relationships. The main gradients are estimated by PCA and constrained to be linear combination of environmental descriptors (**X**) in RDA. In the real world, linear responses are rarely observed. The main exception relates to the sampling of a small part of the gradient, leading to the modelling of a partial response curve:

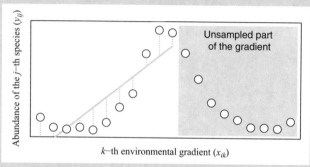

Several widely used statistical methods consider that species responses on gradient are symmetric and bell shaped (i.e., Gaussian curves) but some more flexible techniques are available to deal with asymmetric curves (Oksanen and Minchin 2002). In this context, response of species j to the environmental gradient k can be easily summarised by the species optimum (niche position or centroid, μ_{jk}), maximum (h_{jk}) and niche width (tolerance, t_{jk}):

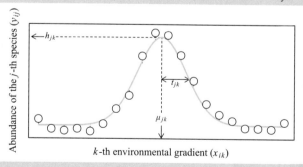

Under the assumption of Gaussian response, the method of weighted averaging (Whittaker 1956) allows to estimate the niche centroid (μ_{jk}) by

(continued)

Box 6.1 (continued)
computing the average environmental condition where the species is present
(weighted by the abundances):

$$\hat{\mu}_{jk} = \frac{\sum_{i=1}^{n} y_{ij} x_{ik}}{\sum_{i=1}^{n} y_{ij}}$$

If $\mathbf{D}_m$ is an $m \times m$ diagonal matrix with the total abundances of species,
then $\mathbf{YD}_m^{-1}$ is the table of species profiles containing relative abundances
$(y_{ij} / \sum_{i=1}^{n} y_{ij})$. Optima for all species on all environmental variables are then
simply computed by the matrix product $(\mathbf{YD_m^{-1}})^\top \mathbf{X}$. Hence, all methods that
transform raw data into species profiles implicitly assume that species have
unimodal responses that can be summarised by their optima.

Among these methods, Correspondence Analysis (CA) and Canonical
Correspondence Analysis (CCA, Sect. 8.4.2) are based on the reciprocal averaging algorithm, an iterative procedure based on the successive estimations
of site and species scores by weighted averaging (Hill 1973). They provide
estimates for the position of the niche centroids on the main gradients and
maximise their separation (ter Braak 1985; ter Braak and Looman 1986).
These gradients are estimated by CA (latent gradients) and constrained to
be a linear combination of the environmental variables ($\mathbf{X}$) in CCA. As these
methods maximise the separation of niche positions, they are also particular
cases of Discriminant Analysis (ter Braak and Verdonschot 1995; Lebreton
et al. 1988a).

6.2   Correspondence Analysis (CA)

Correspondence analysis (CA) is designed to analyse two-way contingency tables.
These tables contain counts of individuals belonging to categories of two categorical
variables. In **R**, the `table` function allows to build such table by crossing two
`factor` objects. For instance, the frequency distribution of 70 species (from the
`carniherbi49` data set of **ade4**) according to their order and diet is obtained by:

```
library(ade4)
data(carniherbi49)
(tab <- table(carniherbi49$taxo$ord, carniherbi49$tab2$clade))
```

```
                Carnivore Herbivore
Artiodactyla            0        24
Carnivora              19         0
Perissodactyla          0         6
```

By definition, a contingency table contains only positive values and its rows and columns play the same role as they both correspond to categories. It is possible to compute marginal (i.e., by row and column) and grand totals:

```
rowSums(tab)
```

```
 Artiodactyla        Carnivora Perissodactyla
           24               19              6
```

```
colSums(tab)
```

```
Carnivore Herbivore
       19        30
```

```
sum(tab)
```

```
[1] 49
```

The association between the two categorical variables can be evaluated by a χ^2 test. The statistics of this test measures the deviation between observed counts and those expected under the hypothesis of independence between the two variables. Here, we used a randomisation version of the test:

```
chisq.test(tab, simulate.p.value = TRUE)
```

```
        Pearson's Chi-squared test with simulated p-value
        (based on 2000 replicates)
data:   tab
X-squared = 49, df = NA, p-value = 5e-04
```

A sites × species table is not a contingency table *sensu stricto* as the sampling unit is the site. However, it can be treated as a contingency table by considering that individuals have been sampled and two categorical variables (namely, the species and the site) have been measured. This would correspond to sample a number of individuals so that the list of species is simply the result of the exploration of the biological diversity of the environment, and the list of sites is simply the result of the exploration of the spatial extent of the study area.

We considered the doubs data set (see Sect. 5.2). In this data set, the doubs$fish data frame contains the number of fish of 27 species that were found in the 30 sites along the Doubs river. In this case, summing values by row, columns or both makes sense as it produces the number of fishes sampled in each site, the number of fishes for each species and the total number of fishes:

```
data(doubs)
fish <- doubs$fish
rowSums(fish)
```

```
  1  2  3  4  5  6  7  8  9 10 11 12 13 14 15 16 17 18 19 20 21 22 23
  3 12 16 21 34 21 16  0 14 14 11 18 19 28 33 40 44 42 46 56 62 72  4
 24 25 26 27 28 29 30
 15 11 43 63 70 87 89
```

```
 colSums(fish)
```

```
Cogo Satr Phph Neba Thth Teso Chna Chto Lele Lece Baba Spbi Gogo Eslu
  15   57   68   73   15   19   18   26   43   56   43   27   55   40
Pefl Rham Legi Scer Cyca Titi Abbr Icme Acce Ruru Blbj Alal Anan
  36   33   29   21   25   45   26   18   38   63   31   57   27
```

```
 sum(fish)
```

```
[1] 1004
```

Several books were dedicated to CA, see, for example, Nishisato (1980) and Greenacre (1984). The theory of CA in the framework of the duality diagram is summarised in Box 6.2. In **ade4**, CA is computed with the dudi.coa function. The first argument of this function is the data frame containing species counts. Additional arguments scannf and nf work as in the dudi.pca function to choose the number of axes on which scores and loadings are computed (see Sect. 5.2). All the outputs of this function are grouped in a dudi object (subclass coa), and Box 6.3 recalls the corresponding output elements.

```
coa1 <- dudi.coa(fish, scannf = FALSE, nf = 2)
```

Correspondence Analysis allows to summarise the structure of a contingency table by identifying associations between categories of both variables (sites and species). The initial data transformation for a CA is different from the transformation used for a PCA (centring and standardisation). In CA, counts are first transformed into frequencies (see Box 6.2). These frequencies are then turned into relative frequencies, dividing them by marginal frequencies, and they are finally centred. This transformation means that CA is based on relative composition (for both species and sites) so that quantitative differences are removed contrary to PCA that works on abundance values. This difference is illustrated with a simulated data set where the abundance of 3 species are generated for sites using a Gaussian response model (Box 6.1). Curves for species 1 and species 2 differ only by their maximum abundance whereas curves for species 2 and 3 differ only for the niche position.

```
fgauss <- function(x = 1:20, mu, t, h) h * exp(-(x - mu)^2/
    (2 * t^2))
sp1 <- fgauss(mu = 10, t = 5, h = 35)
sp2 <- fgauss(mu = 10, t = 5, h = 10)
sp3 <- fgauss(mu = 13, t = 5, h = 10)
sim <- round(cbind(sp1, sp2, sp3))
```

PCA and CA are applied on this simulated data set and distances among species are then computed on data transformed by these two methods.

```
ADEgS(list(g1, g2, g3), layout = matrix(c(rep(1, 4), 2, 3), 2))
```

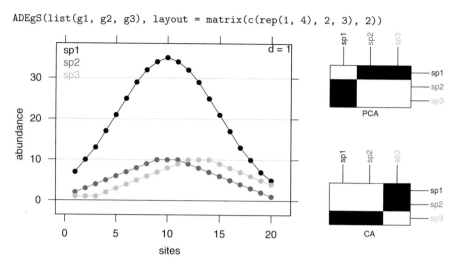

Fig. 6.2 Simulation of the response curves of 3 species for 20 sites. On the right, distances among species are computed in the case of PCA or CA and represented by heatmaps. Black cells correspond to high distances, white cells to low distances.

```
dpca <- dist.dudi(dudi.pca(sim, scale = FALSE, scannf = FALSE),
    amongrow = FALSE)
dcoa <- dist.dudi(dudi.coa(sim, scannf = FALSE), amongrow = FALSE)
g1 <- sld.curves(sim, pld.hori = FALSE, paxes.draw = TRUE,
    plines.col = 1:3, ppoints.col = 1:3, xlab = "sites",
    ylab = "abundance", key = list(space = "inside",
        text = list(lab = colnames(sim), col = 1:3)),
    plot = FALSE)
g2 <- table.image(dpca, axis.text = list(col = 1:3),
    xlab = "PCA", plot = FALSE)
g3 <- table.image(dcoa, axis.text = list(col = 1:3),
    xlab = "CA", plot = FALSE)
```

In PCA, species 2 and 3 are the closest as their absolute abundances in sites are similar (Fig. 6.2). In CA, the values themselves have no influence, it is the shape of the profiles that matters. Hence, species 1 and 2 are the closest as they have the same niche positions. Hence, CA should be used only when the study should focus on relative composition and not consider difference in abundance. This is the case in gradient analysis where species should be ordered by their niche positions on an environmental or a latent gradient.

The same rationale holds for sites. We consider three sites of the simulated data set:

```
sim3 <- sim[c(1, 10, 20), ]
rownames(sim3) <- c(1, 10, 20)
sim3
```

```
   sp1 sp2 sp3
1    7   2   1
10  35  10   8
20   5   1   4
```

When PCA is applied, absolute abundances are considered and site 1 is thus more similar to site 20 than to site 10:

```
dist.dudi(dudi.pca(sim3, scale = FALSE, scannf = FALSE))
```

```
        1      10
10 29.950
20  3.742 31.575
```

On the other hand, site 1 is much more similar to site 10 than to site 20 when CA is applied:

```
dist.dudi(dudi.coa(sim3, scannf = FALSE))
```

```
        1      10
10 0.1332
20 0.7897 0.6576
```

These patterns are due to the fact that CA works on relative compositions and the high proportion of species 1 in sites 1 and 10 (around 70% of the individuals) explains the high level of similarity between these two sites:

```
prop.table(sim3, 1)
```

```
       sp1     sp2     sp3
1   0.7000 0.2000 0.1000
10 0.6604 0.1887 0.1509
20 0.5000 0.1000 0.4000
```

These differences between PCA and CA are due to different parametrisation for data transformation ($tab), sites ($lw) and species weights ($cw) which imply different ways to compute distances among sites: CA uses the χ^2 distance whereas PCA is based on Euclidean distance.

Lastly, note that CA is a symmetric method (see Box 6.2), while PCA is intrinsically asymmetric. In PCA, rows and columns play a very different role: columns are variables and rows are observations. The PCA of a table and the PCA of the transpose of this table give very different results (see, for example, R-mode and Q-mode PCA, Legendre and Legendre 1998). Conversely, rows and columns have the same role in CA, and the CA of the transpose of a table gives exactly the same results as the CA of the table itself. This means that, *a priori*, CA should be used on tables where rows and columns play the same role.

Figure 6.3 shows the first two axes factor maps of CA applied on the doubs$fish data set. Fish species (left) and sampling sites (right) positions are drawn with the s.label function.

The fish species factor map (Fig. 6.3, left) shows very clearly that three zones can be distinguished along the stream. The first one is the trout zone (lower left corner), where the most frequent species are brown trout (Satr), minnow (Phph) and stone loach (Neba). The second one is the grayling zone (upper left corner), where grayling (Thth), blageon (Teso) and european bullhead (Cogo) are also present, while the first three species are decreasing. The last one (on the right of the figure) is the downstream zone, where all other species are present.

```
sl1 <- s.label(coa1$co, plabels.optim = TRUE, ppoints.cex = 0.5,
    plot = FALSE)
sl2 <- s.label(coa1$li, plabels.optim = TRUE, ppoints.cex = 0.5,
    plot = FALSE)
ADEgS(list(sl1, sl2))
```

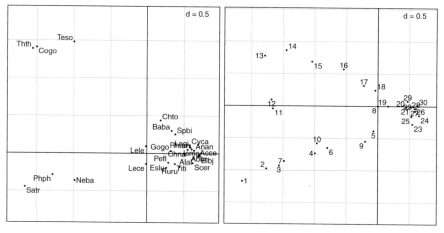

Fig. 6.3 Correspondence Analysis of the Doubs fish species data table. Left: fish species factor map, right: sampling sites factor map.

The sites factor map shows (Fig. 6.3, right) the sites that belong to the three zones. The trout zone extends from site 1 to site 10 (with the exception of site 8), the grayling zone goes from site 11 to site 18, and all other sites belong to the downstream zone. This typology is in good agreement with what is known about the biology of these species in this region (Verneaux 1973) and with the Huet zonation.

There is however a problem with the results of this CA: the high pollution peak that was detected at sites 23 to 26 by the PCA of water physico-chemical parameters (see Fig. 5.6) does not seem to have any effect on fish species distribution. This is strange, as many fish species are very sensitive to water pollution.

And indeed, looking at the raw fish counts (Fig. 6.4) shows that the effect of this pollution on fish numbers is obvious.

Figure 6.4 was drawn using the `table.value` function. This function plots the whole data table, with black squares proportional to the number of fishes (27 species in columns and 30 sites in row). The trout zone and the grayling zone are clearly visible on the left of the figure, but the downstream zone is obviously cut in two parts, just after site 22. At site 23, all species show a dramatic decrease, with only three species still present: `Lece` (chub), `Ruru` (roach) and `Alal` (bleak). This effect of pollution persists along sites 24 to 26. Fish numbers increase downstream, as the stream restoration process takes place and pollution slowly disappears. As CA considers relative and not absolute abundances, the decrease of abundances due to pollution cannot be identified with this method.

```
table.value(fish, ppoints.cex = 0.5)
```

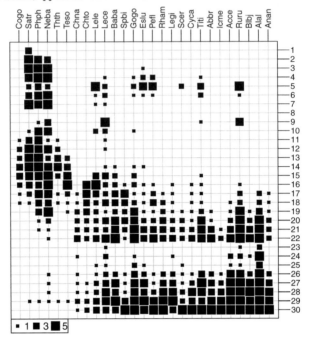

Fig. 6.4 Number of fish of the 27 species (columns) found in the 30 sites (rows) of the doubs data set. The area of black squares is proportional to the number of fishes.

Biplot can be produced for CA using the `biplot` or `scatter` functions. In **ade4**, three types of biplots can be produced (Boxes 6.2 and 6.3) using the argument `method` (Oksanen 1987). If `method = 2`, species are positioned by a unit-variance score (`$c1`) and sites by weighted averaging (`$li`). If `method = 3`, sites are positioned by a unit-variance score (`$l1`) and species by weighted averaging (`$co`). Figure 6.5 illustrates this representation. By default, (`method = 1`) corresponds to a compromise between these two representations (`$li` and `$co`).

Box 6.2 Correspondence Analysis: Basic Mathematical Definitions

Let $\mathbf{Y} = [y_{ij}]$ be a contingency table with n rows and m columns. From the table of frequencies $\mathbf{P} = [p_{ij}] = [y_{ij}/y_{\bullet\bullet}]$ (where $y_{\bullet\bullet}$ is the grand total of the contingency table), two vectors $\mathbf{n} = \mathbf{P}\mathbf{1}_m = (p_{1\bullet} \cdots p_{n\bullet})^\top$ and $\mathbf{m} = \mathbf{P}^\top\mathbf{1}_n = (p_{\bullet 1} \cdots p_{\bullet m})^\top$ of row and column sums are derived. The diagonal matrices of the row and column weights are:

$$\mathbf{D}_n = \mathrm{diag}(\mathbf{n}) \quad \text{and} \quad \mathbf{D}_m = \mathrm{diag}(\mathbf{m})$$

(continued)

Box 6.2 (continued)

Lastly, the matrix $\mathbf{P}$ is doubly centred, such that:

$$\mathbf{P}_0 = \mathbf{P} - \mathbf{D}_n \mathbf{1}_n \mathbf{1}_m^\top \mathbf{D}_m = [p_{ij} - p_{i\bullet} p_{\bullet j}]$$

Correspondence analysis is the analysis of the triplet:

$$\left(\mathbf{D}_n^{-1} \mathbf{P}_0 \mathbf{D}_m^{-1}, \mathbf{D}_m, \mathbf{D}_n\right)$$

and the associated diagram is:

$$
\begin{array}{ccc}
 & \mathbf{D}_m & \\
\mathbb{R}^m & \longrightarrow & \mathbb{R}^{m^*} \\
\mathbf{D}_m^{-1}\mathbf{P}_0^\top\mathbf{D}_n^{-1} \Big\uparrow & & \Big\downarrow \mathbf{D}_n^{-1}\mathbf{P}_0\mathbf{D}_m^{-1} \\
\mathbb{R}^{n^*} & \longleftarrow & \mathbb{R}^n \\
 & \mathbf{D}_n &
\end{array}
$$

The total inertia of this triplet is:

$$I_{\left(\mathbf{D}_n^{-1}\mathbf{P}_0\mathbf{D}_m^{-1}, \mathbf{D}_m, \mathbf{D}_n\right)} = \text{Trace}(\mathbf{D}_n^{-1}\mathbf{P}_0\mathbf{D}_m^{-1}\mathbf{D}_m\mathbf{D}_m^{-1}\mathbf{P}_0^\top\mathbf{D}_n^{-1}\mathbf{D}_n)$$

$$= \text{Trace}(\mathbf{D}_n^{-1}\mathbf{P}_0\mathbf{D}_m^{-1}\mathbf{P}_0^\top)$$

$$= \sum_{i=1}^{n}\sum_{j=1}^{m} \frac{(p_{ij} - p_{i\bullet}p_{\bullet j})^2}{p_{i\bullet}p_{\bullet j}}$$

This quantity is equal to the χ^2 statistic computed on the contingency table divided by the number of individuals ($y_{\bullet\bullet}$). The standard χ^2 test evaluates if the distribution of individuals among categories (i.e., rows and columns) is different from a random arrangement. CA decomposes this total inertia and thus identifies which categories deviate the most from a random distribution.

According to Property 3.1 (Box 3.2), CA searches for a principal axis $\mathbf{a}$ maximising:

$$\left\|\mathbf{D}_n^{-1}\mathbf{P}_0\mathbf{D}_m^{-1}\mathbf{D}_m\mathbf{a}\right\|_{\mathbf{D}_n}^2 = \left\|\mathbf{D}_n^{-1}\mathbf{P}_0\mathbf{a}\right\|_{\mathbf{D}_n}^2$$

The matrix $\mathbf{D}_n^{-1}\mathbf{P}_0$ contains the centred row profiles such that the product $\mathbf{D}_n^{-1}\mathbf{P}_0\mathbf{a}$ places rows at the barycentres (weighted averages, see Box 6.1) of the column points, and thus the quantity maximised is simply a variance between rows. Hence, in $\mathbb{R}^m$, columns have a unit-variance score $\mathbf{a}$ that maximises the variance between the row barycentres.

(continued)

Box 6.2 (continued)

In $\mathbb{R}^n$, Property 3.2 (Box 3.2) shows that CA searches for a principal component **b** maximising:

$$\left\|\mathbf{D}_m^{-1}\mathbf{P}_0^{\top}\mathbf{D}_n^{-1}\mathbf{D}_n\mathbf{b}\right\|_{\mathbf{D}_m}^2 = \left\|\mathbf{D}_m^{-1}\mathbf{P}_0^{\top}\mathbf{b}\right\|_{\mathbf{D}_m}^2$$

By symmetry, the matrix $\mathbf{D}_m^{-1}\mathbf{P}_0^{\top}$ contains the centred column profiles such that the product $\mathbf{D}_m^{-1}\mathbf{P}_0^{\top}\mathbf{b}$ places columns at the barycentres (weighted averages) of the row points (**b**). Hence, the rows are placed by a unit-variance score **b** that maximises the variance between column barycentres ($\left\|\mathbf{D}_m^{-1}\mathbf{P}_0^{\top}\mathbf{b}\right\|_{\mathbf{D}_m}^2$).

These two viewpoints show that CA treats the rows and columns of the table simultaneously and in a symmetric manner. Hence, analysing **Y** or $\mathbf{Y}^{\top}$ produces the same results. As CA puts rows at the weighted average of columns and simultaneously columns at the weighted average of rows, it is also known under the name of reciprocal averaging (Hill 1973). While CA is achieved in **ade4** using the eigen decomposition of a duality diagram, reciprocal averaging is an iterative algorithm that converges to the CA solution.

Box 6.3 Correspondence Analysis: `dudi` Output Elements

In the **ade4** package, the results of a Correspondence Analysis are stored in an object of class `dudi`, subclass `coa`. This object is a list with 12 elements, including the usual elements of any `dudi`. In this list, elements of particular interest are:

- `$eig`: eigenvalues ($\mathbf{\Lambda}$)
- `$cw`: column weights ($\mathbf{D}_m$)
- `$lw`: row weights ($\mathbf{D}_n$)
- `$tab`: centred relative frequencies table ($\mathbf{D}_n^{-1}\mathbf{P}_0\mathbf{D}_m^{-1}$)
- `$c1`: unit-variance column scores ($\mathbf{A}$)
- `$li`: row scores as weighted averages ($\mathbf{L} = \mathbf{D}_n^{-1}\mathbf{P}_0\mathbf{A}$)
- `$l1`: unit-variance row scores ($\mathbf{B}$)
- `$co`: column scores as weighted averages ($\mathbf{C} = \mathbf{D}_m^{-1}\mathbf{P}_0^{\top}\mathbf{B}$)
- `$N`: total sum ($y_{\bullet\bullet}$)

Three types of biplot can be drawn with these coordinates, using the couples (`$li`, `$c1`), (`$l1`, `$co`) and (`$li`, `$co`). A fourth type (reciprocal scaling, Thioulouse and Chessel 1992) can be drawn using the `reciprocal.coa` and `score` functions.

```
sc1 <- scatter(coa1, method = 3, posieig = "none", plot = FALSE)
sv1 <- s.value(coa1$l1, fish[, 5], col = 1:2, plegend.drawKey = FALSE,
      symbol = "circle", centerpar = TRUE)
sd1 <- s.distri(coa1$l1, fish[, 5, drop = FALSE], col = "red",
      ellipseSize = 0, ppoints.cex = 0, plot = FALSE)
cbindADEg(sc1, sv1 + sd1, plot = TRUE)
```

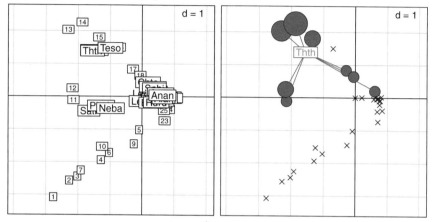

Fig. 6.5 CA of Doubs fish data table. Left: CA biplot (method = 3) where sites are positioned by a unit-variance score ($l1) and species by weighted averaging ($co). Right: principles of weighted averaging illustrated for the grayling (Thth). Sites are represented using the s.value function with symbols proportional to the abundance of grayling. The positions are given by $l1. Then, the function s.distri is used to position the grayling by weighted averaging. The species is represented by a star linking the species to all the sites where it occurs.

6.3 Centred PCA (cPCA)

CA outputs do not show the effect of the pollution peak on fishes and the loss of almost all species. This is because CA works on profiles, and therefore removes quantitative differences between sites and between species. CA compares the shape of the profiles, which means that sites (or species) with different fish numbers but with the same profile shape will seem identical. Pollution, by killing almost all the fishes indistinctly has no influence on the shape of the profiles, since all the species are affected in the same way.

If a quantitative effect must be evidenced, then a PCA should be used instead. However, as explained in Sect. 5.2, the difference of variance between species should not be removed, which means that a covariance matrix PCA (also called "centred PCA") should be preferred to a correlation matrix PCA.

Figure 6.6 shows the results of a covariance matrix PCA on the fish count table. The species factor map shows that the three zones (trout, grayling and downstream) are still detected and ordered on the first principal component from left to right. On the sites factor map, downstream sites are on the right, with the exception of sites 23, 24 and 25, which are on the left, near sites 1 and 8. What is the common point

```
cpca <- dudi.pca(fish, scale = FALSE, scannf = FALSE, nf = 2)
sl1 <- s.label(cpca$co, plabels.optim = TRUE, plot = FALSE)
sl2 <- s.label(cpca$li, plabels.optim = TRUE, plot = FALSE)
ADEgS(list(sl1, sl2))
```

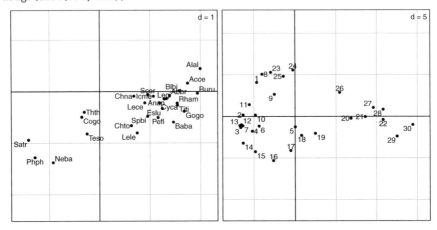

Fig. 6.6 Centred PCA of Doubs fish data table. Left: fish species factor map, right: sites factor map.

between sites 1, 8, and 23, 24, 25? It is simply a very low number of fishes, or even the absence of any fish in site 8 (see Fig. 6.7).

6.4   Standardised and Non-centred PCA

The choice of centring and standardisation in PCA is very important, and the corresponding analyses can give very different results. Restricting the choice to the usual dichotomy "same units ⇒ covariance matrix PCA" and "different units ⇒ correlation matrix PCA" can be inadequate. There are other types of centring and standardisation: non-centred PCA, de-centred PCA, block-standardised PCA, etc., that can prove very useful.

Figures 6.8 and 6.9 show the differences between a correlation matrix PCA (also called "standardised PCA") and a non-centred PCA (ncPCA) on the Doubs fish counts table.

The sites factor map of the normed PCA (Fig. 6.8, right) is very similar to the sites factor map of the centred PCA. But the correlation circle of the normed PCA shows that the standardisation has almost completely removed the distinction between the trout zone and the grayling zone. All the species have been rescaled to unit variance, and some important information about species distribution has been lost. In this analysis, all the species have equal importance. In centred PCA, on the other hand, species with high variations of abundance (and thus high variance) would have more importance than species with low variation of abundances.

```
plot(rowSums(doubs$fish), xlab = "Sites", ylab = "Fish number")
```

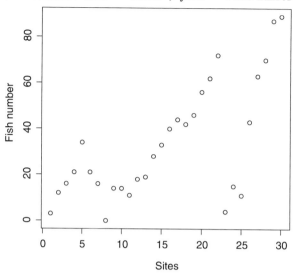

Fig. 6.7 Total number of fishes in the 30 sites of the doubs$env data set.

```
pca <- dudi.pca(fish, scannf = FALSE, nf = 2)
sc1 <- s.corcircle(pca$co, plot = FALSE)
sl1 <- s.label(pca$li, plabels.optim = TRUE, plot = FALSE)
ADEgS(list(sc1, sl1))
```

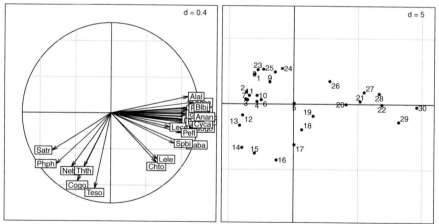

Fig. 6.8 Normed PCA of Doubs fish data table. Left: fish species correlation circle, right: sites factor map.

Conversely, the non-centred PCA (ncPCA) keeps the distinction between the two zones, and puts the empty site (8) at the origin (0, 0) in Fig. 6.9 (just like CA). In centred PCA, the origin corresponds to the average composition of the study area.

```
ncpca <- dudi.pca(fish, scale = FALSE, center = FALSE, scannf = FALSE)
sl1 <- s.label(ncpca$co, plabels.optim = TRUE, plot = FALSE)
sl2 <- s.label(ncpca$li, plabels.optim = TRUE, plot = FALSE)
ADEgS(list(sl1, sl2))
```

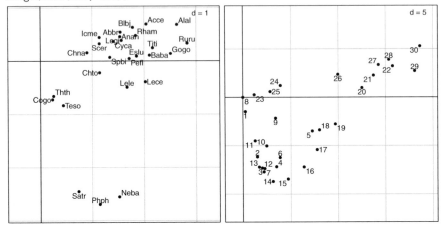

Fig. 6.9 Non-centred PCA of Doubs fish data table. Left: fish species factor map, right: sites factor map.

This example illustrates the fact that the choice of a data analysis method should not be based only on the type of data. The usual shortcuts "quantitative variables ⇒ PCA" and "count tables ⇒ CA" may lead to very bad results. PCA and CA are very different methods that should be used with caution. The choice must be based on the adequacy of the mathematical properties of the method with the aims of the study.

6.5   Principal Coordinate Analysis (PCoA)

Different multivariate methods induce different ways to compute distances among sites (Euclidean distance for PCA, χ^2 distance for CA, see Sect. 6.2). Many distance measures have been defined in particular situations (genetic data, presence-absence, etc.), with special properties well adapted to these situations. See Chap. 7 of Legendre and Legendre (1998) for a detailed analysis and comparison of the ways to measure resemblance between sites (or species) in Ecology. It is therefore desirable to be able to introduce these particular distance measures in multivariate data analysis methods. Principal Coordinate Analysis (PCoA, Gower 1966) takes distance matrix as input and returns coordinates for individuals in a low-dimensional space that best preserve the original distances.

The advantage of PCoA over PCA or CA is that it allows to choose a particular distance measure between sites (or species). A drawback is that it focuses either on individuals or variables, not both. Hence, only one viewpoint (cloud) of the duality diagram theory is considered (see Box 3.1).

Principal Coordinate Analysis can be useful in two different situations:

- when the rectangular (individuals × variables) data table is not available for some reason, for example when the experimental design implies a direct measure of distances instead of measuring parameters on sampling units,
- when the rectangular measures table is available but a particular distance, more appropriate to the data set must be used.

The goal of the analysis is to give Euclidean representations (factor maps) that display individuals, starting from a matrix of Euclidean distances between these individuals. The use of the `dudi.pco` function should thus be restricted to Euclidean distance matrices. It can be tested using the `is.euclid` function. If a non-Euclidean distance matrix is used, PCoA will return negative eigenvalues because the method is not able to return a configuration of individuals that strictly preserve the distances. An alternative is to approximate the distance matrix by a Euclidean one with a simple transformation (see `cailliez` or `lingoes`).

A very useful characteristic of the `dudi.pco` function is that it allows to introduce distance matrices into the duality diagram framework by returning an object of class `dudi`. This means that a `dudi` of class `pco` can, for example, be coupled with another data table with a Coinertia Analysis (Sect. 8.3). This can be used to analyse the relationships between a distance matrix and a table of environmental variables, like in db-RDA (Borcard et al. 2011; Legendre and Anderson 1999). An example of application in the field of microbiology and using Coinertia Analysis instead of Redundancy Analysis is given by Jarraud et al. (2002).

The basic properties and the mathematical notations of PCoA are summarised in Box 6.4.

Box 6.4 PCoA: Basic Mathematical Definitions

Let $\Delta = [\delta_{ij}]$ be a Euclidean distance matrix between n individuals. Principal coordinate analysis (PCoA, Gower 1966) aims to find a configuration of individuals in a multidimensional space that preserves these distances. We consider the possibility to assign weights to individuals as proposed by Gower (1984) and Gower and Legendre (1986) by defining $\mathbf{D}$ a diagonal matrix of weights (this functionality is provided by the function `dudi.pco` of **ade4**).

Let $\mathbf{\Phi} = [-\frac{1}{2}\delta_{ij}^2]$ and m_i, m_j denote the weighted means of the rows and columns of $\mathbf{\Phi}$ and m its global weighted mean. The matrix $\mathbf{\Omega}$ is the doubly centred (by rows and columns) version of $\mathbf{\Phi}$:

$$\mathbf{\Omega} = [\omega_{ij}] = \left[-\frac{1}{2}\delta_{ij}^2 - m_i - m_j + m \right]$$

(continued)

Box 6.4 (continued)

Using matrix notation, we have $\Omega = \mathbf{H}\Phi\mathbf{H}^\top$ where $\mathbf{H} = (\mathbf{I}_n - \mathbf{1}_n\mathbf{1}_n^\top\mathbf{D})$ is the centring operator and $\mathbf{1}_n$ is a vector of ones (of length n).

PCoA consists in the following diagonalisation:

$$\mathbf{D}^{\frac{1}{2}}\mathbf{H}\Phi\mathbf{H}^\top\mathbf{D}^{\frac{1}{2}} = \mathbf{U}\Lambda\mathbf{U}^\top$$

After left and right multiplications by $\mathbf{D}^{-\frac{1}{2}}$, it can be rewritten as:

$$\Omega = \mathbf{H}\Phi\mathbf{H}^\top = \mathbf{D}^{-\frac{1}{2}}\mathbf{U}\Lambda\mathbf{U}^\top\mathbf{D}^{-\frac{1}{2}} = \mathbf{X}\mathbf{X}^\top$$

The matrix $\mathbf{X} = \mathbf{D}^{-\frac{1}{2}}\mathbf{U}\Lambda^{\frac{1}{2}}$ contains the coordinates of individuals in the multidimensional space and it is possible to compute the distances d_{ij} between two individuals i and j in this new space. Let $\mathbf{x}_i$ and $\mathbf{x}_j$ be the vectors of coordinates (i-th and j-th rows of $\mathbf{X}$), the squared distance is equal to (see Appendix A.2):

$$d_{ij}^2 = \left\|\mathbf{x}_i - \mathbf{x}_j\right\|_{\mathbf{D}}^2 = \left\|\mathbf{x}_i\right\|_{\mathbf{D}}^2 + \left\|\mathbf{x}_j\right\|_{\mathbf{D}}^2 - 2\langle\mathbf{x}_i|\mathbf{x}_j\rangle_{\mathbf{D}} = \omega_{ii} + \omega_{jj} - 2\omega_{ij}$$

By definition, $\omega_{ij} = -\frac{1}{2}\delta_{ij}^2 - m_i - m_j + m$ and the distance of an individual with itself is null ($\delta_{ii} = 0$). Hence, $\omega_{ii} = -2m_i + m$ and $\omega_{jj} = -2m_j + m$ and the previous equation simplifies to:

$$d_{ij}^2 = \delta_{ij}^2$$

Hence, as expected, the configuration of individuals obtained by PCoA ($\mathbf{X}$) preserves the original distance matrix. If only few dimensions are kept (few columns in $\mathbf{X}$), the original distances are not strictly preserved but PCoA provides the best approximation. If Δ is not Euclidean, the full representation of the distance is not possible and the diagonalisation step of PCoA will return negative eigenvalues and complex eigenvectors.

All the outputs of the `dudi.pco` function are grouped in a `dudi` object (subclass `pco`), and Box 6.5 recalls the corresponding output elements.

The first argument to the `dudi.pco` function must be an object of class `dist` containing a Euclidean distance matrix. Other arguments are similar to arguments of the other `dudi` functions, except the `full` and `tol` arguments. `full = TRUE` means that all dimensions should be kept in returned objects. `tol`, the tolerance threshold, is used to test whether the distance matrix is Euclidean: an eigenvalue is considered positive if it is larger than `-tol * lambda1` where `lambda1` is the largest eigenvalue.

Box 6.5 PCoA: `dudi` Output Elements

In the **ade4** package, the results of a PCoA are stored in an object of class `dudi`, subclass `pco`. This object is a list with 11 elements, including the usual elements of any `dudi`. In this list, standard outputs of PCoA are provided:

- `$eig`: eigenvalues ($\mathbf{\Lambda}$)
- `$lw`: weights for individuals ($\mathbf{D}$)
- `$li`: coordinates for individuals ($\mathbf{X} = \mathbf{D}^{-\frac{1}{2}}\mathbf{U}\mathbf{\Lambda}^{\frac{1}{2}}$)
- `$l1`: principal components ($\mathbf{D}^{-\frac{1}{2}}\mathbf{U}$)

Some other elements are added to the returned object. This allows to use objects of subclass `pco` as argument to other functions that deal with `dudi` objects:

- `$cw`: weights for "variables" ($\mathbf{I}$)
- `$co`: coordinates for "variables" ($\mathbf{\Lambda}^{\frac{1}{2}}$)
- `$tab`: individuals by "variables" table ($\mathbf{X} = \mathbf{D}^{-\frac{1}{2}}\mathbf{U}\mathbf{\Lambda}^{\frac{1}{2}}$)

Note that the number of columns of `$tab` is equal to rank of the distance matrix whereas it is the number of axes that have been kept by the user (using the `nf` argument) for `$li`.

We used PCoA on the `doubs$fish` data set. The first step consists in computing a distance matrix between the rows of the data frame (sites). The `dist.binary` function computes the Jaccard index (s) between sites after presence/absence transformation. The distances are then computed as $\sqrt{1 - s}$. The `dudi.pco` function is then used to perform the PCoA:

```
dfishJ <- dist.binary(fish, method = 1)
(pcoJ <- dudi.pco(dfishJ, scannf = FALSE))


Duality diagram
class: pco dudi
$call: dudi.pco(d = dfishJ, scannf = FALSE)

$nf: 2 axis-components saved
$rank: 26
eigen values: 0.1023 0.03547 0.03034 0.02503 0.02042 ...
  vector length mode    content
1 $cw     26      numeric column weights
2 $lw     30      numeric row weights
3 $eig    26      numeric eigen values

  data.frame nrow ncol content
1 $tab        30   26  modified array
2 $li         30   2   row coordinates
3 $l1         30   2   row normed scores
4 $co         26   2   column coordinates
5 $c1         26   2   column normed scores
other elements: NULL
```

`s.label(pcoJ$li, plabels.optim = TRUE)`

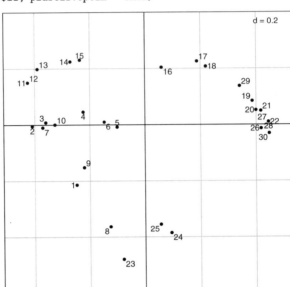

Fig. 6.10 Principal Coordinate Analysis of the Doubs fish species data table.

Other packages contain useful functions to compute ecological (di)similarity indices, distance measures and standardising transformations, like **vegan** (`vegdist` and `decostand` functions) and **labdsv** (`dsvdis` function).

Figure 6.10 shows the same upstream-downstream ordination of sites as with previous analyses, and the same exceptional position of sites 23, 24 and 25 (absence of fish due to pollution, see Fig. 6.6), near site 8 (zero fish between the trout zone and the grayling zone) and site 1 (near the source, with only 3 trouts).

6.6   Other Simple Methods

The **ade4** package provides other methods for the analysis of one species table (see the first part of Table 3.2), but we are not going to detail them here. Here is the list of the functions and the corresponding methods (see the online documentation for more information on how to use them and examples of application):

- `dudi.dec`: Decentred Correspondence Analysis. This analysis can be used when a particular column profile is available. This profile will be used as a reference in a Correspondence Analysis type analysis.

- `dudi.nsc`: Non-Symmetric Correspondence Analysis. This analysis is a Correspondence Analysis with *uniform column weights* (but keeping usual CA *row weights*). See Sect. 14.2.

Chapter 7
Taking into Account Groups of Sites

Abstract This chapter shows how the partitioning of sites can be taken into account during the analysis of an ecological data table. We present the Between-Class and Within-Class Analyses and Discriminant Analysis. Then we present several examples of use of these methods on a small data set with simple structures. The chapter ends with a comparison between Discriminant Analysis and Between-Class Analysis.

7.1 Introduction

Taking into account the existence of groups of sites (or "samples") is achieved by decomposing a data table into two additive components. The first relates to the differences between groups and its analysis aims to describe the main characteristics of the groups. The second component contains only within-groups variations and its analysis focuses on the characteristics of the residuals (i.e., the data variability if groups did not exist).

Groups are to be taken here in a very broad sense. They can, for example, represent space-time structures, like sites belonging to the same geographic region, or to the same period of time. They can also correspond to an experimental design, with groups representing different treatments. One of the advantages of the duality diagram framework used in the **ade4** package is that all the simple methods that have been described in Chaps. 5 and 6 can be used here, which means that the effect of groups can be analysed in any type of data table (quantitative, qualitative or mixed tables, counts, presence/absence, row percentages, etc.).

Two types of analyses, called Between-Class and Within-Class Analysis are implemented in **ade4**. The corresponding generic functions are named bca (formerly between) and wca (formerly within) and several methods are provided:

```
library(ade4)
methods(bca)
```

```
[1] bca.coinertia* bca.dpcoa*    bca.dudi*    bca.rlq*
see '?methods' for accessing help and source code
```

© Springer Science+Business Media, LLC, part of Springer Nature 2018
J. Thioulouse et al., *Multivariate Analysis of Ecological Data with ade4*,
https://doi.org/10.1007/978-1-4939-8850-1_7

```
methods(wca)
```

```
[1]  wca.coinertia*  wca.dpcoa*       wca.dudi*       wca.rlq*
see '?methods' for accessing help and source code
```

Between-Class Analysis models the differences between groups by computing the group means, and the resulting means table is then analysed. Conversely, Within-Class Analysis removes the group effect by computing the residuals between observed data and group means, and analyses the table of these differences (see Box 7.1).

The first analysis can be used to visually check the existence of groups, to describe the main characteristics of the differences between the groups (for example, which variables are best related to which groups?), and to test their statistical significance using a permutation test. The second one tries to find out whether other structures remain in the data table that can be revealed after removing a strong group effect.

Box 7.1 Partitioning the Total Inertia

Let us consider an $n \times p$ matrix $\mathbf{X}$ with the measurements of p variables for n individuals (sites). This data table is treated by a simple multivariate analysis thus defining a statistical triplet $(\mathbf{X}, \mathbf{Q}, \mathbf{D})$ where $\mathbf{D} = \mathrm{diag}(w_1 \cdots w_n)$ is the $n \times n$ diagonal matrix of site weights.

We consider a categorical variable with g categories (groups), namely $G_1, \ldots, G_k, \ldots, G_g$, measured on the n individuals (colours in figure below). This variable can be coded as an $n \times g$ matrix $\mathbf{H} = [h_{ik}]$ of dummy variables (see Appendix A.7), with:

$$h_{ik} = \begin{cases} 1 \text{ if } i \in G_k \\ 0 \text{ if } i \notin G_k \end{cases}$$

Let $\mathbf{P_H} = \mathbf{H}(\mathbf{H}^\top \mathbf{D}\mathbf{H})^{-1}\mathbf{H}^\top \mathbf{D}$ be the projection operator on the dummy variables, the table $\mathbf{X}$ can be decomposed in two additive parts:

$$\mathbf{X} = \mathbf{P_H}\mathbf{X} + (\mathbf{I}_n - \mathbf{P_H})\mathbf{X} = \mathbf{X}_B + \mathbf{X}_W$$

The $n \times p$ matrix $\mathbf{X}_B$ contains groups means (computed using weights in $\mathbf{D}$), repeated inside each group ($\mathbf{X}_B = \left[\bar{x}_j^k\right]$ for $i \in G_k$) where $\bar{x}_j^k = \sum_{i \in G_k} w_i x_{ij}$ is the mean of the j-th variable for group k. The $n \times p$ matrix $\mathbf{X}_W$ contains differences between observed values and group means ($\mathbf{X}_W = \left[x_{ij} - \bar{x}_j^k\right]$).

This partitioning is illustrated here:

(continued)

Box 7.1 (continued)

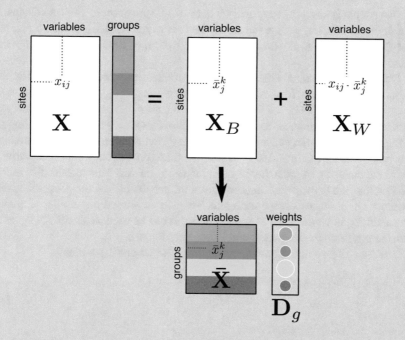

The total inertia (see Box 3.3) of the analysis of $(\mathbf{X}, \mathbf{Q}, \mathbf{D})$ can be decomposed as follows:

$$I_{(\mathbf{X},\mathbf{Q},\mathbf{D})} = \mathrm{Trace}(\mathbf{X}^\top \mathbf{D}\mathbf{X}\mathbf{Q})$$
$$= \mathrm{Trace}((\mathbf{X}_B + \mathbf{X}_W)^\top \mathbf{D}\,(\mathbf{X}_B + \mathbf{X}_W)\,\mathbf{Q})$$

so that

$$I_{(\mathbf{X},\mathbf{Q},\mathbf{D})} = I_{(\mathbf{X}_B,\mathbf{Q},\mathbf{D})} + I_{(\mathbf{X}_W,\mathbf{Q},\mathbf{D})}$$

The first element measures the inertia explained by the differences among groups (between-class inertia). Between-Class Analysis (see Box 7.2) focuses on these differences and is the analysis of the triplet $(\mathbf{X}_B, \mathbf{Q}, \mathbf{D})$. On the other hand, the second element measures differences within groups (within-class inertia). Within-Class Analysis (see Box 7.4) removes differences among groups and focuses on $(\mathbf{X}_W, \mathbf{Q}, \mathbf{D})$.

If we consider $\mathbf{D}_g = \mathbf{H}^\top \mathbf{D}\mathbf{H}$ the $g \times g$ diagonal matrix of groups weights (obtained by summing individual weights per group), we can define $\bar{\mathbf{X}} = \mathbf{D}_g^{-1}\mathbf{H}^\top\mathbf{X}$ the $g \times p$ matrix of group means. Then, Between-Class Analysis corresponds also to the analysis of $(\bar{\mathbf{X}}, \mathbf{Q}, \mathbf{D}_g)$.

7.2 An Environmental Situation

We have already used the `meaudret` data set (Pegaz-Maucet 1980) in Chaps. 2, 3 and 4. In this chapter, we use the `meau` data set which has been chosen by Dolédec and Chessel (1987) to illustrate the first description of Between-Class and Within-Class Analyses.

Both data sets contain the same kind of data, physico-chemical parameters measured four times (four seasons) at several sites along a small stream called the Méaudret (South-East of France). But in the `meaudret` data set, the `oxygen` variable has been removed because it takes the same values in all the sampling sites during winter. This can cause an error in some situations (particularly in multiway analyses). The `meaudret$env` data frame therefore contains only nine variables, while the `meau$env` data frame contains ten variables. The second difference is the fact that the `meaudret` data set gives the results of five sampling sites, while the `meau` data set includes a sixth site. This site is located on another stream, the Bourne river, into which the Méaudret flows. It can be used as a control site, as it is situated upstream the Méaudret and Bourne confluence.

The `meau$env` data frame therefore has 24 rows and 10 columns:

```
library(ade4)
library(adegraphics)
data(meau)
env <- meau$env
dim(env)
```

```
[1] 24 10
```

The ten columns correspond to ten environmental variables: water temperature, flow, pH, conductivity, oxygen, biological oxygen demand (BDO5), oxidability, ammonium, nitrates, and phosphorus.

```
names(env)
```

```
[1] "Temp" "Flow" "pH"   "Cond" "Oxyg" "Bdo5" "Oxyd" "Ammo"
[9] "Nitr" "Phos"
```

The 24 rows correspond to the six sites, sampled four times (sp = spring, su = summer, au = autumn, and wi = winter):

```
row.names(env)
```

```
 [1] "sp_1" "sp_2" "sp_3" "sp_4" "sp_5" "sp_6" "su_1" "su_2"
 [9] "su_3" "su_4" "su_5" "su_6" "au_1" "au_2" "au_3" "au_4"
[17] "au_5" "au_6" "wi_1" "wi_2" "wi_3" "wi_4" "wi_5" "wi_6"
```

The `meau` data set also contains the description of the sampling design coded as two categorical variables (`factor`):

```
(seasons <- meau$design$season)
```

```
[1] spring spring spring spring spring spring summer summer
[9] summer summer summer summer autumn autumn autumn autumn
[17] autumn autumn winter winter winter winter winter winter
Levels: spring summer autumn winter
```

```
(sites <- meau$design$site)
```

```
[1] S1 S2 S3 S4 S5 S6 S1 S2 S3 S4 S5 S6 S1 S2 S3 S4 S5 S6
[19] S1 S2 S3 S4 S5 S6
Levels: S1 S2 S3 S4 S5 S6
```

The aim of the study is to analyse the variations of physico-chemical parameters along the stream and during the year (spatial and temporal components). We first apply a normed PCA on the environmental data table.

```
(envpca <- dudi.pca(env, scannf = FALSE, nf = 3))
```

```
Duality diagram
class: pca dudi
$call: dudi.pca(df = env, scannf = FALSE, nf = 3)

$nf: 3 axis-components saved
$rank: 10
eigen values: 5.745 1.43 1.084 0.6761 0.5244 ...
  vector length mode      content
1 $cw    10      numeric column weights
2 $lw    24      numeric row weights
3 $eig   10      numeric eigen values

  data.frame nrow ncol content
1 $tab         24   10  modified array
2 $li          24    3  row coordinates
3 $l1          24    3  row normed scores
4 $co          10    3  column coordinates
5 $c1          10    3  column normed scores
other elements: cent norm
```

Figure 7.1 shows the PCA of the Méaudret environmental data table. The correlation circle shows that the first axis corresponds to a pollution gradient, with high levels of pollution toward the right and absence of pollution on the left. The second axis is a temperature and flow gradient and underlines the particular behaviour of nitrates (compared to other pollution parameters). The analysis of the sites factor map is not easy, as many labels are superimposed, and spatial and temporal structures are mixed.

Interpretation is easier in Fig. 7.2, where the four seasons are grouped using a star and an ellipse for each site. It is easy to see that site 2 is more polluted than the others (because it is located on the right of the figure). Sites 3, 4 and 5 are less and less polluted, and site 5 is in fact comparable to site 1. Site 6 (control site located on the Bourne river) is on the left of site 1, denoting even lower levels of chemical pollution.

Figure 7.3 shows the same factor map, with the six sampling sites grouped for each season, but the temporal structure is less easy to interpret than the succession of the six sites along the stream.

Here, we show that applying a simple PCA and then using graphical functions allows to display differences among sites or seasons. However, this approach is

```
g1 <- s.corcircle(envpca$co, plot = FALSE)
g2 <- s.label(envpca$li, plot = FALSE)
ADEgS(list(g1, g2))
```

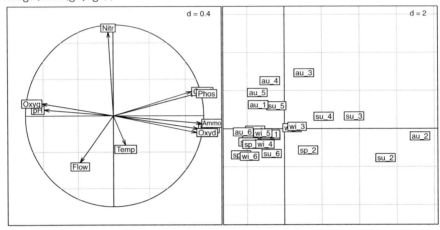

Fig. 7.1 Correlation matrix PCA of the Méaudret environmental data table. Left: parameters correlation circle, right: sites factor map.

```
s.class(envpca$li, meau$design$site, xlim = c(-4, 8), ylim = c(-2, 4),
        col = TRUE)
```

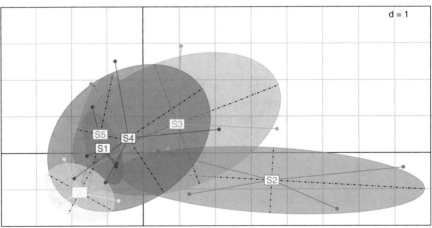

Fig. 7.2 PCA sites factor map, with the four samples grouped for each site.

not optimal. Indeed, the spatial structures can be analysed by computing the mean of the four dates for all the parameters (between-sites analysis), and conversely the temporal structures can be assessed by computing the mean of the six sites (between-dates analysis). It is also possible to try to remove the spatial effect using a within-site analysis and see if temporal structures appear more clearly.

```
s.class(envpca$li, meau$design$season, xlim = c(-4, 8), ylim = c(-2, 4),
        col = TRUE)
```

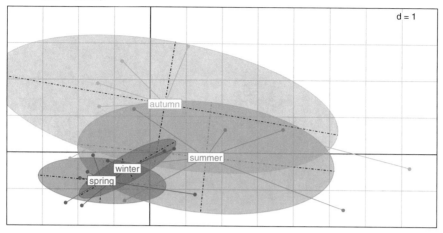

Fig. 7.3 PCA sites factor map, with the six sampling sites grouped for each season.

7.3   Between-Class Analysis: Analysing Differences Between Groups

Between-Class Analyses (BCA, Dolédec and Chessel 1987; Culhane et al. 2002) are methods to separate groups of sites, given a set of variables. There are several types of Between-Class Analyses, corresponding to the initial analysis after which Between-Class Analysis is computed (e.g., Principal Component Analysis, Correspondence Analysis, or Multiple Correspondence Analysis).

BCA is the analysis of a table of group means. Box 7.2 gives the basic definitions of Between-Class Analysis in the framework of the duality diagram.

Box 7.2 Between-Class Analysis: Basic Mathematical Definitions
Using notations defined in Box 7.1, Between-Class Analysis is the analysis of triplet $(\mathbf{X}_B, \mathbf{Q}, \mathbf{D})$ or equivalently $(\bar{\mathbf{X}}, \mathbf{Q}, \mathbf{D}_g)$. It corresponds to the following duality diagram:

$$
\begin{array}{ccc}
 & \mathbf{Q} & \\
\mathbb{R}^p & \longrightarrow & \mathbb{R}^{p^*} \\
\bar{\mathbf{X}}^\mathsf{T} \uparrow & & \downarrow \bar{\mathbf{X}} \\
\mathbb{R}^{g^*} & \longleftarrow & \mathbb{R}^g \\
 & \mathbf{D}_g &
\end{array}
$$

(continued)

Box 7.2 (continued)

Between-Class Analysis is therefore the analysis of the group means table, leading to the diagonalisation of $\bar{\mathbf{X}}^\top \mathbf{D}_g \bar{\mathbf{X}} \mathbf{Q}$. Note that the rank of this matrix is defined by $r = \min(p, g - 1)$. The total inertia of this analysis equals to between-class inertia.

According to Property 3.1 (Box 3.2), the Between-Class Analysis searches for a principal axis $\mathbf{a}$ maximising $\left\| \bar{\mathbf{X}} \mathbf{Q} \mathbf{a} \right\|_{\mathbf{D}_g}^2$. Hence, the analysis seeks coefficients ($\mathbf{a}$) to compute a linear combination of variables ($\bar{\mathbf{X}} \mathbf{Q} \mathbf{a}$) which best separates the groups by maximising the between-class inertia. Sites (i.e., rows of the initial table) can be projected on the principal axes and their coordinates are given by $\mathbf{X} \mathbf{Q} \mathbf{A}$.

The main function to compute a Between-Class Analysis in the **ade4** package is the `bca` function. All the outputs of this function are grouped in a `dudi` object (subclass `between`), and Box 7.3 recalls the corresponding output elements.

The `bca` function takes two main arguments: an analysis of the initial table (a `dudi` object) and a categorical variable (an object of class `factor`). In **ade4**, the user must first perform a simple analysis to identify the main variations in the data table and then use the `bca` function to introduce the partitioning in groups. This two-step implementation has a pedagogical aim by forcing users to interpret simple structures before analysing differences among groups. The outputs of both analyses can then be compared to evaluate the role of the categorical variable. The last two arguments (`scannf` and `nf`) have the same meaning as in the other analysis functions.

As underlined in Sect. 8.4.3.3, Between-Class Analysis is a particular case of analysis on instrumental variables when only one explanatory categorical variable is considered. The main advantage to use `bca` function is that several methods (`plot`, `summary`) are optimised to summarise the results of the analysis.

Box 7.3 Between-Class Analysis: `dudi` Output Elements

In the **ade4** package, the results of a Between-Class Analysis are stored in an object of class `dudi`, subclass `between`. This object is a list with 14 elements, including the usual elements of any `dudi`. In this list, elements of particular interest are:

- `$tab`: table of group means ($\bar{\mathbf{X}}$)
- `$lw`: group weights ($\mathbf{D}_g$)
- `$c1`: principal axes ($\mathbf{A}$)
- `$li`: scores for the groups ($\bar{\mathbf{X}} \mathbf{Q} \mathbf{A}$)

(continued)

> **Box 7.3** (continued)
> - $1s: projection of the rows of the initial data table (sites) onto the BCA axes (**XQA**)
> - $as: projection of the axes of the initial analysis of **X** onto the BCA axes
> - $ratio: ratio of the between-class to total inertia
>
> The row scores of the initial data table ($1s) can be superimposed to the row scores of the Between-Class Analysis ($1i). This gives an idea of the within-class *vs.* between-class variability.
>
> **Permutation test:** The statistical significance of these differences can be tested by a permutation test, with a criterion equal to the ratio of between-class inertia divided by total inertia. In this test, sites are randomly assigned to the groups. As the total inertia is invariant to rows permutation, this test is strictly equivalent to a test based on between-class inertia.

7.3.1 Between-Site Analysis

As explained at the beginning of this chapter, a Between-Class Analysis is the analysis of the table of class means. So the between-site analysis is the analysis of the table of site means. The between-site analysis `betsite` is computed using the `bca` function, and the table of site means is stored in the `betsite$tab` data frame. We can check that the dimensions of the `betsite$tab` data frame are six rows (six sites) and 10 columns (10 physico-chemical parameters), and that the mean of the standardised temperature in site 1 during the four seasons is equal to -0.1834:

```
betsite <- bca(envpca, sites, scannf = FALSE)
dim(betsite$tab)
```

```
[1]   6 10
```

```
betsite$tab[1:3, 1:5]
```

```
        Temp     Flow      pH    Cond     Oxyg
S1 -0.183449 -0.9966  0.1163 -0.2449  0.39460
S2 -0.039880 -0.4293 -0.8805  1.1023 -1.56390
S3  0.007976 -0.1725 -0.3821  0.5818 -0.06673
```

```
mean(envpca$tab$Temp[sites == "S1"])
```

```
[1] -0.1834
```

```
betsite
```

```
Between analysis
call: bca.dudi(x = envpca, fac = sites, scannf = FALSE)
class: between dudi

$nf (axis saved) : 2
$rank:   5
$ratio:  0.4413

eigen values: 3.335 0.6156 0.4027 0.04589 0.01407

   vector length mode     content
1 $eig    5        numeric eigen values
2 $lw     6        numeric group weights
3 $cw    10        numeric col weigths

   data.frame nrow ncol content
1 $tab        6    10   array class-variables
2 $li         6    2    class coordinates
3 $l1         6    2    class normed scores
4 $co        10    2    column coordinates
5 $c1        10    2    column normed scores
6 $ls        24    2    row coordinates
7 $as         3    2    inertia axis onto between axis
```

The plot function can be used to display the main components of the betsite analysis (Fig. 7.4). It provides a composite plot made of six elementary graphs. The main one (top-right, labeled Row scores and classes) shows the row scores of the initial data table ($ls data frame). The four sampling seasons for each site are grouped with a star and an ellipse. Each star and ellipse is labeled with the site name (S1 to S6), located at the gravity centre of the star (centre of the ellipse).

The bottom-right graph (Classes) shows the scores for the groups of the Between-Class Analysis ($li data frame). It contains only six points, corresponding to the six sites.

The following graph on the left (Unconstrained axes) shows the projection of the first three axes of the initial analysis (envpca) onto the Between-Class Analysis. It contains only 3 arrows, as this is the number of axes kept in the envpca analysis. This graph provides a convenient way to understand the relationships between the initial PCA that focuses on total variation and the Between-Class Analysis. Here, we can see that the first two axes of the simple PCA are nearly equivalent (apart from the sign) to the first two axes of the between-site analysis.

The lower-left graph is labeled Eigenvalues; this is the usual eigenvalues bar-chart. The last two graphs on the left are labeled Loadings and Columns. They both show the ten physico-chemical parameters, and they should be comparable. Large differences between these two graphs would imply that the analysis is not coherent. The first one (Loadings) gives the coefficients of the linear combination that maximise the between-class inertia ($c1 data frame). The second one (Columns) shows the scores of the variables ($co data frame).

We can see that the first axis of the Between-Class Analysis is very similar to the first axis of the simple PCA (pollution gradient) indicating that the main structures (identified by PCA) are also the main differences among groups. The factor map of row scores in the simple PCA (Fig. 7.2) is very similar to the factor map of the Between-Class Analysis (Fig. 7.4, Row scores and classes graph). And the correlation circle of parameters (Fig. 7.1) in the simple PCA is very similar to the

```
plot(betsite, row.pellipses.col = adegpar()$ppalette$quali(6))
```

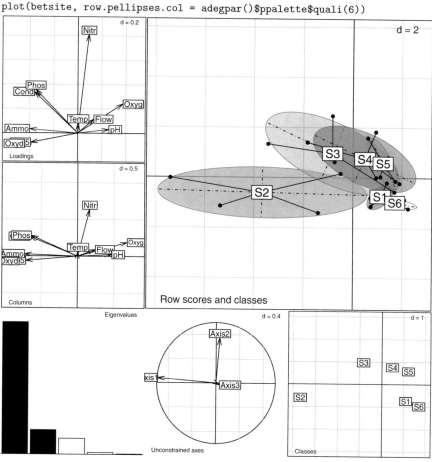

Fig. 7.4 Plot of the `betsite` analysis. This is a composite plot made of six graphs (see text for an explanation of the six graphs).

`Columns` graph in the between-site analysis (Fig. 7.4). This is because the between-site structure is very strong in this data set, and the first axis of the simple PCA already identified it.

The `randtest` function can be used to check the statistical significance of the differences between sites. The criterion used in this test is the ratio of the between-class inertia to the total inertia. The simulated *p*-value and the observed criterion can be obtained by displaying the `rtbetsite` object. By default, 999 permutations are performed.

```
(rtbetsite <- randtest(betsite))

Monte-Carlo test
Call: randtest.between(xtest = betsite)
```

```
plot(rtbetsite)
```

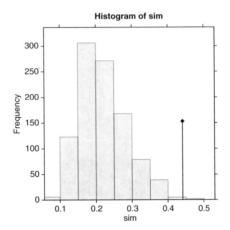

Fig. 7.5 Plot of the `rtbetsite` Monte-Carlo test.

```
Observation: 0.4413

Based on 999 replicates
Simulated p-value: 0.003
Alternative hypothesis: greater

    Std.Obs Expectation      Variance
   3.361814    0.220270      0.004323
```

The observed value of the criterion is equal to 0.4413, which means that 44% of the total inertia comes from the differences between sites. The simulated p-value is equal to 0.003, which means that the difference between sites is highly significant.

The histogram displayed in Fig. 7.5 shows the distribution of the values of the criterion computed on permuted tables. The observed value for the unpermuted table (0.4413) is plotted on the graph with a vertical bar and a black diamond sign.

The main characteristic of the spatial structure of physico-chemical parameters revealed by these analyses is the pollution gradient. Site 1 is not polluted, it is located opposite of the pollution parameters (phosphates, ammonium, oxidability, biological oxygen demand) on the factor maps. Site 2 is the most polluted, while sites 3, 4 and 5 are less and less polluted, as the restoration process takes place downstream along the stream. Site 6 is a control on the Bourne river, and it is not polluted. This particular structure is explained by the fact that the Autrans holiday resort is located between sites 1 and 2. The high tourist activity at this place leads to an overflow of water treatment capacity.

7.3.2   Between-Season Analysis

The between-season analysis gives a more interesting insight into the `meau` data set. Indeed, the simple PCA did not provide a very convincing picture of the seasonal structure of physico-chemical parameters (Fig. 7.3). The between-season analysis is computed using the `bca` function, and we can check the dimension of the `betseason$tab` data frame:

```
betseason <- bca(envpca, seasons, scannf = FALSE)
dim(betseason$tab)
```

```
[1]   4 10
```

The generic `plot` function can be used as in the previous section to display the main components of the `betseason` analysis. The seasonal structure of the physico-chemical parameters is much clearer in Fig. 7.6: we see that the temperature plays a key role in the opposition between warm (spring, summer) and cold (autumn, winter) seasons on the second axis. The first axis is still a pollution gradient (high levels of pollution toward the left), and opposes summer to spring in warm seasons and autumn to winter for cold seasons. This is easy to understand, as Autrans is a well-known summer resort, with high tourist activity during summer holidays.

In the between-season analysis, the values of each parameter are averaged across the six sites. This removes the spatial component of the data set, and makes the seasonal structure much more apparent. Another way to achieve the same result (underline the seasonal effect) is to explicitly remove the spatial component using a within-site analysis.

7.4   Within-Class Analysis: Removing Differences Between Groups of Sites

Within-Class Analysis (Dolédec and Chessel 1987) is the analysis of the residuals between observed data and group means. This means that the differences between groups have been removed from the data set, and we are looking for other structures remaining in the table.

Like in Between-Class Analysis, there is no constraint on the number of sites compared to the number of variables, and no problem with numerous and/or correlated variables.

Box 7.4 gives the basic definitions of a Within-Class Analysis in the framework of the duality diagram.

```
plot(betseason, row.pellipses.col = adegpar()$ppalette$quali(4))
```

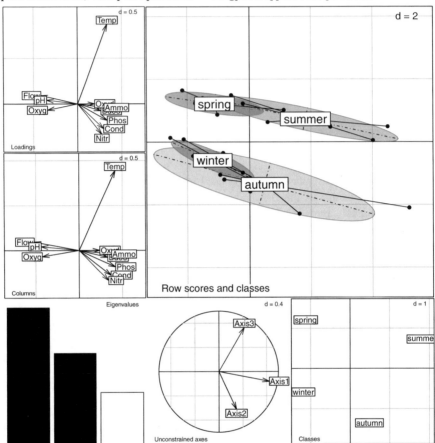

Fig. 7.6 Plot of the betseason analysis.

Box 7.4 Within-Class Analysis: Basic Mathematical Definitions
Using notations defined in Box 7.1, Within-Class Analysis is the analysis of
triplet $(\mathbf{X}_W, \mathbf{Q}, \mathbf{D})$. It corresponds to the following duality diagram:

$$
\begin{array}{ccc}
 & \mathbf{Q} & \\
\mathbb{R}^p & \longrightarrow & \mathbb{R}^{p^*} \\
\mathbf{X}_W{}^\top \uparrow & & \downarrow \mathbf{X}_W \\
\mathbb{R}^{n^*} & \longleftarrow & \mathbb{R}^n \\
 & \mathbf{D} &
\end{array}
$$

(continued)

Box 7.4 (continued)

Within-Class Analysis is therefore the analysis of the matrix of the residuals obtained by eliminating the between-class effect. It is useful when looking for the main features of a data table after removing an unwanted characteristic. It leads to the diagonalisation of matrix $\mathbf{X}_W^{\mathsf{T}} \mathbf{DX}_W \mathbf{Q}$. The total inertia of this analysis equals to within-class inertia.

According to Property 3.1 (Box 3.2), the Within-Class Analysis searches for a principal axis $\mathbf{a}$ maximising $\|\mathbf{X}_W \mathbf{Qa}\|_{\mathbf{D}}^2$. Hence, the analysis seeks coefficients ($\mathbf{a}$) to compute a linear combination of variables ($\mathbf{X}_W \mathbf{Qa}$) which best separates the sites after removing the differences among groups by maximising the within-class inertia.

In the **ade4** package, the `wca` function is used to compute Within-Class Analysis. All the outputs of this function are grouped in a `dudi` object (subclass `within`), and Box 7.5 recalls the corresponding output elements. The arguments of the `wca` function are the same as those of the `bca` function: the `dudi` object, the factor describing the groups, and the `scannf` and `nf` usual arguments. A generic `plot` function is also available in **adegraphics** to summarise the outputs of a `wca` analysis.

Box 7.5 Within-Class Analysis: `dudi` Output Elements

In the **ade4** package, the results of a Within-Class Analysis are stored in an object of class `dudi`, subclass `within`. This object is a list with 16 elements, including the usual elements of any `dudi`. In this list, elements of particular interest are:

- `$tab`: table of differences between observed data and groups means ($\mathbf{X}_W$)
- `$c1`: principal axes of the WCA ($\mathbf{A}$)
- `$li`: scores for the sites ($\mathbf{X}_W \mathbf{QA}$)
- `$ls`: projection of the rows of the initial data table (sites) onto the WCA axes ($\mathbf{XQA}$)
- `$as`: projection of the axes of the initial analysis of $\mathbf{X}$ on the WCA axes
- `$tabw`: weights of groups (useful for K-table analyses)
- `$fac`: factor defining the groups
- `$ratio`: ratio of the within-class to total inertia

The within-site analysis on the Méaudret data set is computed using the `wca` function. This function calculates the residuals between the environmental data table and the site means, and performs the analysis on these residuals:

```
witsite <- wca(envpca, sites, scannf = FALSE)
```

```
g1 <- s.corcircle(witsite$co, plot = FALSE)
g2 <- s.class(witsite$li, sites, col = TRUE, plot = FALSE)
ADEgS(list(g1, g2))
```

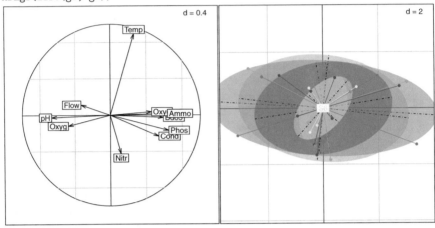

Fig. 7.7 Plot of the witsite analysis. Left: correlation circle of parameter scores, right: row coordinates (grouped by sites).

It is easy to check that the site effect has been removed, by plotting the row scores of the within-site analysis. Figure 7.7 shows that these row scores are centred by site (all six labels are superimposed at the centre of the graph).

Seasonal variations can be exposed by drawing the same row scores (witsite$li), but grouped by season (Fig. 7.8).

The same effect as in the between-season analysis (Fig. 7.6) is visible in Fig. 7.8, with a seasonal effect on the second axis (spring and summer *vs.* autumn and winter) and a pollution gradient on the first axis (summer *vs.* spring and autumn *vs.* winter).

Note that the information contained in the original PCA (envpca) is fully decomposed by the Between- and Within-Class Analyses:

```
sum(envpca$eig)
```

```
[1] 10
```

```
sum(betsite$eig) + sum(witsite$eig)
```

```
[1] 10
```

And the ratios provided by the analysis are simply obtained by:

```
sum(betsite$eig) / sum(envpca$eig)
```

```
[1] 0.4413
```

```
sum(witsite$eig) / sum(envpca$eig)
```

```
s.class(witsite$li, seasons, col = TRUE)
```

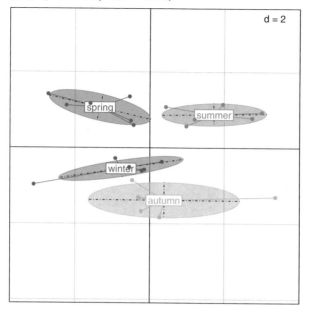

Fig. 7.8 Plot of the `witsite` analysis.

```
[1]  0.5587

 betsite$ratio

[1]  0.4413

 witsite$ratio

[1]  0.5587

 betsite$ratio + witsite$ratio

[1]  1
```

7.5   Discriminant Analysis

The aim of Discriminant Analysis and Between-Class Analysis is the same: highlighting the differences between groups. However, the constraints associated to these analyses differ so that both methods do not maximise the same criteria. Whereas Between-Class Analysis maximises the between-class inertia,

Discriminant Analysis maximises the between-class inertia relative to the total inertia. Box 7.6 describes the basis of Discriminant Analysis.

Box 7.6 Discriminant Analysis: Basic Mathematical Definitions
Using notations defined in Box 7.1, Discriminant Analysis is the analysis of triplet $(\mathbf{X}_B, (\mathbf{X}^\top \mathbf{D}\mathbf{X})^{-1}, \mathbf{D})$. It corresponds to the following duality diagram:

$$
\begin{array}{ccc}
 & (\mathbf{X}^\top\mathbf{D}\mathbf{X})^{-1} & \\
\mathbb{R}^p & \longrightarrow & \mathbb{R}^{p^*} \\
\mathbf{X}_B{}^\top \uparrow & & \downarrow \mathbf{X}_B \\
\mathbb{R}^{n^*} & \longleftarrow & \mathbb{R}^n \\
 & \mathbf{D} &
\end{array}
$$

Hence, Discriminant Analysis shares many similarities with Between-Class Analysis and the only difference is that it uses the Mahalanobis metrics $(\mathbf{X}^\top\mathbf{D}\mathbf{X})^{-1}$ instead of $\mathbf{Q}$ in $\mathbb{R}^p$.

According to Property 3.1 (Box 3.2), Discriminant Analysis searches for a principal axis $\mathbf{a}$ maximising $\left\| \mathbf{X}_B \left(\mathbf{X}^\top\mathbf{D}\mathbf{X}\right)^{-1} \mathbf{a} \right\|_{\mathbf{D}}^2$. If we consider the principal factor instead of the principal axis, we have $\mathbf{a}^* = \left(\mathbf{X}^\top\mathbf{D}\mathbf{X}\right)^{-1} \mathbf{a}$ and the criteria maximised becomes $\|\mathbf{X}_B\mathbf{a}^*\|_{\mathbf{D}}^2$. By definition, $\|\mathbf{a}^*\|_{(\mathbf{X}^\top\mathbf{D}\mathbf{X})}^2 = 1$ which can be rewritten as $\left\|\mathbf{X}\mathbf{a}^*\right\|_{\mathbf{D}}^2 = 1$. Hence, the analysis seeks coefficients $(\mathbf{a}^*)$ to compute a linear combination of variables $(\mathbf{X}_B\mathbf{a}^*)$ which best separates the groups by maximising the between-class inertia with the constraint that the total inertia is equal to 1 ($\left\|\mathbf{X}\mathbf{a}^*\right\|_{\mathbf{D}}^2 = 1$).

This viewpoint refers to maximisation of the correlation ratio (See Appendix A.7) by maximising the between-inertia with the additional constraint that the total inertia is equal to 1.

In the **MASS** package (lda function), the constraint is based on the F-ratio, i.e., the constraint is that the within-class inertia is equal to 1.

The discrimin function of the **ade4** package is used to compute a Discriminant Analysis. All the outputs of this function are grouped in a discrimin object, and Box 7.7 recalls the corresponding output elements. The arguments of the discrimin function are the same as those of the bca function: the first argument is the dudi object corresponding to the preparatory analysis of the data table. The second argument is a factor describing the groups of rows. The last two arguments (scannf and nf) have the same meaning as in the other analysis functions.

> **Box 7.7 Discriminant Analysis: `dudi` Output Elements**
>
> In the **ade4** package, the results of a Discriminant Analysis are stored in an object of class `discrimin`. This object is a list with 8 elements. In this list, elements of particular interest are:
>
> - `$fa`: loadings for variables ($\mathbf{A}^*$)
> - `$li`: scores for sites ($\mathbf{XA}^*$)
> - `$va`: link between the variables of **X** and the scores for sites ($\mathbf{X}^\mathsf{T}\mathbf{DXA}^*$)
> - `$cp`: link between the principal components of the initial analysis of **X** and the scores for sites
> - `$gc`: scores for groups ($\mathbf{X}_B\mathbf{A}^*$)
>
> **Permutation test:** The statistical significance of these differences can be tested by a permutation test, with a criterion equal to the ratio of between-class inertia divided by total inertia. Here, total inertia is computed using $\left(\mathbf{X}^\mathsf{T}\mathbf{DX}\right)^{-1}$ as a metric in $\mathbb{R}^p$. In this test, sites are randomly assigned to the groups. As the total inertia is invariant to rows permutation, this test is strictly equivalent to a test based on between-class inertia.

Discriminant Analysis is applied to study the seasonal structure of physico-chemical parameters:

```
discseason <- discrimin(envpca, seasons, scannf = FALSE)
```

The `plot` function can be used to display the main components of the `discseason` analysis (Fig. 7.9). It provides a composite plot made of six elementary graphs. The main one (top-right, labeled `Row scores and classes`) shows the projections of the sites onto the plane defined by the axes of the Discriminant Analysis (`$li` data frame). The six sampling sites for each season are grouped with a star and an ellipse. Each star and ellipse is labeled with the season name, located at the gravity centre of the star (centre of the ellipse). The bottom-right graph (`Class scores`) shows the group scores (`$gc` data frame). It contains only four points, corresponding to the four seasons. The following graph on the left (`Unconstrained axes`) shows the projection of the axes of the initial Principal Component Analysis (`$cp` data frame) to understand the relationships between the initial PCA and the Discriminant Analysis. Here, we can see that the third axis of the simple PCA—temperature—is equivalent (apart from the sign) to the first axis of the Discriminant Analysis. The lower-left graph (`Eigenvalues`) is the usual eigenvalues barchart. The last two graphs on the left are labeled `Loadings` and `Columns`. The first one represents the coefficients of the variables (`$fa` data frame). The second one represents the covariances between the ten physico-chemical parameters (`$va` data frame) and the axes of the analysis.

The first axis of the Discriminant Analysis is linked to the water temperature and the second axis to the flow. The seasons define a strong structure where the pollution component disappeared.

```
plot(discseason, row.pellipses.col = adegpar()$ppalette$quali(4))
```

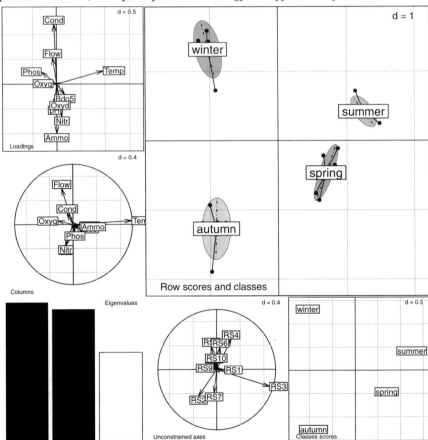

Fig. 7.9 Plot of the `discseason` analysis. This is a composite plot made of six graphs (see text for an explanation).

The `randtest` function can be used to check the statistical significance of the differences between seasons. The criterion used in this test is the ratio of the between-class inertia to the total inertia. The simulated p-value and the observed criterion can be obtained by displaying the `rtdiscseason` object. By default, 999 permutations are performed.

```
(rtdiscseason <- randtest(discseason))

Monte-Carlo test
Call: randtest.discrimin(xtest = discseason)

Observation: 0.2552

Based on 999 replicates
Simulated p-value: 0.001
Alternative hypothesis: greater
```

```
    Std.Obs Expectation      Variance
   5.7955146   0.1306748   0.0004615
```

The observed value of the criterion is equal to 0.2552, which means that 26% of the total inertia comes from the differences between seasons. The simulated *p*-value is equal to 0.001, which means that the difference between seasons is highly significant.

The histogram displayed in Fig. 7.10 shows the distribution of the values of the criterion computed on permuted tables. The observed value for the unpermuted table (0.2552) is plotted on the graph with a vertical bar and a black diamond sign.

The main characteristic of the temporal structure of physico-chemical parameters revealed by this analysis is the water cycle, the pollution gradient is eliminated.

Between-Class Analyses and Discriminant Analyses highlight differences between groups of observations but are not based on the same constraints (see Boxes 7.2 and 7.6). This implies that Between-Class Analysis maximises the between-class inertia whereas Discriminant Analysis maximises the between-class inertia relative to the total inertia. This theoretical difference has important practical implications. Between-Class Analyses can work on tables with few individuals compared to the number of variables and is able to deal with collinearities among variables. On the other hand, Discriminant Analysis requires a high number of individuals compared to the number of variables. An another important difference is illustrated by the Row scores and classes graph of the between-season analysis (Fig. 7.6). On this plot, all the seasons present an elongated ellipse associated to the pollution gradient kept on the first axis of the analysis. Hence, BCA maximises the distance between the centres of the ellipses (i.e., the between-class inertia) but does not control for the size of the ellipses (i.e., the total inertia).

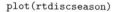

plot(rtdiscseason)

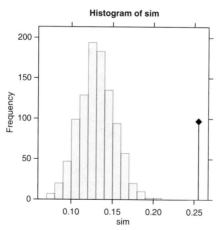

Fig. 7.10 Plot of the rtdiscseason Monte-Carlo test.

On the other hand, Discriminant Analysis tries to maximise the between-class inertia while minimising the total inertia. In the Row scores and classes graph of the Discriminant Analysis (Fig. 7.9), the ellipses of seasons are thus much smaller. All the sites gathered to the gravity centre of the seasons, highlighting the seasonal cycle.

7.6   Conclusion

The main structure of the meau data set is the spatial structure of the pollution along the six sites. There is a strong pollution peak between sites 1 and 2, and the restoration process takes place downstream along sites 3, 4 and 5. The simple PCA of the data table shows this spatial structure very clearly (Figs. 7.1 and 7.2) and it can be interpreted using the contributions of the ten physico-chemical parameters. The between-site analysis does not bring much more information (Fig. 7.4).

There is also a strong seasonal structure, which is not very clearly taken into account by the simple PCA (Fig. 7.3). This structure opposes warm and cold seasons. In the warm season, pollution is lower in spring than in summer because stream flow is higher in spring and pollutants are more diluted. Moreover, tourism is much higher in summer, which still increases pollution. In the cold season, pollution is higher in autumn because stream flow is at its minimum, so the concentration of pollutants is maximum, although most tourists have gone. This structure is adequately revealed by both the between-season analysis (Fig. 7.6) and the within-site analysis (Fig. 7.8). However, this pollution structure disappeared in the Discriminant Analysis (Fig. 7.9) because of the supplementary constraint on the physico-chemical variables keeping only the water cycle (temperature and flow).

These analyses work differently. The between-season and discriminant analyses compute the mean of each parameter among the six sites, so that the spatial effect is removed and the seasonal effect is revealed. The within-site analysis computes the residuals between the raw data table and the spatial model (means by site), thus removing the spatial effect and revealing the seasonal effect.

Chapter 8
Description of Species-Environment Relationships

Abstract This chapter shows how direct and indirect gradient analysis can be handled in the **ade4** package, with a special emphasis on three direct ordination methods: Coinertia Analysis, Redundancy Analysis and Canonical Correspondence Analysis.

8.1 Introduction

Simple methods presented in Chaps. 5 and 6 describe environmental or species structures independently. However, an important question in Ecology is the analysis of the relationships between these two structures with the aim of understanding if/how the organisation of ecological communities is linked to environmental variations. In this chapter, we focus on the case where a number of sites are described by environmental variables and species composition. This leads to consider two tables with the same rows (i.e., the sites). Historically, ecologists have first used indirect approaches for interpreting the structures of species assemblages (structural information extracted by the analysis of the species data) in relation to environmental variability. Site scores along the ordination axes, which are composite indices of species abundances were compared *a posteriori* to environmental variables (*indirect ordination, indirect gradient analysis*). Progressively, new techniques were developed to constrain the ordination according to the table of explanatory environmental variables (*direct ordination, direct gradient analysis*).

8.2 Indirect Ordination

The doubs data set has been described in Chaps. 5 and 6. In indirect ordination methods, community data are first summarised and then interpreted in the light of environmental information. For instance, we apply a centred PCA on the species data while the environmental table is treated by a standardised PCA. Two axes are kept for each analysis.

```
library(ade4)
library(adegraphics)
data(doubs)
pca.fish <- dudi.pca(doubs$fish, scale = FALSE, scannf = FALSE, nf = 2)
pca.env <- dudi.pca(doubs$env, scannf = FALSE, nf = 2)
```

To interpret the outputs of the species ordination, correlations between the axes kept in the two analyses can be computed:

```
cor(pca.env$li, pca.fish$li)
```

```
          Axis1   Axis2
Axis1   0.5682  0.3483
Axis2  -0.4679  0.6309
```

The two ordinations are strongly linked. The first two axes of the fish ordination (columns) are linked to the two main environmental gradients (first two axes of PCA of the environmental table). To facilitate the interpretation, correlations can be computed between original environmental variables and species ordination scores:

```
cor(doubs$env, pca.fish$li)
```

```
          Axis1        Axis2
dfs    0.81691    0.113670
alt   -0.67742    0.001439
slo   -0.57155    0.093089
flo    0.78476   -0.013730
pH    -0.04933   -0.252402
har    0.44764    0.038390
pho    0.11486    0.537131
nit    0.46860    0.309248
amm    0.08400    0.557866
oxy   -0.40336   -0.655908
bdo    0.08548    0.702449
```

The first axis is mainly correlated to geomorphological variables (distance from the source, flow, altitude, slope) whereas the second axis is more linked to chemical processes (biological demand for oxygen, dissolved oxygen, ammonium and phosphate). Note that the computation of these correlations is exactly equivalent to the projection, as supplementary elements, of the standardised environmental variables on the factorial map of the fish ordination. This projection step can be performed by the supcol function.

```
supcol.env <- supcol(pca.fish, pca.env$tab)
head(supcol.env$cosup)
```

```
          Comp1        Comp2
dfs    0.81691    0.113670
alt   -0.67742    0.001439
slo   -0.57155    0.093089
flo    0.78476   -0.013730
pH    -0.04933   -0.252402
har    0.44764    0.038390
```

These correlations can also be depicted on a correlation circle (Fig. 8.1).

```
s.corcircle(supcol.env$cosup)
```

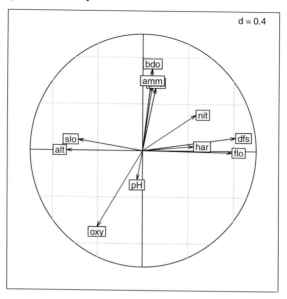

Fig. 8.1 Correlations between environmental variables and sites scores on the first two axes of the PCA of fish species data.

Symmetrically, **ade4** also offers the possibility to represent supplementary sites (which have not been involved in the computation of an analysis) using the `suprow` function. This can be useful for prediction purposes, allowing to compute an analysis on a number of reference sites and then using this model to evaluate the position for new sites.

It is usually assumed that environmental variables influence the distribution of species. In this context, it would be more appropriate to use a regression model to explain the fish species composition by environmental explanatory variables (e.g., `lm(pca.fish$li[, 1] ~ as.matrix(doubs$env))`). A variable selection procedure can be used to avoid overfitting and multicollinearity issues due to the high number (relative to the number of statistical units, i.e., sites) of correlated explanatory variables.

The main advantage of indirect ordination is its simplicity. Its main drawback is its lack of optimality: species ordination reveals the main patterns of community assemblage but does not guarantee that these structures are linked to environmental gradients. If a study focuses on species-environment relationships, two-table methods, that consider both environmental and species tables simultaneously, should be preferred.

8.3   Coinertia Analysis

As shown above, simple multivariate analyses are useful to identify the main environmental and species structures separately. Coinertia Analysis (Dolédec and Chessel 1994; Dray et al. 2003) aims to reveal the main co-structures (i.e., the structures common to both data sets) by combining these separate ordinations into a single analysis. This two-table method is based on the computation of a crossed array (cross-covariance matrix) that measures the relationships between the variables of both data sets. Box 8.1 gives the basic definitions of Coinertia Analysis in the framework of the duality diagram.

Box 8.1 Coinertia Analysis: Basic Mathematical Definitions

In Coinertia Analysis, two sets of variables are measured on the same set of n individuals. This information is stored in two tables and each set of variables is treated by a simple multivariate analysis thus defining two statistical triplets $(\mathbf{X}, \mathbf{Q}, \mathbf{D})$ and $(\mathbf{Y}, \mathbf{M}, \mathbf{D})$ where $\mathbf{X}$ and $\mathbf{Y}$ are $n \times p$ and $n \times m$ matrices, respectively. Note that $\mathbf{D}$ is common to the two triplets because we consider the same individuals in the two analyses. Coinertia Analysis combines these two analyses into a single one to identify which structures are common to both data sets (i.e., co-structures):

The above diagram can be rewritten as follows:

Coinertia Analysis (Dolédec and Chessel 1994; Dray et al. 2003) is the analysis of this diagram and thus is defined by the triplet $(\mathbf{Y}^{\top}\mathbf{DX}, \mathbf{Q}, \mathbf{M})$. The total inertia associated to this triplet is equal to:

$$I_{(\mathbf{Y}^{\top}\mathbf{DX}, \mathbf{Q}, \mathbf{M})} = \mathrm{Trace}(\mathbf{Y}^{\top}\mathbf{DXQX}^{\top}\mathbf{DYM})$$

(continued)

Box 8.1 (continued)

This quantity is a measure of the concordance between the two data sets and is equal to the numerator of the RV coefficient (Box 9.6, Escoufier 1973), a multivariate generalisation of the squared correlation coefficient. Coinertia Analysis decomposes this vectorial covariance onto orthogonal axes, and the general properties of the diagram (Box 3.2) lead to the maximisation of the following inner product:

$$\left\langle \mathbf{Y}^\mathsf{T}\mathbf{D}\mathbf{X}\mathbf{Q}\mathbf{a}|\mathbf{b}\right\rangle_{\mathbf{M}} = \mathbf{b}^\mathsf{T}\mathbf{M}\mathbf{Y}^\mathsf{T}\mathbf{D}\mathbf{X}\mathbf{Q}\mathbf{a} = \langle\mathbf{X}\mathbf{Q}\mathbf{a}|\mathbf{Y}\mathbf{M}\mathbf{b}\rangle_{\mathbf{D}} = \sqrt{\lambda}$$

If $\mathbf{X}$ and $\mathbf{Y}$ contain centred variables, the total inertia is simply a sum of squared covariances between all combinations of variables of the two data sets ($\sum_{i=1}^{p}\sum_{j=1}^{m}\text{cov}^2(\mathbf{x}^i, \mathbf{y}^j)$). In this case, Coinertia Analysis finds two vectors of coefficients $\mathbf{a}$ and $\mathbf{b}$ to obtain linear combinations of the variables of $\mathbf{X}$ and $\mathbf{Y}$ of maximal covariance ($\langle\mathbf{X}\mathbf{Q}\mathbf{a}|\mathbf{Y}\mathbf{M}\mathbf{b}\rangle_{\mathbf{D}} = \text{cov}(\mathbf{X}\mathbf{Q}\mathbf{a}, \mathbf{Y}\mathbf{M}\mathbf{b})$). This covariance can be decomposed as a product of three terms:

$$\text{cov}(\mathbf{X}\mathbf{Q}\mathbf{a}, \mathbf{Y}\mathbf{M}\mathbf{b}) = \text{cor}(\mathbf{X}\mathbf{Q}\mathbf{a}, \mathbf{Y}\mathbf{M}\mathbf{b}) \cdot \|\mathbf{X}\mathbf{Q}\mathbf{a}\|_{\mathbf{D}} \cdot \|\mathbf{Y}\mathbf{M}\mathbf{b}\|_{\mathbf{D}}$$

The first term ($\text{cor}(\mathbf{X}\mathbf{Q}\mathbf{a}, \mathbf{Y}\mathbf{M}\mathbf{b})$) is optimised by Canonical Correlation Analysis (Hotelling 1936). The second ($\|\mathbf{X}\mathbf{Q}\mathbf{a}\|_{\mathbf{D}}$) is maximised by the analysis of $\mathbf{X}$ that aims to identify the main structures in this data set. The last term ($\|\mathbf{Y}\mathbf{M}\mathbf{b}\|_{\mathbf{D}}$) corresponds to the simple analysis of $\mathbf{Y}$. Hence, Coinertia Analysis can be viewed as a compromise between the three analyses aiming to find linear combinations of the two data sets with maximal co-structure. Unlike Canonical Correlation Analysis, that requires more individuals than variables, Coinertia Analysis is based on covariances and thus allows to deal with tables in which the number of individuals is less than the number of variables.

In the **ade4** package, the `coinertia` function is used to compute a Coinertia Analysis. All the outputs of this function are grouped in a `dudi` object (subclass `coinertia`), and Box 8.2 recalls the corresponding output elements.

The first two arguments of the `coinertia` function are the two `dudi` objects corresponding to the analyses of the two data tables. The two other arguments, `scannf` and `nf`, have the same meaning as in the other analysis functions (see Sect. 5.2).

Box 8.2 Coinertia Analysis: dudi Output Elements
In the **ade4** package, the results of a Coinertia Analysis are stored in an object
of class dudi, subclass coinertia. This object is a list with 18 elements,
including the usual elements of any dudi. In this list, elements of particular
interest are:

- $tab: covariances between original variables ($\mathbf{Y}^\top\mathbf{DX}$)
- $eig: eigenvalues ($\mathbf{\Lambda}$)
- $l1: coefficients (loadings) for the variables of **Y** (**B**)
- $c1: coefficients (loadings) for the variables of **X** (**A**)
- $aX: projection of the axes of the analysis of **X** on coinertia axes
- $aY: projection of the axes of the analysis of **Y** on coinertia axes
- $lX: scores of individuals obtained from table **X** (**XQA**)
- $lY: scores of individuals obtained from table **Y** (**YMB**)
- $mX: normed version of scores of individuals obtained from table **X**
- $mY: normed version of scores of individuals obtained from table **Y**

Permutation test: the randtest function can be used to test the statistical
significance of the Coinertia Analysis. The criterion used in this test is the RV
coefficient between the two tables. If the simulated *p*-value given by this test is
not significant, then the Coinertia Analysis outputs should not be interpreted.

Species and environmental tables should be analysed separately and then the
coinertia function can be applied to compute the Coinertia Analysis:

```
(coia.doubs <- coinertia(pca.fish, pca.env, scannf = FALSE))


Coinertia analysis
call: coinertia(dudiX = pca.fish, dudiY = pca.env, scannf = FALSE)
class: coinertia dudi

$rank (rank)      : 11
$nf (axis saved)  : 2
$RV (RV coeff)    : 0.4506

eigenvalues: 119 13.87 0.7566 0.5278 0.2709 ...

  vector length mode      content
1 $eig    11         numeric Eigenvalues
2 $lw     11         numeric Row weights (for pca.env cols)
3 $cw     27         numeric Col weigths (for pca.fish cols)

    data.frame nrow ncol
1  $tab        11   27
2  $li         11   2
3  $l1         11   2
4  $co         27   2
5  $c1         27   2
6  $lX         30   2
7  $mX         30   2
8  $lY         30   2
9  $mY         30   2
10 $aX         2    2
11 $aY         2    2
   content
```

```
 1  Crossed Table (CT): cols(pca.env) x cols(pca.fish)
 2  CT row scores (cols of pca.env)
 3  Principal components (loadings for pca.env cols)
 4  CT col scores (cols of pca.fish)
 5  Principal axes (loadings for pca.fish cols)
 6  Row scores (rows of pca.fish)
 7  Normed row scores (rows of pca.fish)
 8  Row scores (rows of pca.env)
 9  Normed row scores (rows of pca.env)
10  Corr pca.fish axes / coinertia axes
11  Corr pca.env axes / coinertia axes
```

CT rows = cols of pca.env (11) / CT cols = cols of pca.fish (27)

The `plot` function can be used to display the main outputs of the analysis (Fig. 8.2). The barplot of eigenvalues (bottom-left) clearly indicates that two dimensions should be used to interpret the main structures of fish-environment relationships.

Coinertia Analysis computes coefficients for environmental variables (`$l1`) and fish species (`$c1`) which are represented on the two graphs at the bottom of the plot (**Y** and **X** loadings). Hence, it is possible to interpret the different axes and identify relationships between variables of both data sets. The three groups (trout, grayling and downstream) are identified and their position is linked to the geomorphological variables on the first axis and to chemical variables on the second axis. For instance, the three species of the trout group (`Satr`, `Phph` and `Neba`) are present in upstream sites (high altitude and slope, low flow, etc.) where the oxygen concentration is high and the ammonium and phosphate concentrations are low. These loadings are used to compute two sets of site scores allowing to position sites by their species composition (`$lX`) or by their environmental conditions (`$lY`). Coinertia Analysis maximises the squared covariances between these two sets of scores.

The top-right graph of the plot represents sites by normed versions of these scores (`$mX` and `$mY`). Each site corresponds to an arrow (the start corresponds to its species score and the head to its environmental score). A short arrow reveals a good agreement between the environmental conditions of a site and its species composition while a long arrow indicates a discrepancy. For instance, the long arrows for sites 1, 8, 23, 24 and 25 reveal that these sites have few species and similar composition (the start of the arrows are close and located at the opposed direction of the species arrows) but very different environmental conditions (the head of these arrows are spread out). Hence, these sites can be seen as outliers in the global model of species-environment relationships identified by Coinertia Analysis because their species composition did not correspond to their environmental conditions. Indeed, species abundance and richness in these sites are very low due to pollution (see Sect. 6.3) or to the fact that fish richness is also very low near the source of the stream.

Lastly, the two graphs on the left show the projection of the first axes of the two initial simple analyses (`pca.fish` and `pca.env`) onto the coinertia axes. These graphs provide a convenient way to look at the relationships between the main structures of each data set (identified by simple analyses) and the co-structures identified by Coinertia Analysis. For fish species data, the first two axes of the simple PCA are nearly equivalent to the coinertia axes. For environmental data, a rotation has been performed so that a coinertia axis mixes the structures of two PCA axes.

```
plot(coia.doubs)
```

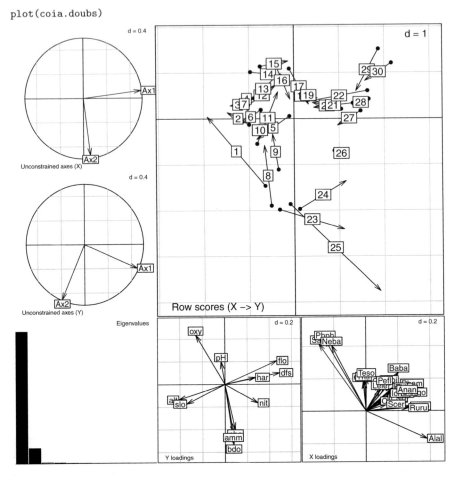

Fig. 8.2 Plot of the outputs of a Coinertia Analysis. This is a composite plot made of six graphs (see text for an explanation of the six graphs).

The summary function provides several useful results about the analysis, especially concerning the criteria maximised:

```
summary(coia.doubs)

Coinertia analysis

Class: coinertia dudi
Call: coinertia(dudiX = pca.fish, dudiY = pca.env, scannf = FALSE)

Total inertia: 134.7

Eigenvalues:
     Ax1       Ax2       Ax3       Ax4       Ax5
119.0194   13.8714    0.7566    0.5278    0.2709

Projected inertia (%):
```

```
      Ax1       Ax2      Ax3      Ax4      Ax5
 88.3570  10.2978   0.5617   0.3918   0.2011

Cumulative projected inertia (%):
     Ax1    Ax1:2    Ax1:3    Ax1:4    Ax1:5
   88.36    98.65    99.22    99.61    99.81

(Only 5 dimensions (out of 11) are shown)

Eigenvalues decomposition:
        eig   covar    sdX    sdY    corr
1  119.02  10.910  6.423  2.326  0.7302
2   13.87   3.724  2.864  1.685  0.7718

Inertia & coinertia X (pca.fish):
     inertia    max    ratio
1     41.25  42.75  0.9650
12    49.45  50.90  0.9714

Inertia & coinertia Y (pca.env):
     inertia    max    ratio
1      5.412  6.322  0.8561
12     8.251  8.553  0.9647

RV:
 0.4506
```

As for any object inheriting from the `dudi` class, the eigenvalues and percentages of (cumulative) projected inertia are returned (see Sect. 3.4). Information on the eigenvalues and their decomposition is also returned. Eigenvalues in Coinertia Analysis are squared covariances between linear combinations of species abundances ($1X) and environmental variables ($1Y). The table `Eigenvalues decomposition` returns the eigenvalues (`eig`) and their square root (`covar`). As shown in Box 8.1, the covariance is equal to the product of the correlation between $1X and $1Y (`corr`), the standard deviation of the environmental score $1Y (`sdY`) and the standard deviation of the species score $1X (`sdX`). The maximal possible values for the standard deviations are produced by the simple analyses of the initial tables (`pca.fish`, `pca.env`) that identify the main structures of each data set. The two tables `Inertia & coinertia` compare the quantity of variance captured by the Coinertia Analysis (`inertia`) to the maximum possible value provided by the simple analysis (`max`). Hence it is possible to ensure that an important proportion of the information contained in each table (structures) is preserved when looking for co-structures (`ratio`).

Lastly, the `summary` function returns the value of the RV coefficient (Box 9.6, Escoufier 1973) that measures the link between two tables. It can been seen as an extension of the bivariate squared correlation coefficient to the multivariate case. It varies between 0 (no correlation) and 1 (perfect agreement) and its significance can be tested by random permutation of the rows of both tables (function `randtest`):

```
randtest(coia.doubs)


Monte-Carlo test
Call: randtest.coinertia(xtest = coia.doubs)

Observation: 0.4506

Based on 999 replicates
Simulated p-value: 0.001
```

```
Alternative hypothesis: greater

    Std.Obs Expectation     Variance
    9.30113      0.08206     0.00157
```

In this case, the link between the composition of species assemblages and environmental conditions is highly significant.

Coinertia Analysis maximises covariances and thus can handle tables containing more variables than individuals. Its framework is very general and flexible: the `coinertia` function takes two `dudi` objects as arguments and thus can be used to link tables containing quantitative variables (`dudi.pca`), qualitative variables (`dudi.acm`), mix of both (`dudi.hillsmith`), fuzzy variables (`dudi.fca`), distance matrices (`dudi.pco`), etc. The only restriction is that rows (i.e., individuals) of the two tables are identical and that the same row weights are used in the two separate analyses. This implies to take some precautions, especially when Correspondence Analysis (CA) is used because this method is based on the computation of particular row weights (Sect. 6.2). In this case, CA row weights should be introduced in the analysis of the second table:

```
coa.fish <- dudi.coa(doubs$fish, scannf = FALSE, nf = 2)
pca.env2 <- dudi.pca(doubs$env, row.w = coa.fish$lw,
       scannf = FALSE, nf = 2)
coia.doubs2 <- coinertia(coa.fish, pca.env2, scannf = FALSE, nf = 2)
```

As CA row weights have been computed using species abundance contained in the `doubs$fish` table, the permutation procedure should keep the association between the row weights and the rows of the first table. This is achieved using the `fixed` argument of the `randtest` function, thus permuting only the rows of the second table:

```
randtest(coia.doubs2, fixed = 1)
```

```
Warning: non uniform weight. The results from permutations
are valid only if the row weights come from the fixed table.
The fixed table is table X : doubs$fish
Monte-Carlo test
Call: randtest.coinertia(xtest = coia.doubs2, fixed = 1)

Observation: 0.6363

Based on 999 replicates
Simulated p-value: 0.001
Alternative hypothesis: greater

    Std.Obs Expectation     Variance
    11.306596    0.105778   0.002202
```

8.4 Analysis on Instrumental Variables

In species-environment studies, it is often assumed that environmental conditions influence species distributions. Coinertia Analysis is based on a covariance criteria and thus does not take into account this asymmetric relationship. Methods based on instrumental variables (also known as constrained/canonical ordination) consider explicitly that a table contains response variables that must be explained by a second table of explanatory (instrumental) variables. They allow to identify the main structures of the first table that are explained by the variables in the second table. In **ade4**, this way to go is provided by the `pcaiv` function. Redundancy Analysis (RDA, Rao 1964; van den Wollenberg 1977) and Canonical Correspondence Analysis (CCA ter Braak 1986) are two particular cases of such approach.

The `pcaivortho` function performs an analysis on orthogonal instrumental variables that focuses on the structures of the response variables that are *not* explained by the instrumental variables (Rao 1964). They are equivalent to pRDA and pCCA, i.e. partial CCA and RDA. Box 8.3 gives the basic definitions of these methods in the framework of the duality diagram.

Box 8.3 Analysis on Instrumental Variables: Basic Mathematical Definitions

We consider two sets of variables measured on the same set of n individuals. The first table $\mathbf{X}$ contains p explanatory variables and the second table (response variables) is treated by a simple multivariate analysis, defining the statistical triplet $(\mathbf{Y}, \mathbf{Q}, \mathbf{D})$ where $\mathbf{Y}$ is an $n \times m$ matrix. Let $\widehat{\mathbf{Y}} = \mathbf{P_X Y}$ where $\mathbf{P_X} = \mathbf{X}(\mathbf{X^T D X})^{-1}\mathbf{X^T D}$ is the projection operator onto $\mathbf{X}$ (See Appendix A.8). The analysis on instrumental variables is defined by the triplet $(\widehat{\mathbf{Y}}, \mathbf{Q}, \mathbf{D})$ and corresponds to the following diagram:

$$
\begin{array}{ccc}
\mathbb{R}^m & \xrightarrow{\ \mathbf{Q}\ } & \mathbb{R}^{m^*} \\
{\scriptstyle \widehat{\mathbf{Y}}^T}\big\uparrow & & \big\downarrow{\scriptstyle \widehat{\mathbf{Y}}} \\
\mathbb{R}^{n^*} & \xleftarrow[\ \mathbf{D}\ ]{} & \mathbb{R}^n
\end{array}
$$

Table $\widehat{\mathbf{Y}}$ contains predicted values computed by a multivariate linear regression (weighted by $\mathbf{D}$) of $\mathbf{Y}$ on $\mathbf{X}$. This is equivalent to regress each individual column of $\mathbf{Y}$ on $\mathbf{X}$ and then stack all the fitted vectors in the matrix $\widehat{\mathbf{Y}}$. While the initial simple analysis corresponding to the triplet $(\mathbf{Y}, \mathbf{Q}, \mathbf{D})$ identifies the main structures, the analysis on instrumental variables focuses on the structures of $\mathbf{Y}$ that are explained by $\mathbf{X}$. The total inertia of this analysis is equal to:

$$I_{(\widehat{\mathbf{Y}}, \mathbf{Q}, \mathbf{D})} = \text{Trace}(\widehat{\mathbf{Y}}^T \mathbf{D} \widehat{\mathbf{Y}} \mathbf{Q})$$

The ratio $R_{\mathbf{Y}|\mathbf{X}} = I_{(\widehat{\mathbf{Y}}, \mathbf{Q}, \mathbf{D})}/I_{(\mathbf{Y}, \mathbf{Q}, \mathbf{D})}$ varies between 0 and 1 and measures the proportion of the total inertia of the initial analysis that is explained by the instrumental variables (Miller and Farr 1971; Miller 1975; Peres-Neto et al. 2006). It is thus the multivariate equivalent of the regression coefficient of determination R^2. The $R_{\mathbf{Y}|\mathbf{X}}$ statistic can be used in a randomisation testing

(continued)

> **Box 8.3** (continued)
>
> procedure to evaluate if the instrumental variables ($\mathbf{X}$) explain a significant part of the variation contained in the response table ($\mathbf{Y}$).
>
> The general properties of a duality diagram (Box 3.2) show that the principal axes maximise the quantity $\left\| \widehat{\mathbf{Y}} \mathbf{Qa} \right\|^2_{\mathbf{D}}$ and the principal components maximise $\left\| \widehat{\mathbf{Y}}^{\mathsf{T}} \mathbf{Db} \right\|^2_{\mathbf{Q}}$. These quantities can have different meanings according to the initial analysis performed on $\mathbf{Y}$ (see Boxes 8.4 and 8.6).

8.4.1 Redundancy Analysis

Redundancy Analysis (RDA) is a particular analysis on instrumental variables corresponding to the case where the table of response variables (i.e., species abundances) is treated by a PCA (see Box 8.4 for details).

> **Box 8.4 Redundancy Analysis: Basic Mathematical Definitions**
>
> The case where a centred PCA is applied on $\mathbf{Y}$ (see Box 8.3) leads to the triplet $\left(\mathbf{Y}, \mathbf{I}_m, \frac{1}{n}\mathbf{I}_n \right)$. The corresponding analysis on instrumental variable, associated to the triplet $\left(\widehat{\mathbf{Y}}, \mathbf{I}_m, \frac{1}{n}\mathbf{I}_n \right)$, is known as Principal Component Analysis on Instrumental Variables (Rao 1964, PCAIV) or Redundancy Analysis (van den Wollenberg 1977, RDA).
>
> The principal axis $\mathbf{a}$ maximises the quantity:
>
> $$\left\| \widehat{\mathbf{Y}} \mathbf{a} \right\|^2_{\frac{1}{n}\mathbf{I}_n} = \left\| \mathbf{P}_{\mathbf{X}} \mathbf{Y} \mathbf{a} \right\|^2_{\frac{1}{n}\mathbf{I}_n} = \mathrm{var}(\widehat{\mathbf{Y}}\mathbf{a})$$
>
> RDA seeks coefficients ($\mathbf{a}$) to construct a linear combination of the variables of $\mathbf{Y}$. This linear combination $\mathbf{Ya}$ maximises the variance explained by $\mathbf{X}$.
>
> On the other hand, the principal component $\mathbf{b}$ maximises:
>
> $$\left\| \frac{1}{n} \widehat{\mathbf{Y}}^{\mathsf{T}} \mathbf{b} \right\|^2_{\mathbf{I}_m} = \sum_{j=1}^{m} \mathrm{cov}^2(\mathbf{b}, \mathbf{y}_j)$$
>
> If we decompose the duality diagram, we can show that RDA finds coefficients ($\mathbf{e}$) for the explanatory variables ($\mathbf{X}$). The linear combination $\mathbf{b} = \mathbf{Xe}$ is a principal component (or constrained component, Obadia 1978) that maximises the sum of squared correlations (if $\mathbf{Y}$ is treated by a standardised PCA) or covariances (in the case of a centred PCA) with the response variables ($\mathbf{Y}$).

In practice, RDA is the PCA of a table containing the predicted values of species abundances by environmental variables.

In **ade4**, the `pcaiv` function is used to compute an RDA. All the outputs of this function are grouped in a `dudi` object (subclass `pcaiv`), and Box 8.5 recalls the corresponding outputs elements.

The `pcaiv` function takes two main arguments: an analysis of the response table (a `dudi` object) and a table of explanatory variable (an object of class `data.frame`). In **ade4**, the user must first use the `dudi.pca` function to identify the main variations in species composition and then use the `pcaiv` function to introduce environmental variables. This two-step implementation has a pedagogical aim by forcing users to interpret simple (unconstrained) structures before analysing structures explained by external variables. The outputs of the constrained and unconstrained analyses can then be compared to evaluate the role of explanatory variables.

Box 8.5 Redundancy Analysis: `dudi` Output Elements

In the **ade4** package, the results of a Redundancy Analysis are stored in an object of class `dudi`, subclass `pcaiv`. This object is a list with 17 elements, including the usual elements of any `dudi`. In this list, elements of particular interest are:

- `$tab`: predicted table ($\widehat{\mathbf{Y}}$)
- `$eig`: eigenvalues ($\mathbf{\Lambda}$)
- `$c1`: coefficients (loadings) for the variables of $\widehat{\mathbf{Y}}$ ($\mathbf{A}$)
- `$as`: projection of the axes of the initial analysis of $\mathbf{Y}$ on the instrumental variables analysis axes
- `$li`: row scores as linear combination of the explanatory variables ($\mathbf{P_X Y Q A}$)
- `$ls`: projection of the rows of $\mathbf{Y}$ on the principal axes ($\mathbf{Y Q A}$)
- `$fa`: coefficients (loadings) for the explanatory variables of $\mathbf{X}$ ($\mathbf{E}$)
- `$l1`: constrained principal component ($\mathbf{B} = \mathbf{X E}$)
- `$co`: projections of the variables of $\mathbf{Y}$ on the principal components ($(\mathbf{P_X Y})^{\top}\mathbf{D B}$)
- `$cor`: correlations between the variables of $\mathbf{X}$ and the principal components

Permutation test: the `randtest` function can be used to test the statistical significance of the RDA analysis. The criterion used in this test is the $R_{\mathbf{Y}|\mathbf{X}}$ coefficient (see Box 8.3). If the simulated p-value given by this test is not significant, then the RDA outputs should not be interpreted.

RDA is performed by applying the `pcaiv` function with the `pca.fish` object as first argument:

```
rda.doubs <- pcaiv(pca.fish, doubs$env, scannf = FALSE, nf = 2)
```

The object `rda.doubs` inherits from the class `dudi`. In `rda.doubs$tab`, the original fish table (`pca.fish$tab`) has been replaced by the abundance values predicted by environmental variables:

```
head(rda.doubs$tab[, 1])
```

```
[1] -0.7111 -0.9018 -0.1837 -0.2879 -0.3884 -0.4447
```

```
head(predict(lm(pca.fish$tab[, 1] ~ as.matrix(doubs$env))))
```

```
      1       2       3       4       5       6
-0.7111 -0.9018 -0.1837 -0.2879 -0.3884 -0.4447
```

The `plot` function displays the main outputs of the analysis (Fig. 8.3).

There are two ways to interpret RDA outputs. In the first interpretation, the analysis computes loadings for the fish species (`$c1`) which are represented on the bottom-right graph. The three groups of species are identified. These loadings are then used to compute scores (`$ls`) for the sites. These site scores are thus linear combinations of species abundances maximising the variance explained by environmental variables. Fitted values of these scores predicted by environmental variables are contained in `$li`. Sites are positioned by two sets of score: the first set is based on the species composition (`$ls`) and the second relates to the environmental conditions (`$li`). Both sets are plotted simultaneously on the top-right graph of the plot. Residuals of the global species-environment model are represented by arrows (each site is an arrow and the start corresponds to its fitted environmental score and the head to its composition). A short arrow reveals a good agreement between the species composition of a site and its prediction by environmental conditions while a long arrow indicates a discrepancy.

In the second interpretation, the analysis seeks loadings for environmental variables (`$fa`) which are represented on the top-left graph, to compute a constrained principal component (linear combination of environmental variables stored in `$l1`). In this example, the first constrained principal component is mainly defined by the distance from the source (`dfs`) that corresponds to the highest loading. The constrained principal component maximises the sum of squared covariances with the fish species. Species are thus represented by these covariances (`$co`). Correlations between the constrained principal component and environmental variables are stored in `$cor` and plotted on the middle-left graph. The first constrained principal component is mainly correlated to geomorphological variables (positively with distance from the source and flow, negatively with altitude and slope). While the first dimension is mainly built with the distance from the source, it is strongly correlated with several other environmental descriptors. This lack of agreement between loadings and correlations is due to collinearity among variables (Dormann

plot(rda.doubs)

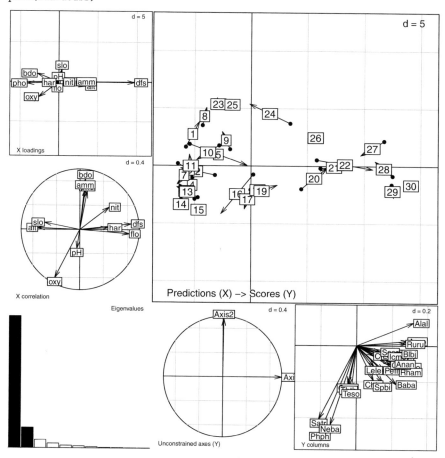

Fig. 8.3 Plot of the outputs of a Redundancy Analysis. This is a composite plot made of six graphs (see text for an explanation of the six graphs).

et al. 2013) so that one variable (distance from the source) is sufficient to explain the effect of all geomorphological variables. The use of correlations should thus be preferred to interpret the different dimensions. This sensitivity of coefficients to collinearity is a major difference between RDA and Coinertia Analysis (Dray et al. 2003).

Lastly, the middle-bottom graph shows the projection of the first axes of the initial simple analysis (pca.fish) onto the RDA axes. This graph provides a convenient way to look at the relationships between the unconstrained structures and the structures explained by environmental variables. Here, there is a perfect agreement indicating that the main patterns of variation in species composition are fully explained by the environmental descriptors included in the analysis.

The summary function provides several useful results about the analysis, especially concerning the criteria maximised:

```
summary(rda.doubs)

Principal component analysis with instrumental variables

Class: pcaiv dudi
Call: pcaiv(dudi = pca.fish, df = doubs$env, scannf = FALSE,
      nf = 2)

Total inertia: 50.26

Eigenvalues:
     Ax1       Ax2      Ax3      Ax4      Ax5
 38.4177    5.9540   2.4162   1.3387   0.7431

Projected inertia (%):
     Ax1       Ax2      Ax3      Ax4      Ax5
  76.441    11.847    4.808    2.664    1.478

Cumulative projected inertia (%):
     Ax1    Ax1:2    Ax1:3    Ax1:4    Ax1:5
   76.44    88.29    93.10    95.76    97.24

(Only 5 dimensions (out of 11) are shown)

Total unconstrained inertia (pca.fish): 66.08

Inertia of pca.fish explained by doubs$env (%): 76.06

Decomposition per axis:
    iner inercum inerC inercumC ratio    R2 lambda
1 42.75   42.7  42.59    42.6 0.996 0.902  38.42
2  8.16   50.9   7.76    50.4 0.989 0.767   5.95
```

As for any object inheriting from the dudi class, the eigenvalues and percentages of (cumulative) projected inertia are returned (see Sect. 3.4). The function returns also the total inertia (variation) of the unconstrained analysis (i.e., pca.fish) and the percentage explained by the explanatory variables. In this example, 76.06% of the variation in species composition is explained by the environment. The function randtest is based on this quantity and allows to evaluate its statistical significance by randomly permuting the rows of the explanatory table:

```
randtest(rda.doubs)

Monte-Carlo test
Call: randtest.pcaiv(xtest = rda.doubs)

Observation: 0.7606

Based on 99 replicates
Simulated p-value: 0.01
Alternative hypothesis: greater

     Std.Obs Expectation    Variance
    4.782390    0.392281    0.005931
```

Lastly, the `summary` function also returns information on the eigenvalues and their decomposition. The initial analysis (`pca.fish`) seeks linear combination of the variables with maximal variance. These variances and their cumulative sum are reported in the `iner` and `inercum` columns, respectively.

```
## iner
pca.fish$eig[1]
```

```
[1] 42.75
```

```
sum(pca.fish$li[, 1]^2 * pca.fish$lw)
```

```
[1] 42.75
```

In Redundancy Analysis, eigenvalues (`lambda`) measure amounts of variance in species composition explained by the environmental variables. Hence, each eigenvalue corresponds to the product of a variance (`inerC`) by a coefficient of determination (`R2`).

```
## lambda
rda.doubs$eig[1]
```

```
[1] 38.42
```

```
sum(rda.doubs$li[, 1]^2 * rda.doubs$lw)
```

```
[1] 38.42
```

```
## inerC
sum(rda.doubs$ls[, 1]^2 * rda.doubs$lw)
```

```
[1] 42.59
```

```
## R2
summary(lm(rda.doubs$ls[, 1] ~ as.matrix(doubs$env)))$r.squared
```

```
[1] 0.9019
```

```
summary(lm(rda.doubs$ls[, 1] ~ rda.doubs$li[, 1]))$r.squared
```

```
[1] 0.9019
```

RDA (which maximises the explained variance) can thus be seen as a PCA (which maximises the variance) with an additional constraint of prediction by the environmental variables. As RDA considers a compromise (product variance by coefficient of determination), the maximisation of the variance is not optimal and we can thus measure the effect of the environmental constraint by computing the ratio (`ratio`) between the variance obtained in RDA and the maximal value obtained in PCA.

```
## ratio
sum(rda.doubs$ls[, 1]^2 * rda.doubs$lw) / pca.fish$eig[1]
```

```
[1] 0.9965
```

8.4.2 Canonical Correspondence Analysis

Correspondence Analysis on Instrumental Variables (CAIV) corresponds to the case where the species response table is treated by Correspondence Analysis (CA). This method is known by ecologists under the name of Canonical Correspondence Analysis (CCA). CCA is probably the mostly widely used method for direct gradient analysis. In **ade4**, it is performed using the general `pcaiv` function applied on a CA `dudi` object created by the `dudi.coa` function.

Box 8.6 Canonical Correspondence Analysis: Basic Mathematical Definitions

The case where a CA is applied on $\mathbf{Y}$ leads to the triplet $(\mathbf{Z}, \mathbf{D}_m, \mathbf{D}_n)$ where $\mathbf{Z} = \mathbf{D}_n^{-1}\mathbf{P}_0\mathbf{D}_m^{-1}$ (see Box 6.2 for details). The corresponding analysis on instrumental variable is associated to the triplet $(\mathbf{P_X Z}, \mathbf{D}_m, \mathbf{D}_n)$ where $\mathbf{P_X} = \mathbf{X}(\mathbf{X}^\top\mathbf{D}_n\mathbf{X})^{-1}\mathbf{X}^\top\mathbf{D}_n$. It is known as Correspondence Analysis on Instrumental Variables (Lebreton et al. 1988a,b) or Canonical Correspondence Analysis (CCA, ter Braak 1986, 1987). As CCA is a particular analysis on instrumental variables, it can be interpreted in the general framework presented above.

In community ecology, the success of CCA is due to its close relationships with the ecological niche theory and the unimodal response model (see Box 6.1). In CCA, the principal component is a linear combination of environmental variables ($\mathbf{b} = \mathbf{X}\mathbf{e}$) that maximises:

$$\left\|(\mathbf{P_X Z})^\top\mathbf{D}_n\mathbf{b}\right\|_{\mathbf{D}_m}^2 = \mathbf{b}^\top\mathbf{D}_n\mathbf{P_X}\mathbf{Z}\mathbf{D}_m(\mathbf{P_X Z})^\top\mathbf{D}_n\mathbf{b}$$

The projector $\mathbf{P_X}$ is $\mathbf{D}_n$-symmetric (i.e., $\mathbf{D}_n\mathbf{P_X} = \mathbf{P_X}^\top\mathbf{D}_n$) and by definition, we have $\mathbf{b} = \mathbf{X}\mathbf{e}$ and $\mathbf{P_X}\mathbf{b} = \mathbf{b}$. The previous equation can thus be rewritten as:

$$\left\|(\mathbf{P_X Z})^\top\mathbf{D}_n\mathbf{b}\right\|_{\mathbf{D}_m}^2 = \mathbf{b}^\top\mathbf{D}_n\mathbf{Z}\mathbf{D}_m\mathbf{Z}^\top\mathbf{D}_n\mathbf{b} = \left\|\mathbf{Z}^\top\mathbf{D}_n\mathbf{b}\right\|_{\mathbf{D}_m}^2$$

As $\mathbf{Z} = \mathbf{D}_n^{-1}\mathbf{P}_0\mathbf{D}_m^{-1}$, we obtain:

$$\left\|(\mathbf{P_X Z})^\top\mathbf{D}_n\mathbf{b}\right\|_{\mathbf{D}_m}^2 = \left\|\mathbf{D}_m^{-1}\mathbf{P}_0^\top\mathbf{b}\right\|_{\mathbf{D}_m}^2 = \mathrm{var}_{\mathbf{D}_m}(\mathbf{D}_m^{-1}\mathbf{P}_0^\top\mathbf{b})$$

The matrix $\mathbf{D}_m^{-1}\mathbf{P}_0^\top\mathbf{b}$ contains the centred positions of species, computed by weighted averaging (see Box 6.1) on the environmental gradient ($\mathbf{b}$). Hence, CCA looks for a site score, linear combination of environmental variables ($\mathbf{b} = \mathbf{X}\mathbf{e}$) that maximises the separation (weighted variance)

(continued)

Box 8.6 (continued)

of species means. In this context, it perfectly fits the ecological theory by assuming Gaussian response curves of species and by identifying the environmental gradients that maximise the separation of niche centroids. In this viewpoint, CCA inherits from Green's Discriminant Analysis (Green 1971, 1974) and also maximises the separation of niche positions. The only difference is that CCA considers that environmental features are measured for sites while Discriminant Analysis focuses on individuals (ter Braak and Verdonschot 1995; Lebreton et al. 1988a). This equivalence is detailed in Sect. 8.4.3.2.

On the other hand, principal axis **a** maximises:

$$\|\mathbf{P_X Z D}_m \mathbf{a}\|^2_{\mathbf{D}_n} = \left\|\mathbf{P_X D}_n^{-1}\mathbf{P_0 a}\right\|^2_{\mathbf{D}_n} = \mathrm{var}_{\mathbf{D}_n}(\mathbf{P_X D}_n^{-1}\mathbf{P_0 a})$$

CCA seeks a unit-variance species score (**a**). Sites are positioned by weighted averaging ($\mathbf{D}_n^{-1}\mathbf{P_0 a}$) so that a site is at the average of the species that are present in it. This score is usually denoted WA-score in the literature and maximises the weighted-variance explained by **X**. The predictions of the WA-score by the environmental variables are given by $\mathbf{P_X D}_n^{-1}\mathbf{P_0 a}$ and usually named LC-score (LC for linear combination). Hence, CCA finds a species score to position sites by weighted averaging so that the prediction of this score by the environmental variables is maximised.

These interpretations show that two steps of weighted averaging (for species and sites) are performed in CCA. Whereas our presentation is based on the eigen decomposition, CCA can also be performed by adding a multiple regression step in the iterative reciprocal averaging algorithm (ter Braak 1986).

CCA is a particular analysis on instrumental variables, thus all interpretations of the outputs described for RDA remain valid. As it is based on CA, the principal characteristic of CCA is that it relates to weighted-averaging principle and thus provides an estimation of niche unimodal response to environmental gradient (see Boxes 6.1 and 8.6 for details). We will focus on this aspect in this chapter. As RDA, CCA is simply performed using the `pcaiv` function:

```
cca.doubs <- pcaiv(coa.fish, doubs$env, scannf = FALSE, nf = 2)
```

The `cca.doubs` object inherits from the `dudi` class (see Box 8.7). As for other two-table methods, the `plot` function displays the main outputs of the analysis. According to the niche viewpoint, CCA seeks loadings for environmental variables (`cca.doubs$fa`) that are used to compute a site score (`cca.doubs$ll`, see Fig. 8.4).

```
cca.coef <- s.arrow(cca.doubs$fa, plot = FALSE)
cca.site <- s.label(cca.doubs$ll, plot = FALSE)
ADEgS(list(cca.site, cca.coef), positions = matrix(c(0, 0.6,
       0.4, 1, 0.3, 0, 1, 0.7), byrow = TRUE, nrow = 2))
```

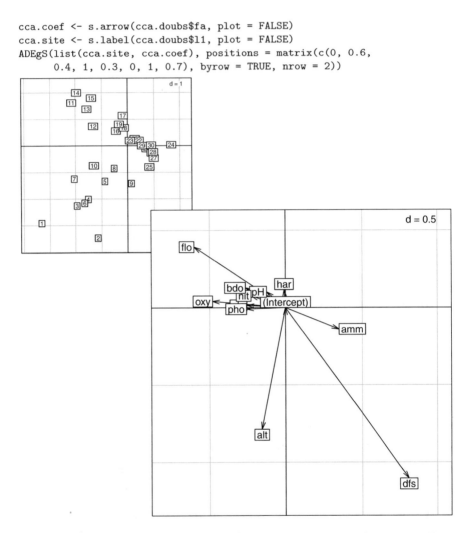

Fig. 8.4 Plot of the outputs of a Canonical Correspondence Analysis. Site scores as linear combination of environmental variables ($ll) and loadings for the environmental variables ($fa).

Box 8.7 Canonical Correspondence Analysis: dudi Output Elements
In the **ade4** package, the results of a Canonical Correspondence Analysis are stored in an object of class dudi, subclass pcaiv. This object is a list with 17 elements, including the usual elements of any dudi. In this list, elements of particular interest are:

- $eig: eigenvalues ($\Lambda$)

(continued)

Box 8.7 (continued)
- $fa: coefficients (loadings) for the explanatory variables of **X** (**E**)
- $l1: unit-variance site scores, linear combinations of environmental variables (**B** = **XE**)
- $co: species scores obtained by weighted averaging ($\mathbf{D}_m^{-1}\mathbf{P}_0^\top\mathbf{B}$)
- $c1: unit-variance species scores (**A**)
- $ls: site scores (WA) obtained by weighted averaging ($\mathbf{D}_n^{-1}\mathbf{P}_0\mathbf{A}$)
- $li: site scores (LC), linear combinations of the explanatory variables ($\mathbf{P_X}\mathbf{D}_n^{-1}\mathbf{P}_0\mathbf{A}$)

Permutation test: the randtest function can be used to test the statistical significance of the CCA. The criterion used in this test is the ratio of the inertia (sum of eigenvalues) of the constrained analysis divided by the inertia of the unconstrained analysis. If the simulated *p*-value given by this test is not significant, then the CCA outputs should not be interpreted.

Then, species score can be computed by weighted averaging. For instance, the brown trout (Satr) is present in the following sites:

```
t(doubs$fish[doubs$fish[, 2] > 0, 2, drop = FALSE])
```

```
     1 2 3 4 5 6 7 10 11 12 13 14 15 16 17 18 29
Satr 3 5 5 4 2 3 5  1  3  5  5  5  4  3  2  1  1
```

Its position on the first two CCA axes can be computed using the weighted.mean function:

```
apply(cca.doubs$l1, 2, weighted.mean, w = doubs$fish[, 2])
```

```
    RS1     RS2
-1.5269 -0.4276
```

The s.distri function can be used to position species on the sites plot (Fig. 8.5). On the plot, the species (brown trout, Satr) is positioned by weighted averaging and segments link the species to the sites where it is present.

The getstats function returns the different statistics computed to produce the plot. Here, we obtain:

```
getstats(cca.Satr)
```

```
$means
        RS1     RS2
Satr -1.527 -0.4276
```

Species scores are directly computed when the cca.doubs object is created and stored in cca.doubs$co:

```
cca.Satr <- s.distri(cca.doubs$l1, doubs$fish[, 2, drop = FALSE],
     ellipseSize = 0, plines.lty = 2, plabels.cex = 2, plot = FALSE)
superpose(cca.Satr, cca.site, plot = TRUE)
```

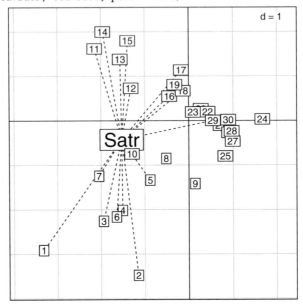

Fig. 8.5 Plot of the outputs of a Canonical Correspondence Analysis. Site scores as linear combination of environmental variables (`$l1`) and species positioned by weighted averaging (here, only the brown trout (`Satr`) is represented).

```
cca.doubs$co[2, ]

        Comp1    Comp2
Satr -1.527  -0.4276
```

Hence, a biplot can be drawn using the `superpose` function to represent simultaneously the site (`$l1`) and the species scores (`$co`) on the same plot (Fig. 8.6).

8.4.3   Related Software and Methods

Links with other methods or software are presented in this paragraph.

8.4.3.1   vegan

The **vegan** package contains the `rda` and `cca` functions and provides many additional functionalities for this type of analysis (significance tests, formula interface, conditional effects, etc.). The links between outputs from **ade4** and **vegan**

```
cca.species <- s.label(cca.doubs$co, plot = FALSE)
superpose(update(cca.site, plabels.cex = 0, plot = FALSE), cca.species,
    plot = TRUE)
```

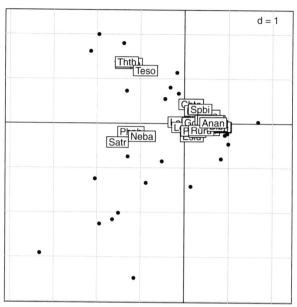

Fig. 8.6 Plot of the outputs of a canonical correspondence analysis. Simultaneous representation of site and species scores.

Table 8.1 Canonical Correspondence Analysis: equivalency between objects created by the **ade4** and **vegan** packages. In **vegan**, the scores for sites and species can be obtained with the scores.cca function.

	ade4	vegan
Eigenvalues	$eig	CCAeig
Site scores (LC)	$li	
Unit-variance site scores	$l1	CCAu
Site scores (WA)	$ls	CCAwa
Unit-variance species scores	$c1	CCAv
Species scores	$co	
Species weights	$cw	$colsum
Site weights	$lw	$rowsum
Correlation with environmental variables	$cor	CCAbiplot

packages are summarised in Table 8.1 in the case of Canonical Correspondence Analysis. The same equivalences exist in the case of Redundancy Analysis but some discrepancies are observed because **vegan** uses unbiased estimates for the variance (i.e., divided by $n - 1$) while **ade4** divides by n to preserve some properties in the geometric viewpoint.

8.4.3.2 Discriminant Analysis

Canonical Correspondence Analysis shares many similarities with Green's Discriminant Analysis (Green 1971, 1974). It can be demonstrated that both methods are identical except in the statistical objects considered in the analysis: they are the sites in CCA and the individuals in Discriminant Analysis. This equivalence between both approaches can be illustrated using **ade4** functionalities. Each non-null cell of the doubs$fish table is associated to a given species, a given site and is characterised by a number of individuals:

```
idx <- which(doubs$fish > 0, arr.ind = TRUE)
nind <- doubs$fish[doubs$fish > 0]
```

It is then possible to inflate the data by duplicating the rows of the original environmental table doubs$env so that each row corresponds to an individual. A vector with the species names is also created to indicate the species identity of each individual:

```
env.ind <- doubs$env[rep(idx[, 1], nind), ]
species.ind <- names(doubs$fish)[rep(idx[, 2], nind)]
sum(doubs$fish)
```

```
[1] 1004
```

```
nrow(env.ind)
```

```
[1] 1004
```

```
length(species.ind)
```

```
[1] 1004
```

Discriminant Analysis is then performed on the inflated tables. The aim of the analysis is to find a linear combination of environmental variables that maximises the separation of species identities.

```
pca.ind <- dudi.pca(env.ind, scannf = FALSE, nf = 2)
dis.ind <- discrimin(pca.ind, factor(species.ind),
    scannf = FALSE, nf = 2)
```

This Discriminant Analysis is equivalent to CCA:

```
dis.ind$eig
```

```
[1] 0.534524 0.121839 0.068703 0.049168 0.027090 0.012941
[7] 0.009867 0.005425 0.003534 0.002166 0.001612
```

```
cca.doubs$eig
```

```
[1] 0.534524 0.121839 0.068703 0.049168 0.027090 0.012941
[7] 0.009867 0.005425 0.003534 0.002166 0.001612
```

In practice, this viewpoint has been developed for the analysis of herbarium data where environmental information is gathered for individuals and not for sites (Gimaret-Carpentier et al. 2003; Pélissier et al. 2003a).

8.4.3.3   Between- and Within-Class Analyses

Between- and Within-Class Analyses are presented in Chap. 7. These methods can
be seen as particular cases of (orthogonal) analysis on instrumental variables where
only one explanatory categorical variable is considered:

```
data(meau)
envpca <- dudi.pca(meau$env, scannf = FALSE, nf = 3)
class(meau$design$season)
```

```
[1] "factor"
```

Analyses performed by the `bca` (respectively `wca`) and `pcaiv` (respectively
`pcaivortho`) functions are similar but the former produce additional outputs
adapted to the analysis of a partition of individuals into groups.

The `bca` function is equivalent to the `pcaiv` when only one categorical variable
is used as explanatory:

```
envbca <- bca(envpca, meau$design$season, scannf = FALSE)
envpcaiv <- pcaiv(envpca, data.frame(meau$design$season),
    scannf = FALSE)
envbca$eig
```

```
[1] 1.5551 1.0390 0.5918
```

```
envpcaiv$eig
```

```
[1] 1.5551 1.0390 0.5918
```

We have the same link between `wca` and `pcaivortho`:

```
envwca <- wca(envpca, meau$design$season, scannf = FALSE)
envpcaivortho <- pcaivortho(envpca, data.frame(meau$design$season),
    scannf = FALSE)
envwca$eig
```

```
[1] 4.650543 0.870064 0.556517 0.390037 0.205465 0.065492
[7] 0.031483 0.022419 0.012484 0.009637
```

```
envpcaivortho$eig
```

```
[1] 4.650543 0.870064 0.556517 0.390037 0.205465 0.065492
[7] 0.031483 0.022419 0.012484 0.009637
```

These outputs are also equivalent to the results obtained with the `rda` function
of the **vegan** package:

```
library(vegan)
n <- nrow(envpca$tab)
eigenvals(rda(envpca$tab ~ meau$design$season),
    "constrained")[1:3]
```

```
 RDA1   RDA2   RDA3
1.6227 1.0841 0.6175
```

```
envpcaiv$eig[1:3] * n/(n - 1)
```

```
[1]  1.6227  1.0841  0.6175
```

```
eigenvals(rda(envpca$tab ~ Condition(meau$design$season)),
        "unconstrained")[1:5]
```

```
   PC1     PC2     PC3     PC4     PC5
4.8527  0.9079  0.5807  0.4070  0.2144
```

```
envpcaivortho$eig[1:5] * n/(n - 1)
```

```
[1]  4.8527  0.9079  0.5807  0.4070  0.2144
```

Chapter 9
Analysing Changes in Structures

Abstract This chapter is a short introduction to the K-table family of methods. We first present some examples of ecological K-table, the structure of the `ktab` object used in the **ade4** package to store a K-table, and the functions that allow to build and manage them. We briefly present three types of methods: STATIS, Multiple Factor Analysis and Multiple Coinertia Analysis. We explain the differences between these three groups of methods, with several examples of use.

9.1 Introduction

When the set of samples (rows of a data table) is split into groups, we have seen in Chap. 7 that several data analysis methods can take into account these groups and model their differences (Between-Class Analysis) or remove these differences (Within-Class Analysis). Another approach consists in considering that the groups correspond to separate tables, with successive tables stacked vertically (Fig. 9.1B). This leads to what is called the K-table structure.

The set of columns (environmental variables or species) can also be split into groups, and this also leads to a K-table structure. One can imagine that, in this case, tables are stacked horizontally (Fig. 9.1A).

The aim of analysing a set of tables instead of just one table is to find out what makes these tables different, or conversely, to find common points among all the tables. Are all the tables structured in the same way? Is the samples typology and the variables/species typology the same across all the tables, or are there some changes from one table to another? These questions are particularly interesting when the series of tables is a time series, with each table corresponding to one date (Fig. 9.1C). But the series of tables can also correspond to other criteria, like taxonomic groups for species, or geographical regions for samples.

© Springer Science+Business Media, LLC, part of Springer Nature 2018
J. Thioulouse et al., *Multivariate Analysis of Ecological Data with ade4*,
https://doi.org/10.1007/978-1-4939-8850-1_9

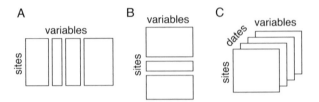

Fig. 9.1 Structures of data of K-table. A: Several sets of variables measured on the same sites. B: A set of variables measured for different groups of sites. C: An example of a data cube with the measurements of the same variables for the same sites repeated at different dates.

9.2 *K*-table Management in ade4

9.2.1 *K-table Examples*

Here are a few examples of K-table data sets taken from **ade4** that correspond to the different cases presented in Fig. 9.1. The friday87 data set (Friday 1987) contains one table (friday87$fau) with 91 macro-invertebrate species sampled in 16 ponds. The 91 species are grouped in 10 taxonomic groups: Hemiptera, Odonata, Trichoptera, Ephemeroptera, Coleoptera, Diptera, Hydracarina, Malacostraca, Mollusca, Oligochaeta. These species data can be considered as a K-table with 10 tables (one for each taxonomic group), each table having 16 rows and a number of columns equal to the number of species in each group (11, 7, 13, 4, 13, 22, 4, 3, 8, 6, respectively). This data set corresponds to the case presented in Fig. 9.1A.

```
data(friday87)
dim(friday87$fau)
```

```
[1] 16 91
```

```
friday87$fau.blo
```

```
    Hemiptera        Odonata   Trichoptera Ephemeroptera
           11              7            13             4
   Coleoptera        Diptera   Hydracarina  Malacostraca
           13             22             4             3
     Mollusca    Oligochaeta
            8              6
```

The second example belongs to the field of hydrobiology. In **ade4**, the data set is called jv73, and it comes from the PhD thesis of J. Verneaux (Verneaux 1973). It is a list with six components. The physico-chemistry table (jv73$phychi) has 92 rows (92 sites located along 12 rivers) and 12 variables. A factor (jv73$fac.riv) gives the name of the stream on which each site is located. This data set corresponds to the case presented in Fig. 9.1B.

```
data(jv73)
names(jv73)
```

```
[1]  "morpho"   "phychi"   "poi"      "xy"        "contour"
[6]  "fac.riv"  "Spatial"
```

```
dim(jv73$phychi)
```

```
[1]  92 12
```

```
table(jv73$fac.riv)
```

Allaine	Audeux	Clauge	Cuisance	Cusancin	Dessoubre
8	5	6	8	4	5
Doubs	Doulonnes	Drugeon	Furieuse	Lison	Loue
16	3	6	9	5	17

The third example comes from a paper by Blondel and Farré (1988) about the influence of vegetation successions on bird communities composition in European forests. The `bf88` data set in the **ade4** package contains the number of birds of 79 species observed in four regions (Burgundy, Provence, Corsica, Poland) along a gradient of six stages of vegetation succession (from 1: "open, bushy growth less than 1 m" to 6: "closed, forest with trees higher than 20 m"). Data are arranged in a list of six data frames, corresponding to the six ecological stages, each data frame having 79 rows (bird species) and four columns (the four regions). This data set corresponds to a data cube as presented in Fig. 9.1C with vegetation stages instead of dates.

```
data(bf88)
names(bf88)
```

```
[1]  "S1" "S2" "S3" "S4" "S5" "S6"
```

```
dim(bf88$S1)
```

```
[1]  79   4
```

9.2.2   Building and Using a K-table

In **ade4**, a *K*-table is stored in an object of class `ktab`. A `ktab` object is a list of data frames that share the same row names (Fig. 9.2) and the following seven additional components:

- `lw`: row weights, common to all the tables (vector)
- `cw`: column weights (vector)
- `blo`: number of columns of each table (vector)
- `TL`: index for rows (data frame: table number, row number)

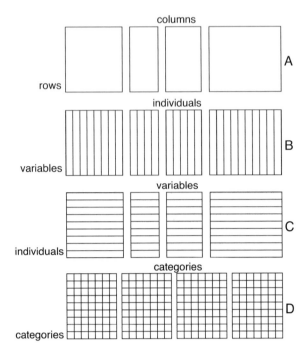

Fig. 9.2 Organisation of a K-table in **ade4**. All the tables of a ktab must have the same rows (they must share the same row names and row weights), but their columns may be different (A). This is an arbitrary choice and it does not mean that only tables with the same individuals and different variables can be used. Indeed, tables having the same variables but different individuals can be transposed to fit in this scheme (B). while tables having the same individuals and different variables can be used 'as is' (C). Of course data cubes with the same rows and the same columns (e.g., three-way contingency tables) can also fit (D). Note that tables that do not have at least one dimension (rows or columns) in common cannot be analysed in the framework of K-table methods.

- TC: index for columns (data frame: table number, column number)
- T4: index for 4 elements of an array (data frame: table number, 1:4), mainly for internal use
- call: function call

The tables must share the same row names and row weights. This means that one can consider the tables of a ktab as stacked horizontally. If the common dimension of the tables is the columns (tables stacked vertically), they must be transposed to have their common dimension as rows.

There are five functions to build a ktab. They differ by the type of objects from which they start:

- ktab.list.df: a list of data frames with the same rows. This function is adapted for cases A and C of Fig. 9.1. It can be used for case B if data frames are firstly transposed.
- ktab.list.dudi: a list of dudi objects with the same rows. This function is adapted for cases A and C of Fig. 9.1. It can be used for case B if dudi objects are firstly transposed.
- ktab.within: an object created by a wca analysis (see Chap. 7.4). This function is adapted for cases A and C of Fig. 9.1.
- ktab.data.frame: a data frame that should be split by columns and a vector indicating the number of columns in each table. This function is adapted for cases B and C of Fig. 9.1. It can be used for case A if the data frame is firstly transposed.
- ktab.match2ktabs: a pair of ktab objects (see Chap. 10) with the same structure.

Note that the transformation of the data table (e.g., centring and standardisation) must be performed during the creation step of the ktab object and that row and column weights must also be set at this stage. Some functions (ktab.list.df, ktab.data.frame) allow to introduce any arbitrary data transformation and row or column weights, while others (ktab.list.dudi, ktab.within, ktab.match2ktabs) use the data transformation and row and column weights of a previous analysis of the data set. In the example presented in Fig. 9.3, the scalewt function is used to standardise the data table and the ktab.list.df function creates a standardised PCA ktab object, with the default uniform row and column weights. In Fig. 9.4, the ktab.within function uses the dudi object created by the withinpca function to perform a "Bouroche transformation" where the ktab object can be partially standardised (standardisation of each table separately) or totally standardised (centring of each table separately and global standardisation).

Several other functions can then be used to manage ktab objects:

- c: concatenates several ktab objects sharing the same rows
- []: selects tables, rows and/or columns in a ktab
- is.ktab: tests if its argument is a ktab
- t: transposes all the tables of a ktab (tables must have the same column names and weights)
- row.names: returns or modifies the vector of row names shared by all the tables
- col.names: returns or modifies the vector of column names
- tab.names: returns or modifies the vector of table names
- ktab.util.names: automatically builds unique row, column and tab names

```
kp1 <- kplot(sep1, posieig = "none", psub.cex = 0, plot = FALSE)
tr1 <- s.traject(sep1$Li, facets = sep1$TL[, 1], plabels.cex = 0,
      col = "red", psub.cex = 2, plot = FALSE)
s1 <- superpose(kp1, tr1)
plot(s1)
```

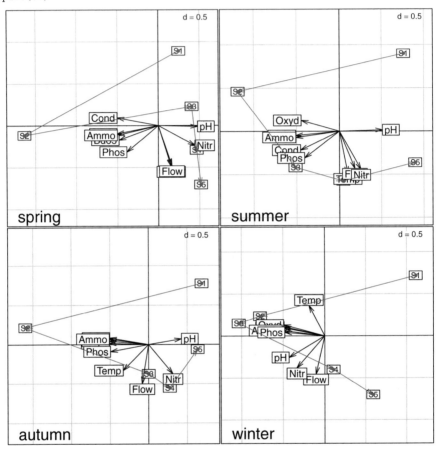

Fig. 9.3 Plot of the four separate PCA (one for each season) of the meaudret data set. Physico-chemical variables are represented by their labels with arrows from the origin, and the five sites (S1 to S5) are linked by upstream-downstream red arrows.

9.2.3 Separate Analyses of a K-table

The simplest way to use a ktab is to do the separate analysis of each table. This can be done automatically for all the tables of a ktab using the sepan function. The exact analysis that is performed depends on the data transformation and on the row and column weights. For example, if a table of quantitative variables is centred and standardised with uniform row and column weights, then the separate analyses are standardised PCAs.

```
wit1 <- withinpca(meaudret$env, meaudret$design$season,
    scannf = FALSE, scaling = "partial")
kta1 <- ktab.within(wit1,
    colnames = rep(c("S1", "S2", "S3", "S4", "S5"), 4))
pta1 <- pta(t(kta1), scannf = FALSE)
```

```
plot(pta1)
```

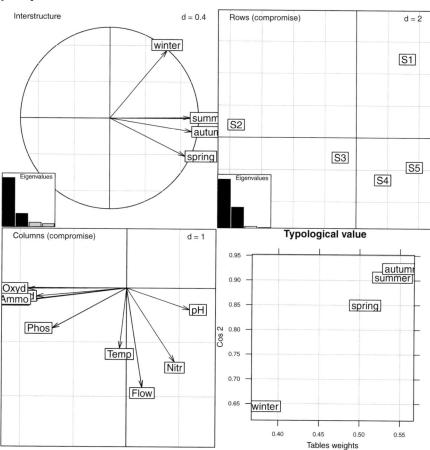

Fig. 9.4 Plot of the PTA of the meaudret data set (Interstructure and Compromise steps).

As an example, we can use again the meaudret data set (Pegaz-Maucet 1980) that we have already seen in Chaps. 2 and 3. We compute the PCA of environmental variables measured in the five sampling sites, but separately for each season. The table of environmental variables meaudret$env is first centred and standardised for each season, using the by and scalewt functions and the meaudret$design$season factor. The by function returns a list of matrices that must be turned into data frames before they can be used in the `ktab.list.df` function. The `ktab` object `ktam` is built and the `sepan` function is used to perform a PCA on each table. The `kplot` function can then be used to plot the four separate biplots (Fig. 9.3).

```
data(meaudret)
env <- by(meaudret$env, meaudret$design$season, scalewt)
ktam <- ktab.list.df(lapply(env, as.data.frame),
      rownames = paste("S", 1:5, sep = ""))
sep1 <- sepan(ktam)
```

We can see that the same structure is reproduced during each season, with the first principal component representing a pollution gradient (highly polluted sites on the left) and the second one showing the upstream-downstream morphological gradient (Flow, Temperature).

The problem with Fig. 9.3 is that each analysis has been computed independently from the three others. This means that they are not at the same scale, they cannot be superimposed or even compared. Indeed nothing guarantees that one axis in one figure will correspond to the same structure in another figure. Axes can be inverted, or even be completely different.

We need a way to have these four figures at the same scale and in the same space and this is the objective of K-table methods.

9.3   Strategies of K-table Methods

According to the structure of the K-table and the type of data, different methods can be used:

- **Partial Triadic Analysis** is restricted to data cubes where all tables have the same individuals and variables
- **Foucart COA** is restricted to three-way contingency tables (i.e., data cubes with counts where rows and columns correspond to categories)
- **STATIS on operators** allows to deal with K-tables with at least the same individuals (STATIS on WD) or at least the same variables (STATIS on VQ)
- **Multiple Factor Analysis** is restricted to K-tables with at least the same individuals
- **Multiple Coinertia Analysis** is originally restricted to K-tables with at least the same individuals but can be applied on K-tables with at least the same variables if they have been firstly transposed.

The first two methods are also named "STATIS on tables". Both "STATIS on tables" and "STATIS on operators" methods share many similarities. All these methods can be decomposed in three steps, called the Interstructure, the Compromise and the Intrastructure (Lavit 1988; Lavit et al. 1994). The Interstructure uses the RV coefficients to compute a matrix of scalar products between the tables that measures their relationships. When all the tables have both the same rows and columns, STATIS, and the associated computation of the RV coefficient, is performed directly on tables (see Box 9.1). Two analyses have been developed in this case: Partial

Triadic Analysis (PTA, Thioulouse and Chessel 1987) and Foucart Correspondence Analysis (Foucart 1978; Pavoine et al. 2007).

When the tables have only one common dimension (rows or columns), the analysis, including the computation of RV coefficients, is performed on Escoufier operators (Escoufier 1973). In this framework, the RV coefficient (see Box 9.6) is a multivariate generalisation of the squared correlation coefficient that allows to measure the link between two tables with only one common dimension (rows or columns). It is used, for example, in Coinertia Analysis (see Box 8.1). The case where the rows (sites or samples) are common to all the tables is called STATIS-WD, while the case where the columns (variables or species) are in common is called STATIS-VQ.

Then, the Compromise is computed as a combination of the K tables, and the Intrastructure projects the elements (rows and columns) of each table onto the analysis of the Compromise. This approach gave rise to many generalisations (see, for example, Abdi et al. 2012).

Box 9.1 The RV Coefficient on Tables

Let $\mathbf{X}_k$ and $\mathbf{X}_\ell$ be two tables with the same n rows and the same p columns.

Let $(\mathbf{X}_k, \mathbf{Q}, \mathbf{D})$ and $(\mathbf{X}_\ell, \mathbf{Q}, \mathbf{D})$ be the two associated statistical triplets. The inner-product between the tables is defined by:

$$\mathrm{Covv}(\mathbf{X}_k, \mathbf{X}_\ell) = \mathrm{Trace}(\mathbf{X}_k^\top \mathbf{D} \mathbf{X}_\ell \mathbf{Q}) = \mathrm{Trace}(\mathbf{X}_\ell^\top \mathbf{D} \mathbf{X}_k \mathbf{Q})$$

The vectorial variance $\mathrm{Vav}(\mathbf{X}_k)$ is equal to:

$$\mathrm{Covv}(\mathbf{X}_k, \mathbf{X}_k) = \mathrm{Trace}(\mathbf{X}_k^\top \mathbf{D} \mathbf{X}_k \mathbf{Q})$$

The vectorial correlation coefficient, or RV coefficient (Rv) is:

$$Rv(\mathbf{X}_k, \mathbf{X}_\ell) = \frac{\mathrm{Covv}(\mathbf{X}_k, \mathbf{X}_\ell)}{\sqrt{\mathrm{Vav}(\mathbf{X}_k)}\sqrt{\mathrm{Vav}(\mathbf{X}_\ell)}}$$

Remark: If the K-table contains only quantitative standardised variables, $\mathrm{Covv}(\mathbf{X}_k, \mathbf{X}_\ell) = \sum_{i=1}^{p} \mathrm{cor}(\mathbf{X}_k^i, \mathbf{X}_\ell^i)$ and $\mathrm{Vav}(\mathbf{X}_k) = p$.

In this case, the RV coefficient (Rv) is the average of the correlations between all the pairs of variables:

$$Rv(\mathbf{X}_k, \mathbf{X}_\ell) = \frac{1}{p} \sum_{i=1}^{p} \mathrm{cor}(\mathbf{X}_k^i, \mathbf{X}_\ell^i)$$

where $\mathbf{X}_k^i$ ($\mathbf{X}_\ell^i$ respectively) are the column vector associated to the i-th variable of the k-th table (ℓ table, respectively).

9.4 Partial Triadic Analysis

The theoretical background of Triadic Analysis was established in the PhD thesis of
Jaffrenou (1978). He showed that it was in fact equivalent to Tucker's Three-Mode
Factor Analysis (Tucker 1966). An application of a particular case (called "Partial
Triadic Analysis") to ecological situations was published by Thioulouse and Chessel
(1987). The extension to the complete case ("Complete Triadic Analysis") was
then explained by Kroonenberg (1989), in the framework of Three-mode Principal
Component Analysis (Kroonenberg 1983).

The main characteristic of PTA is its simplicity: computations can be done with
a simple PCA software, and interpretations are usually easy. One drawback is the
constraint on the number of samples and variables that have to be the same for all
the tables. Several recent examples of application can be found in hydrobiology
(Rolland et al. 2009; Bertrand and Maumy 2010; Mendes et al. 2010; Slimani et al.
2017). Basic definitions are recalled in Box 9.2.

Box 9.2 PTA: Basic Mathematical Definitions

Let $\mathbf{X}_1, \ldots, \mathbf{X}_k, \ldots, \mathbf{X}_K$ be K tables of quantitative variables with the same n
rows (samples) and the same p columns (variables). Let $(\mathbf{X}_1, \mathbf{Q}, \mathbf{D}), \ldots, (\mathbf{X}_k,$
$\mathbf{Q}, \mathbf{D}), \ldots, (\mathbf{X}_K, \mathbf{Q}, \mathbf{D})$ be the K associated statistical triplets.

Partial Triadic Analysis is decomposed in three steps.

Step 1: the Interstructure

For each couple of tables $(\mathbf{X}_k, \mathbf{X}_\ell)$, we can compute the RV coefficient (see
Box 9.1) and put it in the $\mathbf{Rv}$ matrix:

$$\mathbf{Rv} = \begin{pmatrix} Rv(\mathbf{X}_1, \mathbf{X}_1) & \ldots & Rv(\mathbf{X}_1, \mathbf{X}_k) & \ldots & Rv(\mathbf{X}_1, \mathbf{X}_K) \\ \vdots & \ddots & \vdots & \ddots & \vdots \\ Rv(\mathbf{X}_k, \mathbf{X}_1) & \ldots & Rv(\mathbf{X}_k, \mathbf{X}_k) & \ldots & Rv(\mathbf{X}_k, \mathbf{X}_K) \\ \vdots & \ddots & \vdots & \ddots & \vdots \\ Rv(\mathbf{X}_K, \mathbf{X}_1) & \ldots & Rv(\mathbf{X}_K, \mathbf{X}_k) & \ldots & Rv(\mathbf{X}_K, \mathbf{X}_K) \end{pmatrix}$$

The eigenvalues $\mathbf{\Lambda}_B$ and the normed eigenvectors $\mathbf{U}_B$ of the $\mathbf{Rv}$ matrix
are used to compute a score of the tables $\mathbf{S} = \mathbf{U}_B \mathbf{\Lambda}_B^{\frac{1}{2}}$, where the letter
B (Between) refers to the interstructure. These scores can be plotted in a
correlation circle.

Step 2: the Compromise

Let $\mathbf{u}_B^{\top} = (\alpha_1 \ldots \alpha_k \ldots \alpha_K)$ be the first eigenvector of the Interstructure
analysis with $\sum_{k=1}^{K} \alpha_k^2 = 1$. The α_k are used to define the K-table weighting.
The Compromise table is therefore built as a combination of the K tables:

(continued)

Box 9.2 (continued)

$$\mathbf{X} = \sum_{k=1}^{K} \alpha_k \mathbf{X}_k$$

The analysis of the Compromise is the analysis of the triplet $(\mathbf{X}, \mathbf{Q}, \mathbf{D})$ in the sense of a duality diagram (maximisation of the projected inertia, see Boxes 3.1 and 5.1).

The row scores $(\mathbf{L})$ projection of the rows of $\mathbf{X}$ onto the principal axes $(\mathbf{A})$ and the column scores $(\mathbf{C})$ projection of the columns of $\mathbf{X}$ onto the principal components $(\mathbf{B})$ are given by $\mathbf{L} = \mathbf{XQA}$ and $\mathbf{C} = \mathbf{X}^\top\mathbf{DB}$.

An RV coefficient can be calculated between the Compromise table $\mathbf{X}$ and each table $\mathbf{X}_k$: $Rv(\mathbf{X}, \mathbf{X}_k)$. It represents the squared cosine and defines the link between the Compromise and each table.

Step 3: the Intrastructure
Let $\mathbf{\Lambda}$ be the eigenvalues and $\mathbf{A}$ the eigenvectors of the Compromise study $(\mathbf{X}, \mathbf{Q}, \mathbf{D})$. The rows of each table are projected onto the principal axes: $\mathbf{R}_k = \mathbf{X}_k\mathbf{QA}$, and the columns of each table are projected onto the principal components: $\mathbf{C}_k = \mathbf{X}_k^\top\mathbf{DB}$.

Let $\mathbf{A}_k$ be the principal axes ($\mathbf{B}_k$ the principal components) of the separate analysis of the k-th table. These principal axes (principal components) can be projected onto the principal axes $\mathbf{A}$ (principal components $\mathbf{B}$) of the Compromise study: $\mathbf{A}_k^\top\mathbf{QA}$ ($\mathbf{B}_k^\top\mathbf{DB}$).

In the **ade4** package, a PTA can be computed using the `pta` function. All the outputs are grouped in a `dudi` object (subclass `pta`), and Box 9.3 recalls the corresponding output elements.

Box 9.3 PTA: `dudi` Output Elements
In the **ade4** package, the results of a PTA are stored in an object of class `dudi`, subclass `pta`. This object is a list with 25 elements, including the usual elements of any `dudi`. In this list, elements of particular interest are:

Step 1: the Interstructure

- `$RV`: matrix of RV coefficients $(\mathbf{RV})$
- `$RV.eig`: eigenvalues of RV $(\mathbf{\Lambda}_B)$
- `$RV.coo`: scores of tables $(\mathbf{S})$
- `$tab.names`: names of tables

(continued)

Box 9.3 (continued)
Step 2: the Compromise

- $tabw: weights of tables ($\mathbf{u}_B$)
- $cw: column weights (**Q**)
- $lw: row weights (**D**)
- $eig: eigenvalues ($\mathbf{\Lambda}$)
- $cos2: squared cosines between Compromise and tables ($Rv(\mathbf{X}, \mathbf{X}_k)$)
- $tab: Compromise table (**X**)
- $li: row coordinates (**L**)
- $l1: principal components (**B**)
- $co: column coordinates (**C**)
- $c1: principal axes (**A**)

Step 3: the Intrastructure

- $Tli: row coordinates ($\mathbf{R}_k$ stacked vertically)
- $Tco: column coordinates ($\mathbf{C}_k$ stacked vertically)
- $Tcomp: projection of separate principal components ($\mathbf{B}_k^\top\mathbf{DB}$ stacked vertically)
- $Tax: projection of separate principal axes ($\mathbf{A}_k^\top\mathbf{QA}$ stacked vertically)

The results on the `meaudret` data set are shown in Fig. 9.4. The first step uses the `withinpca` function to compute a within-class PCA, with the Bouroche "Partial" standardisation (Bouroche 1975). This means that, after a global centring and standardisation, variables are standardised separately within each table. Variables have therefore a null mean and unit variance in each table. The `ktab` object `kta1` is then built with the `ktab.within` function and the same column names are given to the four tables. The `ktab` is then transposed to have variables in columns, and the PTA is computed with the `pta` function:

```
wit1 <- withinpca(meaudret$env, meaudret$design$season,
      scannf = FALSE, scaling = "partial")
kta1 <- ktab.within(wit1,
      colnames = rep(c("S1", "S2", "S3", "S4", "S5"), 4))
pta1 <- pta(t(kta1), scannf = FALSE)
```

The `plot` function draws Fig. 9.4. The Interstructure graph (top-left) shows that the winter table structure is different from the structure of the three other seasons. The two graphs of the Compromise (Rows = sites plot and Columns = variables plot) show the pollution gradient on the first axis and the upstream-downstream morphology gradient on the second. The `Typological value` graph (bottom-right) gives the importance of each table in the Compromise and shows that winter contributes less than the other seasons to the Compromise structure.

The `kplot` function can then be used to draw the Intrastructure graphs (Fig. 9.5). This figure displays the projection of the rows and columns of the four tables and

```
kplot(pta1)
```

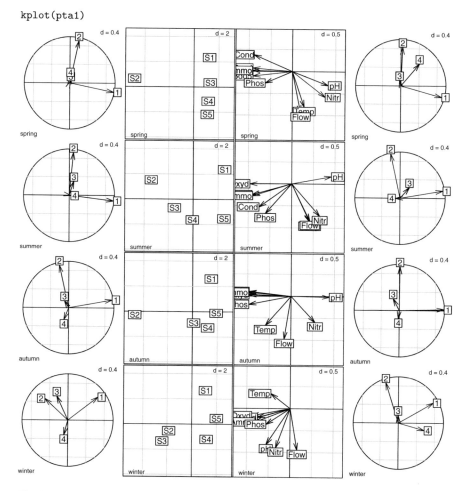

Fig. 9.5 Plot of the PTA of the `meaudret` data set (Intrastructure step). The first column of graphs shows the projection of the principal axes of the PCA of each table into the PTA. The second column shows the factor map of sites. The third column shows the factor map of physico-chemical variables. The fourth column shows the projection of the principal components of the PCA of each table into the PTA.

of the principal axes and components of the four PCA. It shows how the structure of each table (or its principal axes) differs from the structures of the others but interpretation is easier in Fig. 9.6.

Figure 9.6 is the same type of display as Fig. 9.3 (one graph for each season), but it uses the coordinates of the Intrastructure step of the PTA. Compared to Fig. 9.3, the graphs of four seasons are now at the same scale and can be superimposed and compared. All the points are in the same space, so the two axes have the same meaning in all the graphs. In the present case, the interpretation is not changed,

```
ar1 <- s.arrow(pta1$Tco * 3, facets = pta1$TC[, 1], psub.cex = 2,
    labels = pta1$TC[, 2], plot = FALSE)
tr1 <- s.traject(pta1$Tli, facets = pta1$TL[, 1], plabels.cex = 0,
    psub.cex = 0, col = "red", plot = FALSE)
la1 <- s.label(pta1$Tli, facets = pta1$TL[, 1], psub.cex = 0,
    labels = pta1$TL[, 2], plot = FALSE)
s1 <- superpose(tr1, la1)
s2 <- superpose(s1, ar1)
plot(s2)
```

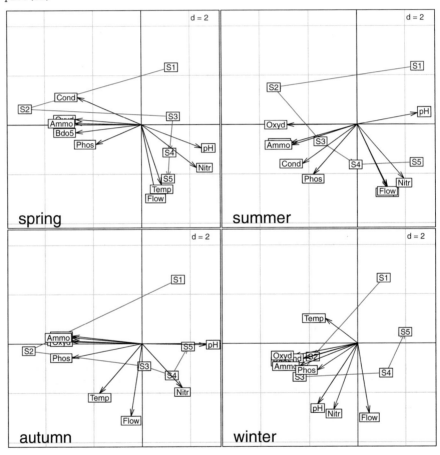

Fig. 9.6 Plot of the PTA of the `meaudret` data set (Intrastructure step) split by season.

because the structures are very strong and the four separate PCA had already given the same picture. But in the case where structures are weaker, or when they are more different across tables, using a K-table approach could help get a better idea of the global structure, and how it is distorted in each table.

9.5 Foucart COA

The aim of Foucart COA is to coordinate the Correspondence Analyses of a series of contingency tables crossing the same two variables (Pavoine et al. 2007). Because of the properties of contingency tables, Foucart COA is even simpler than PTA, both from a theoretical point of view and for the implementation in **ade4**. Indeed, the Compromise table is simply the mean of the frequencies of all the contingency tables, and the `foucart` function in **ade4** simply takes a list of data frames as argument instead of a `ktab`. Basic mathematical definitions are recalled in Box 9.4.

Box 9.4 Foucart Analysis: Basic Mathematical Definitions
Let $\mathbf{X}_1, \ldots, \mathbf{X}_k, \ldots, \mathbf{X}_K$ be K contingency tables with the same I rows and J columns: $\mathbf{X}_k = \left[n_{ij}^k \right]$. Let $(\mathbf{X}_1, \mathbf{D}_J^1, \mathbf{D}_I^1), \ldots, (\mathbf{X}_k, \mathbf{D}_J^k, \mathbf{D}_I^k), \ldots, (\mathbf{X}_K, \mathbf{D}_J^K, \mathbf{D}_I^K)$ be the K associated statistical triplets.

The Foucart Analysis is decomposed in two steps: the Common Structure and the Intrastructure.

Step 1: the Common Structure
Let $\mathbf{P}_k = \left[\frac{n_{ij}^k}{n_{\bullet\bullet}^k} \right]$ be the frequency table associated to the k-th contingency table $\mathbf{X}_k$ where $n_{\bullet\bullet}^k$ is the grand total.

The Common table $\mathbf{P}$ is therefore built as an average contingency table:

$$\mathbf{P} = \frac{1}{K} \sum_{k=1}^{K} \mathbf{P}_k = \left[\frac{1}{K} \sum_{k=1}^{K} \frac{n_{ij}^k}{n_{\bullet\bullet}^k} \right]$$

As for a classical contingency table, we can compute the row and column sums:

$$p_{i\bullet} = \frac{1}{K} \sum_{k=1}^{K} \frac{n_{i\bullet}^k}{n_{\bullet\bullet}^k} \quad \text{and} \quad p_{\bullet j} = \frac{1}{K} \sum_{k=1}^{K} \frac{n_{\bullet j}^k}{n_{\bullet\bullet}^k}$$

These margins define two metrics, $\mathbf{D}_I = \text{diag}(p_{1\bullet} \cdots p_{I\bullet})$ and $\mathbf{D}_J = \text{diag}(p_{\bullet 1} \cdots p_{\bullet J})$.

The Common Structure analysis is the study of the triplet $(\mathbf{Z}, \mathbf{D}_J, \mathbf{D}_I)$ with $\mathbf{Z} = \mathbf{D}_I^{-1} \mathbf{P} \mathbf{D}_J^{-1} - \mathbf{1}_{IJ}$ (see Box 6.2 for more details).

Step 2: the Intrastructure
The rows and columns of the K tables are projected onto the axes of the analysis of the average table (Step 1).

The projection of columns is obtained by $(\mathbf{P}_k^J)^\top \mathbf{B}$ with $\mathbf{P}_k^J = \mathbf{P}_k \left(\mathbf{D}_J^k \right)^{-1}$.

The projection of rows is obtained by $\mathbf{P}_k^I \mathbf{A}$ with $\mathbf{P}_k^I = \left(\mathbf{D}_I^k \right)^{-1} \mathbf{P}_k$.

In the **ade4** package, the `foucart` function is used to compute a Foucart COA. All the outputs of this function are grouped in a `foucart` object and Box 9.5 recalls the corresponding output elements.

Box 9.5 Foucart Analysis: `dudi` Output Elements

In the **ade4** package, the results of a Foucart Analysis are stored in an object of class `dudi`, subclass `coa`, subclass `foucart`. This object is a list with 18 elements, including the usual elements of any `dudi`. In this list, elements of particular interest are:

Step 1: the Common Structure

- `$blocks`: number of columns in each table
- `$tab.names`: names of tables
- `$tab`: transformed average table ($\mathbf{Z}$)
- `$cw`: column weights ($\mathbf{D}_J$)
- `$lw`: row weights ($\mathbf{D}_I$)
- `$c1`: principal axes ($\mathbf{A}$)
- `$co`: column scores as weighted averages ($\mathbf{C} = \mathbf{Z}^\top \mathbf{D}_I \mathbf{B}$)
- `$l1`: principal components ($\mathbf{B}$)
- `$li`: row scores as weighted averages ($\mathbf{L} = \mathbf{Z} \mathbf{D}_J \mathbf{A}$)

Step 2: the Intrastructure

- `$Tco`: column scores ($(\mathbf{P}_k^J)^\top \mathbf{B}$ stacked vertically)
- `$Tli`: row scores ($\mathbf{P}_k^I \mathbf{A}$ stacked vertically)

The `bf88` data set (Sect. 9.2.1, page 169) can be used to illustrate this method:

```
fou1 <- foucart(bf88, scannf = FALSE, nf = 3)
```

Figure 9.7 is a summary of the Common structure and of the Intrastructure of this analysis. The two graphs on the top of the figure are the row and column graphs of the Common structure (mean of the contingency tables). They show the list of bird species (left) and the four regions (right).

The bottom two graphs show the Intrastructure, i.e., the projections of the rows and columns of the six contingency tables into the analysis of the Common structure. They display the projection of the 79 bird species (left) and of the four regions (right) for the six stages of vegetation succession.

The `kplot` function can be used to draw Fig. 9.8. This is also a display of the Intrastructure, but unlike in Fig. 9.7, the six stages of vegetation succession are split in six separate graphs (S1 to S6). The 79 bird species and the four regions are displayed in each graph, showing the changes in bird species composition and relative region positions changes along the vegetation gradient.

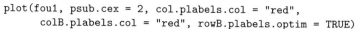

```
plot(fou1, psub.cex = 2, col.plabels.col = "red",
     colB.plabels.col = "red", rowB.plabels.optim = TRUE)
```

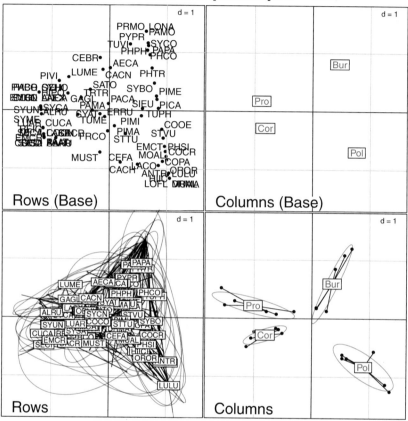

Fig. 9.7 Plot of the Foucart COA of the `bf88` data set.

The final interpretation is made easier in Fig. 9.9, where only the coordinates of the four regions in the Intrastructure is kept. Grey level polygons are used to show the between-regions variability of bird species composition along the gradient of vegetation succession. This variability is high in the first three stages (1–3, light grey polygons), and low in the last three (4–6, dark grey polygons). This corresponds to the bird species composition convergence in forest environments.

9.6 STATIS on Operators

When the tables of a K-table have only one dimension in common, the STATIS method uses the Escoufier operators to compare the tables (see Box 9.6).

```
kplot(fou1, col.plabels = list(cex = 3, col = "red",
      label = fou1$TC[, 2]), row.plabels = list(cex = 2,
      label = fou1$TL[, 2], plabels.boxes.draw = FALSE),
      psub.cex = 3, pgrid.text.cex = 2)
```

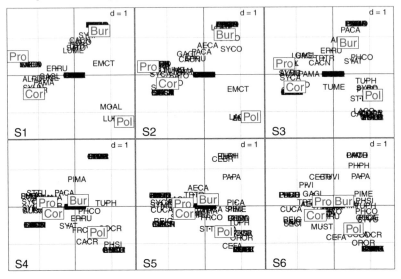

Fig. 9.8 `kplot` of the Foucart COA of the `bf88` data set.

```
pols <- s.class(fou1$Tco, fou1$TC[, 1], ppolygons.col = gray(5:0/6),
      chullSize = 1, starSize = 0, ellipseSize = 0, plabels.cex = 0,
      plegend.drawKey = FALSE)
pols <- s.label(fou1$Tco, add = TRUE)
```

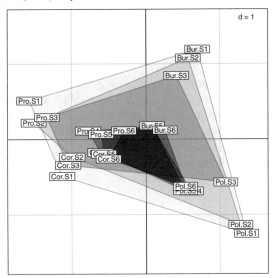

Fig. 9.9 Interpretation of Foucart COA of the `bf88` data set.

Box 9.6 The RV Coefficient on the Escoufier Operators

Let $\mathbf{X}_k$ and $\mathbf{X}_\ell$ be two tables with the same n rows and different columns.

Let $(\mathbf{X}_k, \mathbf{Q}_k, \mathbf{D})$ and $(\mathbf{X}_\ell, \mathbf{Q}_\ell, \mathbf{D})$ be the two associated statistical triplets. The respective analyses of these two triplets lead to two configurations of rows constructed with $\mathbf{X}_k\mathbf{Q}_k\mathbf{X}_k^\top\mathbf{D}$ and $\mathbf{X}_\ell\mathbf{Q}_\ell\mathbf{X}_\ell^\top\mathbf{D}$ also called the Escoufier operators $\mathbf{W}_k\mathbf{D}$ and $\mathbf{W}_\ell\mathbf{D}$. As they have different columns, a way to compare these triplets is to define an inner-product between the operators:

$$\text{COVV}(\mathbf{X}_k, \mathbf{X}_\ell) = \text{Trace}(\mathbf{X}_k\mathbf{Q}_k\mathbf{X}_k^\top\mathbf{D}\mathbf{X}_\ell\mathbf{Q}_\ell\mathbf{X}_\ell^\top\mathbf{D})$$

which can be written using the Escoufier operators

$$\text{COVV}(\mathbf{X}_k, \mathbf{X}_\ell) = \text{Trace}(\mathbf{W}_k\mathbf{D}\mathbf{W}_\ell\mathbf{D})$$

The vectorial variance $\text{VAV}(\mathbf{X}_k)$ is equal to:

$$\begin{aligned}
\text{VAV}(\mathbf{X}_k) &= \text{COVV}(\mathbf{X}_k, \mathbf{X}_k) \\
&= \text{Trace}(\mathbf{X}_k\mathbf{Q}_k\mathbf{X}_k^\top\mathbf{D}\mathbf{X}_k\mathbf{Q}_k\mathbf{X}_k^\top\mathbf{D}) \\
&= \text{Trace}(\mathbf{W}_k\mathbf{D}\mathbf{W}_k\mathbf{D})
\end{aligned}$$

The vectorial correlation coefficient, or RV coefficient is therefore:

$$RV(\mathbf{X}_k, \mathbf{X}_\ell) = \frac{\text{COVV}(\mathbf{X}_k, \mathbf{X}_\ell)}{\sqrt{\text{VAV}(\mathbf{X}_k)}\sqrt{\text{VAV}(\mathbf{X}_\ell)}}$$

also written

$$RV(\mathbf{W}_k\mathbf{D}, \mathbf{W}_\ell\mathbf{D}) = \frac{\text{Trace}(\mathbf{W}_k\mathbf{D}\mathbf{W}_\ell\mathbf{D})}{\sqrt{\text{Trace}((\mathbf{W}_k\mathbf{D})^2)}\sqrt{\text{Trace}((\mathbf{W}_\ell\mathbf{D})^2)}}$$

Property: $0 \leq RV(\mathbf{W}_k\mathbf{D}, \mathbf{W}_\ell\mathbf{D}) \leq 1$

Box 9.7 gives the basic definitions of the STATIS method in the framework of the duality diagram and of the **ade4** package.

Two cases are usually considered: (1) the tables of the series have the same columns (variables) or (2) the same rows (individuals or samples). If tables have different rows *and* different columns, then none of these methods can be used.

When variables are identical across all the tables, then STATIS compares covariance matrices (VQ) and analyses similarities between variables. This is called the "STATIS on VQ" strategy.

The "STATIS on WD" strategy is used when the tables have the same rows. It compares matrices of scalar products between individuals (WD), and analyses similarities between individuals (Box 9.7).

Box 9.7 STATIS Analysis: Basic Mathematical Definitions

Let $X_1, \ldots, X_k, \ldots, X_K$ be K tables containing $p_1, \ldots, p_K$ variables respectively (columns) and the same n rows (samples or individuals). Let $(X_1, Q_1, D), \ldots, (X_k, Q_k, D), \ldots, (X_K, Q_K, D)$ be the K associated statistical triplets.

Let W_k be the following matrix $W_k = X_k Q_k X_k^\top$. Then $W_k D$ is the matrix of the inner product between the individuals of table k. It is also called the Escoufier operator.

STATIS analysis is decomposed in three steps:

Step 1: the Interstructure

For all the pairs of triplets (X_k, Q_k, D) and (X_ℓ, Q_ℓ, D), we can compute the RV coefficients and put them in an **RV** matrix (see Box 9.6, Escoufier operator).

The eigenvalues Λ_B and the normed eigenvectors U_B of the **RV** matrix give a score of the tables $S = U_B \Lambda_B^{\frac{1}{2}}$, where the letter B (Between) refers to the interstructure. This score can be displayed in a correlation circle.

Step 2: the Compromise

Let $u_B^\top = (\alpha_1 \ldots \alpha_k \ldots \alpha_K)$ be the components of the first eigenvector of the Interstructure analysis with $\sum_{k=1}^K \alpha_k^2 = 1$. The α_k are used as weights for table X_k. One can then define the Compromise operator:

$$WD = \sum_{k=1}^K \alpha_k \frac{W_k D}{\sqrt{VAV(X_k)}}$$

Let Λ and U be the eigenvalues of **WD** and the eigenvectors, respectively ($U^\top D U = I$). One can compute the coordinates of all n individuals onto the principal axes $L = WDU\Lambda^{\frac{1}{2}}$.

Step 3: the Intrastructure

One can project the variables of each table onto the Compromise to obtain a score $C_k = X_k^\top D U$.

One can project the scalar product of each k table onto the Compromise $L_k = W_k DU\Lambda^{\frac{1}{2}}$.

In the **ade4** package, these differences are not considered and the `statis` function can be used to analyse both situations. The drawback is that the `ktab` object must take this into account. In all cases, the rows of all the tables must be identical, and the `ktab` must be prepared accordingly. If variables are the same for all the tables and individuals differ (STATIS on VQ), then the tables must be transposed to have the common dimension in rows.

All the outputs of the `statis` function are grouped in a `statis` object, and Box 9.8 recalls the corresponding outputs elements.

Box 9.8 STATIS Analysis: `dudi` Output Elements

In the **ade4** package, the results of a STATIS Analysis are stored in an object of class `statis`. This object is a list with 15 elements. In this list, elements of particular interest are:

Step 1: the Interstructure

- `$RV`: matrix of RV coefficients (**RV**)
- `$RV.eig`: eigenvalues (Λ_B)
- `$RV.coo`: table scores (**S**)
- `$tab.names`: table names

Step 2: the Compromise

- `$RV.tabw`: table weights ($\mathbf{u}_B$)
- `$cos2`: squared cosines between Compromise and tables ($RV(\mathbf{X}, \mathbf{X}_k)$)
- `$C.li`: coordinates of the rows of the Compromise (**L**)

Step 3: the Intrastructure

- `$C.Co`: column coordinates ($\mathbf{C}_k$ stacked vertically)
- `$C.T4`: row scores ($\mathbf{L}_k$ stacked vertically)

In the `friday87` data set, the `fau` data frame containing 91 species grouped in 10 taxa (see Sect. 9.2.1), and one table of environmental variables (`mil`) make up 11 tables with the same rows (16 ponds). The fauna and the environmental data frames are bound together into the `w1` data frame with the `cbind.data.frame` function. The species are centred, and the environmental variables are standardised. The `kta1` K-table is then built with the `ktab.data.frame` function (Fig. 9.10).

Figure 9.10 shows the eigenvalues barcharts of the 11 separate analyses (one for each table). STATIS measures the importance of a table by the sum of the squared eigenvalues, instead of the sum of eigenvalues as it is the case in one-table analyses. This change from the sum (mean) to the sum of squares (variance) is equivalent to the change from abundance to diversity.

The taxa that have the highest importance from this point of view are Diptera, Trichoptera, Mollusca and Ephemeroptera (on two axes). It is interesting to notice that this importance is not related to the richness of taxonomic groups, but to the strength of their structure.

```
w1 <- cbind.data.frame(scalewt(friday87$fau, scale = FALSE),
    scalewt(friday87$mil))
kta1 <- ktab.data.frame(w1, c(friday87$fau.blo, 11),
    tabnames = c(friday87$tab.names, "Environment"))
sep1 <- sepan(kta1)
plot(sep1, psub.cex = 2, paxes.draw = FALSE)
```

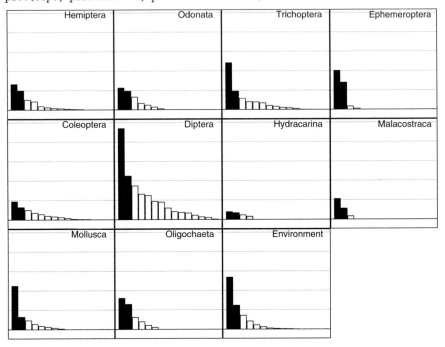

Fig. 9.10 Eigenvalues of the separate analyses of the `friday87` data set.

The STATIS analysis is computed with the `statis` function, and the results are displayed according to the three steps of *K*-table analyses: Interstructure, Compromise and Intrastructure (Figs. 9.11, 9.12, 9.13, 9.14 and 9.15):

```
statis1 <- statis(kta1, scannf = FALSE)
```

In the Interstructure step, the matrix of RV coefficients between operators is diagonalised, and the resulting eigenvalues can be found in `statis1$RV.eig`. This gives the eigenvalues barchart of Fig. 9.11. The components of the first eigenvector are then used as weights in a linear combination of initial operators. This linear combination is called the Compromise, and the corresponding weights can be found in `statis1$RV.tabw`.

The correlation circle of the Interstructure (Fig. 9.11) can be drawn with the coordinates found in `statis1$RV.coo`. This figure shows the importance (`Typological value`) of each table in the Compromise study. Here, we can see that the structure is not very coherent among tables, and that the environment will

```
bc2 <- plotEig(statis1$RV.eig, yax = 1, nf = 1, pbackground.box = TRUE,
      psub = list(text = "Eigenvalues", cex = 2) , plot = FALSE)
cs2 <- s.corcircle(statis1$RV.coo, pbackground.box = FALSE, plot = FALSE)
ADEgS(list(cs2, bc2), rbind(c(0, 0, 1, 1), c(0, 0.55, 0.45, 1)))
```

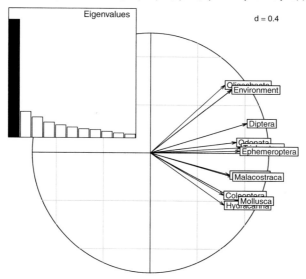

Fig. 9.11 STATIS analysis of the `friday87` data set: eigenvalues barchart and correlation circle of the Interstructure.

not be able to explain the distribution of all taxa. The environmental variables seem to be better related to Oligocheta than to Mollusca, Coleoptera and Hydracarina.

The analysis of the Compromise gives a second eigenvalues barchart (Fig. 9.12) with two prominent eigenvalues. These values can be found in `statis1$C.eig`.

The factor map of the Compromise for the 16 ponds (Fig. 9.12, left) is drawn using the coordinates in `statis1$C.li`. The structure observed in this figure corresponds to a differential distribution of several taxa in some ponds: Trichoptera, Ephemeroptera, Hydracarina, Malacostraca, Mollusca and Oligochaeta are mostly absent from ponds on the left (ponds R, E, J, P, Q).

This structure can be seen directly in the data, in Fig. 9.13. This figure displays the distribution of the 91 species in the 16 ponds. It is drawn with the `s.distri` function and the following code, that builds a new `ktab` object `kta2`, containing only the species data (excluding the environmental variables table).

```
kta2 <- ktab.data.frame(friday87$fau, friday87$fau.blo)
glc <- list()
for (j in 1:length(friday87$fau.blo)) {
      glc <- c(glc, s.distri(statis1$C.li, kta2[[j]],
               plot = FALSE, storeData = TRUE, starSize = 0.5,
               ellipseSize = 0, pellipses.axes.draw = FALSE,
               psub.cex = 2, psub.text = names(kta2)[[j]],
               pgrid.text.cex = 2, plabels.cex = 2))
      }
ADEgS(glc)
```

```
bcC <- plotEig(statis1$C.eig, yax = 2, nf = 2, pbackground.box = TRUE,
    psub = list(text = "Eigenvalues", cex = 2), plot = FALSE)
slC <- s.label(statis1$C.li, plabels.cex = 1.5, plabels.optim = TRUE,
    plot = FALSE)
ccC <- s.corcircle(statis1$C.Co[statis1$TC[, 1] == "Environment", ],
    pbackground.box = FALSE, plot = FALSE)
ADEgS(list(slC, ccC, bcC), rbind(c(0, 0, 0.5, 1), c(0.5, 0, 1, 1),
    c(0.35, 0, 0.65, 0.4)))
```

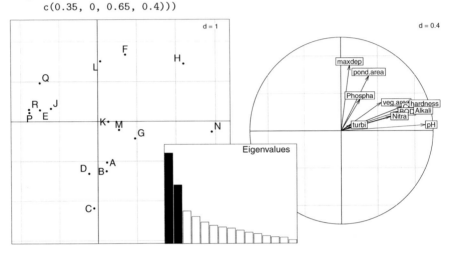

Fig. 9.12 Compromise of the STATIS analysis of the `friday87` data set: eigenvalues barchart (middle), ponds factor map (left), and environmental variables (right).

```
ADEgS(glc)
```

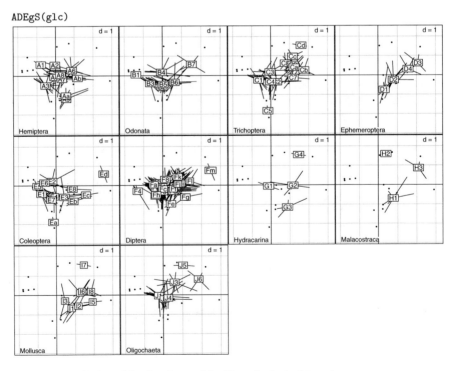

Fig. 9.13 Distribution of the abundance of the 91 species in the 16 ponds.

```
kp1 <- kplot(statis1, plabels.cex = 2, psub.cex = 2)
```

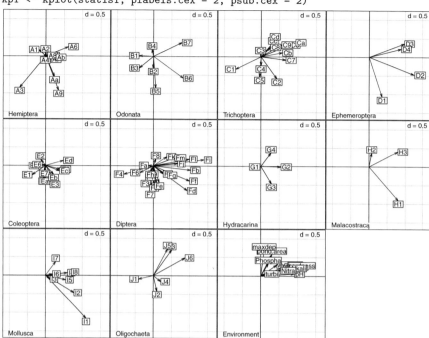

Fig. 9.14 Columns Compromise plot of the STATIS analysis.

The `for` loop operates on the ten tables of the `ktab` (the ten species groups), drawing one graph for each group. The resulting ten graphs are collected in the `glc` list, and plotted with the `ADEgS` function of the **adegraphics** package.

There is one star for each species, with branches that connect the gravity centre of the species to the ponds where it is present. Species are grouped by taxa, and it is easy to see that, for example, Ephemeroptera are present only in ponds on the right (ponds with high pH).

The factor map of the Compromise for variables (species and environmental parameters) can be drawn with the column coordinates (in `statis1$C.co`). Figure 9.12 (right) shows the environmental variables only. Pond size (area and depth) and water pH are the two main factors that explain the variations in species distributions. Large ponds tend to be in the top part of the graph, while ponds with high pH and hardness tend to be on the right.

The factor map of the Compromise for columns can be drawn automatically using the `kplot` function (Fig. 9.14), and the `plot` function can be used to draw the synthetic graph of a `statis` object (Fig. 9.15).

The `kplot` function draws a figure (Fig. 9.14) that has the same organisation as the graph of species distributions (Fig. 9.13), with one graph for each species group. In each group (e.g., Hemiptera), each species is represented by an arrow with

```
plot(statis1)
```

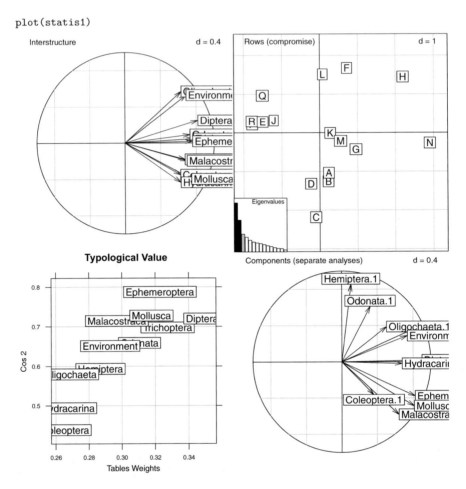

Fig. 9.15 Generic plot of the `statis` analysis of the `friday87` data set.

a label giving the species code. This figure also corresponds to the plot of ponds (Fig. 9.12), and shows which species is more abundant (or which environmental variable is higher) in each pond.

The generic plot of the STATIS analysis (`plot` function, see Fig. 9.15) is a collection made of the Interstructure plot (top-left), the rows (ponds) Compromise plot (top-right), the `Typological value` plot (bottom-left), and the component projection plot (bottom-right). The `Typological value` plot gives the importance of each table in the analysis, and the component projection plot shows the projection of the first principal vector of each table on the Compromise factor map.

9.7   Multiple Factor Analysis

Multiple Factor Analysis (MFA, Escofier and Pagès 1994) was developed by B. Escofier and J. Pages in the early 1980s (INRIA internal research reports). The aim of MFA is to analyse K groups of variables measured on the same individuals. Many variants and extensions have been defined in other situations, for example, tables with mixed quantitative and qualitative variables, variables arranged in a hierarchy, or dual MFA (groups of individuals instead of groups of variables).

Box 9.9 gives the basic definitions of MFA. Row weights are equal to the row weights of separate tables, and column weights are equal to the concatenated column weights of separate tables. Each table is multiplied by a weight that decreases the importance of large tables and increases the one of small tables.

Box 9.9 MFA: Basic Mathematical Definitions

Let $\mathbf{X}_1, \cdots, \mathbf{X}_k, \cdots, \mathbf{X}_K$ be K tables with the same n sampling units (rows). Table k contains p_k variables (columns), and $\sum_{k=1}^{K} p_k = p$. Let $(\mathbf{X}_1, \mathbf{Q}_1, \mathbf{D})$, $\ldots, (\mathbf{X}_k, \mathbf{Q}_k, \mathbf{D}), \ldots, (\mathbf{X}_K, \mathbf{Q}_K, \mathbf{D})$ be the K associated statistical triplets.

The Multiple Factor Analysis is decomposed in two steps:

Step 1: the Reference Structure

A global analysis is performed on the statistical triplet $(\mathbf{X}, \mathbf{Q}, \mathbf{D})$ where $\mathbf{X}$ contains all tables stacked horizontally $\mathbf{X} = [\mathbf{X}_1 | \ldots | \mathbf{X}_k | \ldots | \mathbf{X}_K]$, and $\mathbf{D}$ is the diagonal matrix of row weights.

A table weighting π_k is applied to each table to avoid those with more variables, higher total inertia or with a higher first eigenvalue dominate the global study. Three main propositions can therefore be chosen:

- the inverse of the first eigenvalue of the separate analysis of each table (by default),
- the inverse of the total inertia of the separate analysis of each table,
- a uniform weighting if tables are comparable.

Let $\mathbf{X}$ be the previous one including table weightings:

$$\mathbf{X} = [\pi_1 \mathbf{X}_1 | \ldots | \pi_k \mathbf{X}_k | \ldots | \pi_K \mathbf{X}_K]$$

Let $\mathbf{Q}$ be the diagonal block matrix of column weights:

$$\mathbf{Q} = \begin{pmatrix} \mathbf{Q}_1 & \mathbf{0} & \mathbf{0} \\ \hline \mathbf{0} & \ddots & \mathbf{0} \\ \hline \mathbf{0} & \mathbf{0} & \mathbf{Q}_K \end{pmatrix}$$

MFA finds the principal components $\mathbf{B}$ of the triplet $(\mathbf{X}, \mathbf{Q}, \mathbf{D})$ in the sense of the duality diagram (see Box 3.1). The corresponding analysis is a PCA for

---

(continued)

Box 9.9 (continued)

quantitative variables (see Box 5.1) and an MCA for qualitative variables (see Box 5.3).

Let **A**, **B**, **C** and **L** be the matrices of principal axes, principal components, column scores and row scores, respectively.

Step 2: the Intrastructure

The intrastructure links each table to the Reference Structure by $\left\|\mathbf{X}_k^\top \mathbf{DB}\right\|_{\mathbf{Q}_k}^2$ and computes the projection of the principal components of the separate analysis of a table onto the principal components of the Reference Structure by $\mathbf{B}_k^\top \mathbf{DB}$.

Finally, one can project the n rows of each k table as supplementary rows onto the Reference Structure ($\mathbf{X}_k \mathbf{Q}_k \mathbf{X}_k^\top \mathbf{DB}$).

In **ade4**, the `mfa` function is used to compute an MFA. All the outputs of this function are grouped in an `mfa` object and Box 9.10 recalls the corresponding output elements.

Box 9.10 MFA: `dudi` Output Elements

In the **ade4** package, the results of an MFA are stored in an object of class `mfa`. This object is a list with 19 elements. In this list, elements of particular interest are:

Step 1: the Reference Structure

- `$tab`: grand matrix (**X**)
- `$tab.names`: table names
- `$eig`: eigenvalues
- `$lw`: row weights (**D**)
- `$cw`: column weights (**Q**)
- `$l1`: row normed scores (**B**)
- `$li`: row coordinates (**L**)
- `$c1`: column normed scores (**A**)
- `$co`: column coordinates (**C**)

Step 2: the Intrastructure

- `$link`: link with grand table ($\left\|\mathbf{X}_k^\top \mathbf{DB}\right\|_{\mathbf{Q}_k}^2$ stacked vertically)
- `$T4comp`: component projections ($\mathbf{B}_k^\top \mathbf{DB}$ stacked vertically)
- `$lisup`: row coordinates for each table ($\mathbf{X}_k \mathbf{Q}_k \mathbf{X}_k^\top \mathbf{DB}$ stacked vertically)

```
afm1 <- mfa(kta1, scannf = FALSE, nf = 2)
plot(afm1, comp = list(plabels.boxes.draw = FALSE,
     psub.position = "topright"), pgrid.text.pos = "bottomright")
```

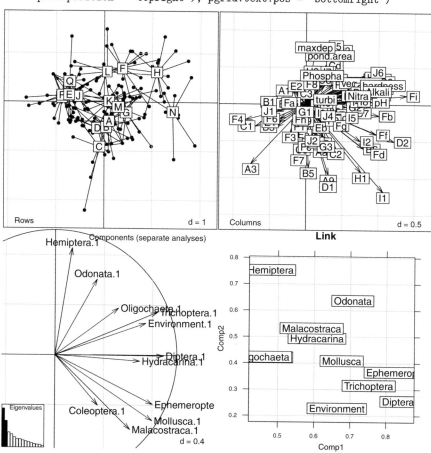

Fig. 9.16 Generic plot of the Multiple Factor Analysis of the `friday87` data set.

Figure 9.16 shows the results of MFA on the `friday87` data set. The eigenvalues barchart is very similar to the eigenvalues barchart of the STATIS Compromise (see Fig. 9.12, middle graph). The rows and columns coordinates are used to draw the top two graphs in Fig. 9.16 (`Rows` = Rows projection and `Columns` = Columns projection). The lower left graph (`Components (separate analyses)`) shows the projection of the principal components of each table into the factor map of MFA. The result is very similar to the same graph in the STATIS analysis (Fig. 9.15). The lower right graph (`Link`) displays the link between each table and the Reference Structure. It shows, for example, that the environmental variables table (`Environment`) has no influence on the second component of the MFA, as opposed to the Hemiptera table (`Hemiptera`).

```
s.label(afm1$li, plabels.optim = TRUE)
```

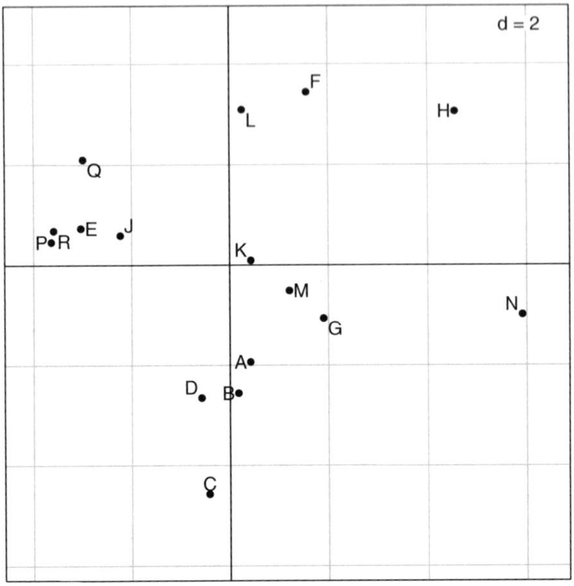

Fig. 9.17 Plot of the 16 ponds in the MFA of the `friday87` data set.

The factor map of the rows (ponds) is displayed in Fig. 9.17. Although computations are completely different, it is also very similar to the Compromise plot of STATIS (Fig. 9.15, top-right graph).

It is possible to draw a map of sites (ponds) for each table (taxa), in the same way as in STATIS trajectories. The coordinates of the rows of each table are in `afm1$lisup`. These coordinates can be used to draw a simultaneous display of ponds and taxa, either with taxa grouped by pond (Fig. 9.18) or with species split by taxa (Fig. 9.19). The first figure underlines the coherence of species composition within each pond, while the second one allows to compare the distribution of species in the ponds for each taxon.

In Fig. 9.18, the coordinates of the rows (ponds) for all the tables (taxa) are grouped by pond. A star and an ellipse are drawn for each pond. For example, for pond N (on the right), the 11 branches of the star link the position of pond N for the eleven tables to their gravity centre. The ellipse is just a graphical summary of the means, variances and the covariance of the 11 coordinates of the pond. This figure shows that the species composition of ponds can be very different, some ponds sheltering particular taxa.

In Fig. 9.19, the same coordinates (`afm1$lisup`, black dots) are used, but they are superimposed to the coordinates of species (`afm1$co`, arrows), and the resulting plot is split by taxa (one graph for each taxon, plus the graph for environmental variables). This figure can be used to compare the distribution of species among the ponds, and it shows very clearly that some taxa prefer particular ponds.

```
s.class(afm1$lisup, afm1$TL[, 2], labels = row.names(afm1$tab))
```

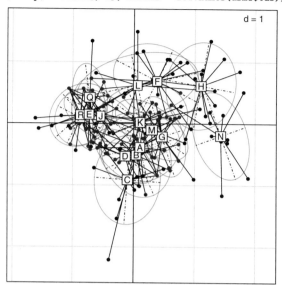

Fig. 9.18 Plot of the 16 ponds for the eleven taxa in the MFA of `friday87` data.

```
kp2 <- kplot(afm1)
```

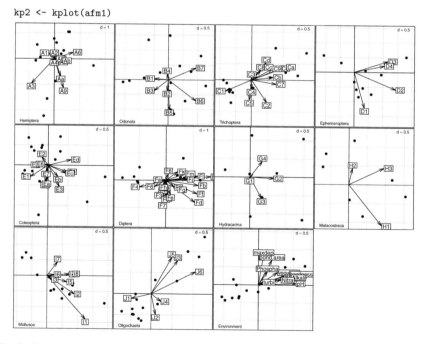

Fig. 9.19 Plot of the 16 ponds for the eleven taxa in the Multiple Factor Analysis of the `friday87` data set. The coordinates of species are split by taxon (plus the set of environmental variables).

9.8 Multiple Coinertia Analysis

We have seen in Chap. 3 (Box 3.1) that one table can be seen as a cloud of variables in $\mathbb{R}^n$, and as a cloud of samples in $\mathbb{R}^p$. In the same way, K tables can be seen as K clouds of variables *in the same space*. This is the point of view of MFA (see Fig. 9.20).

K tables also give K inertia operators and K clouds of samples (or variables) *in the same space*: this is the STATIS point of view.

But K tables can also be seen as K clouds of samples *in K different variable spaces*, and this is the point of view of Multiple Coinertia Analysis. (MCOA, see Box 9.11 for basic mathematical definitions and Fig. 9.21).

The successive steps of MCOA can be summed up as follows:

1. start from K tables with the same rows;
2. K tables define K clouds of points (samples) in K Euclidean spaces. These points are equally weighted in all the clouds. In each space, we look for a normed vector (axis) on which the cloud of points is projected;
3. a unit variance reference code is defined;
4. axes and reference code optimise the weighted sum of squared covariances between the reference code and the coordinates of each projection. Iterate under orthogonality constraint on axes and codes.

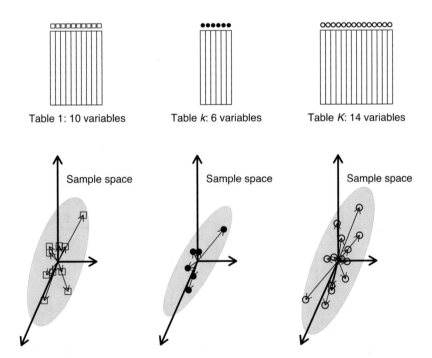

Fig. 9.20 K tables can be seen as K clouds of variables in the same sample space (MFA point of view).

Box 9.11 MCOA: Basic Mathematical Definitions

Let $\mathbf{X}_1, \cdots, \mathbf{X}_k, \cdots, \mathbf{X}_K$ be K tables with the same n sampling units. Table k contains p_k variables and $\sum_{k=1}^{K} p_k = p$.

Let $(\mathbf{X}_1, \mathbf{Q}_1, \mathbf{D}), \ldots, (\mathbf{X}_k, \mathbf{Q}_k, \mathbf{D}), \ldots, (\mathbf{X}_K, \mathbf{Q}_K, \mathbf{D})$ be the K associated statistical triplets.

As for Multiple Factor Analysis, tables with more variables, more inner total inertia or with stronger first eigenvalues could dominate the global study. A table weighting π_k is therefore applied to each table (see more detail in (Box 9.9)) and one can analyse the new following triplet $(\sqrt{\pi_k}\mathbf{X}_k, \mathbf{Q}_k, \mathbf{D})$ for $k = 1, K$.

In MCOA, a Reference Structure is built using an iterative process from the K tables and projections are computed to study the relationships between this Reference and tables.

Step 1: the Reference Structure

1. First step of the iterative process

   We look for K normed vectors $\mathbf{u}_k^1$ in each $\mathbb{R}^{p_k}$ space ($k = 1, K$) and a synthesis variable $\mathbf{v}_1$ of $\mathbb{R}^n$ maximising:

$$g(\mathbf{u}_1^1, \ldots, \mathbf{u}_k^1, \ldots, \mathbf{u}_K^1, \mathbf{v}_1) = \sum_{k=1}^{K} \pi_k \langle \mathbf{X_k Q_k u}_k^1 | \mathbf{v}_1 \rangle_{\mathbf{D}}^2$$

   The solution of $\mathbf{v}_1$ is obtained by the first principal component $\mathbf{b}_1$ of the triplet study $(\mathbf{X}, \mathbf{Q}, \mathbf{D})$ with $\mathbf{X} = \left[\sqrt{\pi_1}\mathbf{X}_1 | \ldots | \sqrt{\pi_k}\mathbf{X}_k | \ldots | \sqrt{\pi_K}\mathbf{X}_K \right]$ and $\mathbf{Q}$ and $\mathbf{D}$ defined as in Box 9.9.

   The solution of the $\mathbf{u}_k^1$ ($k = 1, K$) is obtained by the decomposition of the first principal axis $\mathbf{a}_1$ in K blocks. Each k block is therefore $\mathbf{Q}_k$-normed ($k = 1, K$).

2. Second step of the iterative process

   Let $\mathbf{P}_k^1$ be the $\mathbf{Q}_k$-orthogonal projector on $\mathbf{u}_k^1$ ($k = 1, K$) and $\mathbf{Z}_k = \sqrt{\pi_k}\mathbf{X}_k - \sqrt{\pi_k}\mathbf{X}_k \left(\mathbf{P}_k^1 \right)^{\top}$.

   We look for K normed vectors $\mathbf{u}_k^2$ in each $\mathbb{R}^{p_k}$ space ($k = 1, K$) and a synthesis variable $\mathbf{v}_2$ of $\mathbb{R}^n$.

   The solution of $\mathbf{v}_2$ is obtained by the first principal component $\mathbf{b}_1$ of the triplet study $(\mathbf{Z}, \mathbf{Q}, \mathbf{D})$ with $\mathbf{Z} = [\mathbf{Z}_1 | \ldots | \mathbf{Z}_k | \ldots | \mathbf{Z}_K]$ with $\langle \mathbf{v}_1 | \mathbf{v}_2 \rangle_{\mathbf{D}} = 0$.

   The solution of the $\mathbf{u}_k^2$ ($k = 1, K$) is obtained by the decomposition of the first principal axis $\mathbf{a}_1$ in K blocks. Each k block is therefore $\mathbf{Q}_k$-normed with $\langle \mathbf{u}_k^1 | \mathbf{u}_k^2 \rangle_{\mathbf{Q}_k} = 0$ ($k = 1, K$).

and the process is reiterated s times.

(continued)

Box 9.11 (continued)

The $\mathbf{v}_f$ $(f = 1, s)$ are stored in the $\mathbf{V}$ matrix and defines the Reference Structure. The $\mathbf{u}_k^f$ $(f = 1, s)$ normed vectors are stored in a $\mathbf{U}_k$ matrix and defines the Reference Structure.

Step 2: the Intrastructure

Each table is projected onto the Reference Structure by rows ($\mathbf{L}_k = \sqrt{\pi_k}\mathbf{X}_k\mathbf{Q}_k\mathbf{U}_k$) and by columns ($\mathbf{C}_k = \sqrt{\pi_k}\mathbf{X}_k^\top\mathbf{D}\mathbf{V}$).

The principal axes of each separate analysis can be projected onto the principal axes of the Multiple Coinertia Analysis: $\mathbf{A}_k^\top\mathbf{Q}_k\mathbf{U}_k$.

And, for a f axis, one can compute the squared covariance between the row coordinates of each table $\mathbf{L}_k^f$ and the Reference Structure for a f axis: $\mathbf{v}_f$.

MCOA is therefore, axis by axis, the inertia analysis of each table with matched coordinates using synthesis variables (Chessel and Hanafi 1996). The first coordinate is directly given by the first component of MFA. Further ones are more precise from the point of view of the geometry of clouds, but the optimality of the variables representation is lost.

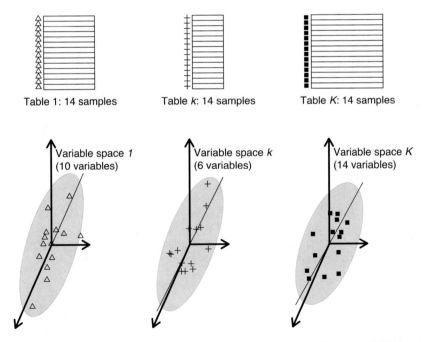

Fig. 9.21 K tables can be seen as K clouds of samples in different variable spaces (MCOA point of view).

In **ade4**, MCOA is computed using the `mcoa` function (Box 9.12):

```
mcoa1 <- mcoa(kta1, scannf = FALSE, nf = 2)
```

Box 9.12 MCOA: `dudi` Output Elements

In the **ade4** package, the results of a Multiple Coinertia Analysis are stored in an object of class `mcoa`. This object is a list with 14 elements. In this list, elements of particular interest are:

- `$pseudoeig`: pseudo eigenvalues
- `$SynVar`: synthetic scores (**V**)
- `$axis`: coinertia axis (**U**$_k$ stacked vertically)
- `$Tli`: coinertia coordinates (**L**$_k$ stacked vertically)
- `$Tl1`: coinertia normed scores
- `$Tax`: inertia axes onto coinertia axis ($\mathbf{A}_k^\top \mathbf{Q}_k \mathbf{U}_k$ stacked vertically)
- `$Tco`: columns onto the synthetic scores (**C**$_k$ stacked vertically)
- `$lambda`: eigenvalues of separate analyses
- `$cov2`: pseudo eigenvalues (synthetic analysis)

The plot of MCOA (Fig. 9.22) is nearly identical to the plot of MFA (Fig. 9.16), except for an inversion of the second axis.

The `kplot` of MCOA (Fig. 9.23) compares the projection of the cloud of points in each space with the synthetic typology (called `Reference` in Fig. 9.23). This strategy can be very useful to link a faunistic K-table to an environmental variables table (Concordance Analysis).

9.9   Conclusion

The K-table data analysis methods that have been broached in this chapter belong to three families: STATIS, MFA and MCOA. When all the tables of the K-table have the same individuals and the same variables, the "STATIS on tables" strategy can be used, with, for example, the PTA and Foucart COA methods. When the tables have only one dimension in common, then the STATIS on WD (same individuals) and STATIS on VQ (same variables) can be used.

When the K-table has the same individuals, MFA provides a point of view oriented to the interpretation of the relationships between the variables, with many possible generalisations.

Lastly, MCOA is a generalisation of Coinertia Analysis. In this example of application, it was used to analyse a K-table including ten faunistic tables and an environmental table. However, in this context, Concordance Analysis (Lafosse and Hanafi 1997; Bady et al. 2004), a generalisation of MCOA to the analysis of $K + 1$

plot(mcoa1)

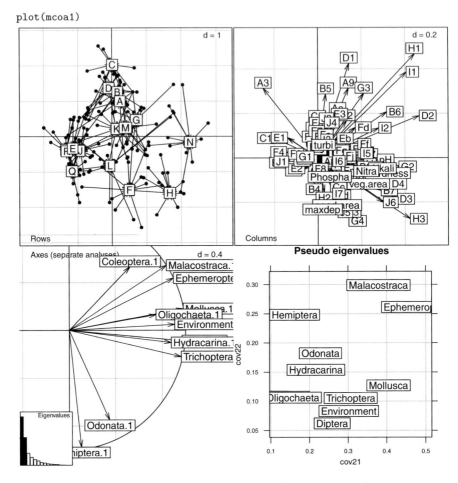

Fig. 9.22 Generic plot of the Multiple Coinertia Analysis of the `friday87` data set.

tables, could be preferred as it considers explicitly the environmental table as a reference table to ordinate the K faunistic tables. Unfortunately, this method is not yet implemented in **ade4**. Two other $K + 1$ methods are available in **ade4**: Multiblock Partial Least Square (PLS) and Multiblock PCAIV (Chap. 8). These two regression-based methods are able to analyse the effect of K explanatory tables on a response table. They are implemented in the `mbpls` and `mbpcaiv` functions (Bougeard and Dray 2018).

Figure 9.24 shows the main K-table data analysis methods available in the **ade4** package. The `ktab` class allows to handle all these methods in the same way and using the same utility functions. The same K-table object can thus be analysed using STATIS, MFA and MCOA and the results of the three methods can be compared easily.

`kplot(mcoa1)`

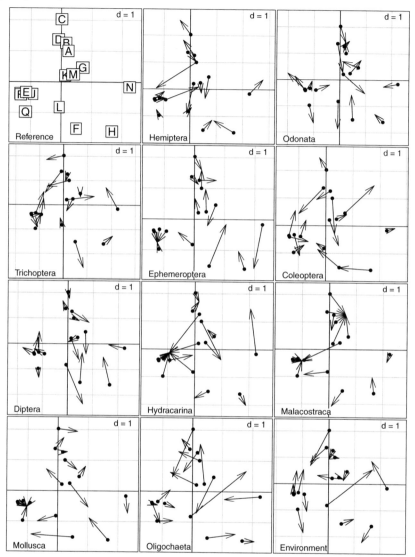

Fig. 9.23 `kplot` of the Multiple Coinertia Analysis of the `friday87` data set.

Two methods are particularly simple and easy to use:

- Partial Triadic Analysis, for series of tables having the same rows and the same columns,
- Multiple Factor Analysis, for tables having the same rows and different sets of variables.

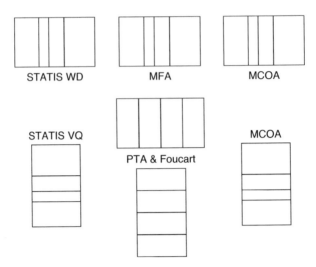

Fig. 9.24 The main K-table data analysis methods available in the **ade4** package.

The use of the RV coefficient is fundamental for coupling two tables. Its generalisation to the simultaneous analysis of K tables is the basis of the methods that have been described in this chapter. The analysis of K *pairs of tables* (see Chap. 10) is also based on this concept.

Chapter 10
Analysing Changes in Co-structures

Abstract This chapter is dedicated to the analysis of the changes in species-environment relationships, through the analysis of a series of pairs of tables. Each pair is made of one species table and one environmental variables table. The rows of both tables are identical and correspond to the samples where measures were made. The series of tables comes from the repetition of these two tables at several occasions. Three methods are compared in the chapter: Between-Class Coinertia Analysis, STATICO and COSTATIS.

10.1 Introduction

A series of pairs of ecological tables can be obtained when species data and environmental data are collected several times in the same locations. This data structure can also be seen as a couple of K-tables: one K-table relates to species data and a second one to environmental data. The study of changes in species-environment relationships can be important, for example, from the point of view of species conservation, or for global change studies.

We have seen previously that one pair of ecological tables can be analysed with many multivariate data analysis methods (also called "Coupling methods", see Chap. 8). We have also seen methods that allow to take into account the existence of groups of samples in a data table (Between-Class and Within-Class Analyses, see Chap. 7). In the previous chapter, we have seen methods that can be used to analyse a K-table (K-table methods, see Chap. 9). Here, we need to mix these three categories of methods in order to be able to analyse one couple of K-tables, or one series of pairs of ecological tables. Figure 10.1 sums up these three categories of methods and presents the three strategies that can be used to mix them: BGCOIA, STATICO and COSTATIS. A comparison of these methods is presented in Thioulouse (2011).

A real-size example of application to the Ecology of aquatic Heteroptera in the Medjerda watershed (Tunisia) can be found in Slimani et al. (2017). In this chapter, we use the `meau` data set (Pegaz-Maucet 1980) that we have already seen in Chap. 7 (see Fig. 10.2).

© Springer Science+Business Media, LLC, part of Springer Nature 2018
J. Thioulouse et al., *Multivariate Analysis of Ecological Data with ade4*,
https://doi.org/10.1007/978-1-4939-8850-1_10

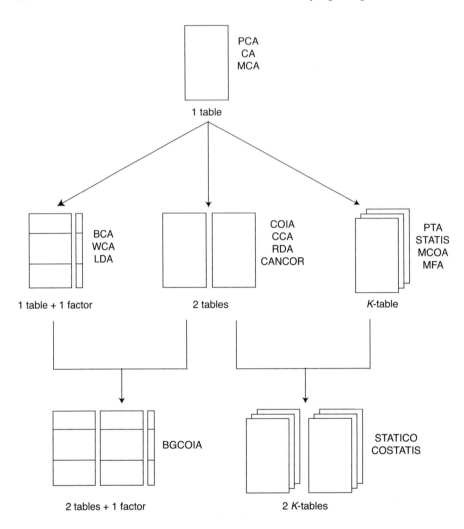

Fig. 10.1 Data structures that lead to two *K*-tables analyses. **One table** methods: PCA (Principal Component Analysis), CA (Correspondence Analysis) and MCA (Multiple Correspondence Analysis). **Two tables** coupling methods: COIA (Coinertia Analysis), CCA (Canonical Correspondence Analysis), RDA (Redundancy Analysis) and CANCOR (Canonical Correlations Analysis). Taking into account **groups of rows**: BCA (Between-Class Analysis), WCA (Within-Class Analysis) and LDA (Linear Discriminant Analysis). *K*-table methods: PTA (Partial Triadic Analysis), STATIS (Structuration des Tableaux A Trois Indices de la Statistique), MCOA (Multiple Coinertia Analysis) and MFA (Multiple Factor Analysis). Analysis of a series of pairs of ecological tables: **BGCOIA** (Between-Group Coinertia Analysis), **STATICO** (STATIS and Coinertia) and **COSTATIS** (Coinertia and STATIS).

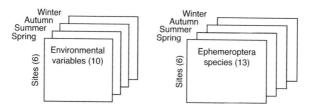

Fig. 10.2 A pair of data cube, or a series of pairs of ecological tables. This example corresponds to the meau data set from the **ade4** package.

10.2 BGCOIA

BGCOIA (Franquet et al. 1995, see Box 10.1 for basic mathematical definitions) is a Between-Group Coinertia Analysis. More precisely, it is obtained by considering each table of the sequence as a group. The mean of the columns in each table is computed and arranged in two new tables, with one row corresponding to one table. There is one table for species data means and one table for environmental variables means. A Coinertia Analysis is then done on this couple of mean tables. In the same way as in K-table analysis methods, the rows of the initial tables can be projected into this analysis to help interpret the results.

Box 10.1 BGCOIA: Basic Mathematical Definitions

Let $\mathbf{X}$ be the centred table of species data, with n rows and p variables, let $\mathbf{Y}$ be the centred table of environmental variables, with n rows and q variables, let $\mathbf{D}_p$ and $\mathbf{D}_q$ be the corresponding matrices of columns weights, and let $\mathbf{D}_n$ be the diagonal matrix of row weights.

The n rows are split into g groups. Let $\bar{\mathbf{X}}$ and $\bar{\mathbf{Y}}$ be the $g \times p$ and $g \times q$ matrices of group means, respectively. Let $\mathbf{D}$ be the diagonal matrix of group weights. The Between-Class Analyses of $\mathbf{X}$ and $\mathbf{Y}$ are the analyses of triplets $(\bar{\mathbf{X}}, \mathbf{D}_p, \mathbf{D})$ and $(\bar{\mathbf{Y}}, \mathbf{D}_q, \mathbf{D})$ (see details in Box 7.2).

A Coinertia Analysis combines theses two analyses into a single one to identify which structures are common to both data sets:

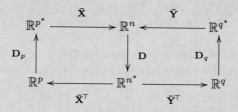

BGCOIA is the analysis of the triplet $(\bar{\mathbf{Y}}^{\mathsf{T}} \mathbf{D} \bar{\mathbf{X}}, \mathbf{D}_p, \mathbf{D}_q)$.

(continued)

Box 10.1 (continued)

When the two tables are analysed by a PCA, then $\mathbf{D}_p = \mathbf{I}_p$, $\mathbf{D}_q = \mathbf{I}_q$ and $\mathbf{D}_n = \frac{1}{n}\mathbf{I}_n$. In this case, BGCOIA is simply the analysis of matrix $\bar{\mathbf{X}}^T\mathbf{D}\bar{\mathbf{Y}}\bar{\mathbf{Y}}^T\mathbf{D}\bar{\mathbf{X}}$. This is therefore the Coinertia Analysis of the two tables of group means (see details in Box 8.1).

The main advantage of this method is its simplicity, from both theoretical and practical points of view. The two data cubes are reduced to two tables by taking the means of each elementary table of the cubes, and Coinertia Analysis is then applied to the two resulting tables.

In the **ade4** package, BGCOIA can be seen as the Between-Class Analysis of a `coinertia` object. The result is a `betcoi` object (bgcoia2), and Box 10.2 recalls the corresponding output elements.

Box 10.2 BGCOIA: dudi Output Elements

In the **ade4** package, the results of a BGCOIA are stored in an object of class dudi, subclass betcoi. This object is a list with 24 elements, including the usual elements of any dudi. In this list, elements of particular interest are:

- $tab: crossed table ($\mathbf{Y}^T\mathbf{DX}$)
- $l1: coefficients (loadings) for the variables of **Y** (**B**)
- $c1: coefficients (loadings) for the variables of **X** (**A**)
- $lX: scores of groups obtained from table **X**
- $lY: scores of groups obtained from table **Y**
- $mX: normed version of group scores obtained from table **X**
- $mY: normed version of group scores obtained from table **Y**
- $aX: projection of the axes of the bca analysis of **X** on coinertia axes
- $aY: projection of the axes of the bca analysis of **Y** on coinertia axes
- $msX: normed version of scores of individuals obtained from table **X**
- $msY: normed version of scores of individuals obtained from table **Y**
- $acX: projection of the coinertia axes of **X** on betcoi axes
- $acY: projection of the coinertia axes of **Y** on betcoi axes

The following code shows how computations can be performed in the first theoretical framework (Coinertia Analysis of two Between-Class Analyses):

```
data(meau)
pca.env <- dudi.pca(meau$env, scannf = FALSE, nf = 4)
pca.spe <- dudi.pca(meau$spe, scale = FALSE, scannf = FALSE, nf = 4)
bet.env <- bca(pca.env, meau$design$site, scannf = FALSE, nf = 2)
bet.spe <- bca(pca.spe, meau$design$site, scannf = FALSE, nf = 2)
bgcoial <- coinertia(bet.env, bet.spe, scannf = FALSE, nf = 3)
names(bgcoial)
```

```
[1]  "tab"   "cw"   "lw"   "eig"  "rank"  "nf"  "ll"   "li"
[9]  "co"    "cl"   "lX"   "mX"   "lY"    "mY"  "aX"   "aY"
[17] "call"  "RV"
```

In that case, supplementary information are missing such as projections of individuals and variables from initial tables **X** and **Y**. The following code shows how computations can be performed in the second theoretical framework (Between-Class Analysis of a Coinertia Analysis):

```
coi <- coinertia(pca.env, pca.spe, scannf = FALSE, nf = 3)
bgcoia2  <- bca(coi, meau$design$site, scannf = FALSE)
names(bgcoia2)
```

```
[1]  "tab"   "cw"   "lw"   "eig"  "rank"  "nf"  "ll"   "li"
[9]  "co"    "cl"   "lX"   "mX"   "lY"    "mY"  "aX"   "aY"
[17] "call"  "RV"   "lsY"  "lsX"  "msX"   "msY" "acY"  "acX"
```

Figure 10.3 shows the results of the BGCOIA on the `meau` data set, with the factor map of Ephemeroptera species, of environmental variables, and of sampling sites. The factor map for sampling sites is double: there is one map for the rows of the table of environmental variables (red labels), and one map for the rows of the Ephemeroptera species (blue labels). Both maps are superimposed, to make comparisons easier.

It is easy to see the pollution gradient (first axis, pollution on the left) and the upstream-downstream physical gradient (second axis, upstream is upward) on the environmental variables map and on the sites map (red labels). This structure is very strong and can be found again for the species on the Ephemeroptera map and on the sites map (blue labels). See Thioulouse (2011) for further interpretations.

10.3 STATICO

The STATICO method was first published in 1999, as a method for the analysis of K pairs of tables (Simier et al. 1999; Thioulouse et al. 2004). The principle of the method is simple: the relations between the two tables of each pair are analysed using Coinertia Analysis (see Chap. 8). During this step, the two tables are crossed, producing a cross-covariance table. In a second step, the series of cross-covariance tables is analysed with a Partial Triadic Analysis (see Chap. 9).

The particular choice of these methods (COIA and PTA) results in constraints on the set of environmental variables, species and sites that can be analysed by STATICO. The environmental variables must be the same in all the environmental tables, and the list of species must be the same in all the species tables too. Some species (but not too many) may be absent from some species tables, as the values in the corresponding columns can be set to zero. The sampling sites (rows of the tables) must be the same for the two tables of one pair, but they may be different among the series.

The Interstructure step of STATICO, like the Interstructure of the STATIS method, gives optimal weights that are used to build a Compromise. The Compromise of STATICO is a weighted mean of the cross-covariance tables. The analysis

```
ar1 <- s.arrow(bgcoia2$l1, plabels.boxes.draw = FALSE,
      plabels.cex = 1.5, plot = FALSE)
ar2 <- s.arrow(bgcoia2$c1, plabels.boxes.draw = FALSE,
      plabels.cex = 1.5, plot = FALSE)
xlim1 <- range(bgcoia2$msX[, 1], bgcoia2$msY[, 1])
ylim1 <- range(bgcoia2$msX[, 2], bgcoia2$msY[, 2])
cl1 <- s.class(bgcoia2$msX, meau$design$site, ellipseSize = 0,
      xlim = xlim1, ylim = ylim1, ppoints = list(pch = 21, fill = "red"),
      plabels = list(cex = 1.5, col = "red"), labels = 1:6, plot = FALSE)
cl2 <- s.class(bgcoia2$msY, meau$design$site, ellipseSize = 0,
      xlim = xlim1, ylim = ylim1, ppoints = list(pch = 21,
      fill = "blue"), plabels = list(cex = 1.5, col = "blue"),
      labels = 1:6, plot = FALSE)
clt <- superpose(cl2, cl1, plot = FALSE)
ADEgS(list(clt, ar1, ar2), rbind(c(0.2, 0, 1, 1), c(0, 0.6, 0.4, 1),
      c(0, 0, 0.4, 0.4)))
```

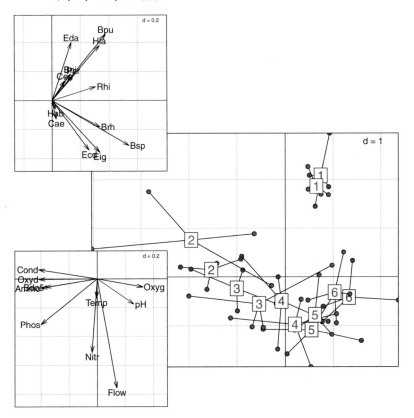

Fig. 10.3 BGCOIA of the `meau` data set. The Ephemeroptera species factor map (top-left) is drawn with the `s.arrow` function and the coordinates in `bgcoia2$l1`. The environmental variables factor map (bottom-left) is drawn with the `s.arrow` function and the coordinates in `bgcoia2$c1`. The sites factor map (middle graph on the right) is drawn with the `s.class` function and the coordinates in `bgcoia2$msX` (sites for environmental variables, red labels) and in `bgcoia2$msY` (sites for Ephemeroptera species, blue labels).

of this Compromise gives a graphical display of the environmental variables and of the species. Finally, the Intrastructure step projects the rows and columns of each table of the sequence in the analysis of the Compromise, with usual supplementary element projection technique (Lebart et al. 1984). This gives a display of the environmental variables at each date, of the species at each date, and two displays of the sampling sites at each date (one from the point of view of environmental variables and one from the point of view of species).

Basic mathematical definitions are recalled in Box 10.3.

In the **ade4** package, the `statico` function is used to compute a STATICO Analysis. All the outputs are grouped in a `dudi` object (subclass `pta`), and Box 10.4 recalls the corresponding output elements.

Box 10.3 STATICO Analysis: Basic Mathematical Definitions

Let $(\mathbf{X}_k, \mathbf{D}_p, \mathbf{D}_{n_k})$ and $(\mathbf{Y}_k, \mathbf{D}_q, \mathbf{D}_{n_k})$ be the pair of triplets at date k for $k = 1, K$.

$\mathbf{X}_k$ is the table of environmental variables measured at date k, and $\mathbf{Y}_k$ is the table of species observed at the same date. $\mathbf{D}_p$ and $\mathbf{D}_q$ are the same for all the dates and $\mathbf{D}_{n_k} = \mathrm{diag}\left(\frac{1}{n_k}\right)$ is the same for both tables of each pair.

Let $\mathbf{Z}_k$ be the k-th cross product table: $\mathbf{Z}_k = \mathbf{Y}_k^{\top}\mathbf{D}_{n_k}\mathbf{X}_k$. Note that the triplet $(\mathbf{Z}_k, \mathbf{D}_p, \mathbf{D}_q)$ corresponds to a Coinertia Analysis (see Box 8.1).

STATICO is the Partial Triadic Analysis of the K-table made by this series of $q \times p$ cross product tables.

Step 1: the Interstructure
The Interstructure step gives optimal weights α_k (see Box 9.2) such that the inertia of the triplet $(\sum_k^K \alpha_k \mathbf{Z}_k, \mathbf{D}_p, \mathbf{D}_q)$ is maximum with the constraint $\sum_{k=1}^{K} \alpha_k^2 = 1$.

Step 2: the Compromise The Compromise of STATICO ($\mathbf{Z}$) is a weighted mean of the cross product tables using weights α_k: $\mathbf{Z} = \sum_k^K \alpha_k \mathbf{Z}_k$ (Simier et al. 1999). The Compromise is the analysis of the triplet $(\mathbf{Z}, \mathbf{D}_p, \mathbf{D}_q)$. It gives a graphical display of the environmental variables (rows of $\mathbf{Z}$) and of the species (columns of $\mathbf{Z}$).

Step 3: the Intrastructure The Intrastructure step is based on usual row and column projections (see details in Box 9.2).

Box 10.4 STATICO Analysis: `dudi` Output Elements
In the **ade4** package, the results of a STATICO Analysis are stored in an object of class `dudi`, subclass `pta`. This object is a list with 28 elements, including

(continued)

Box 10.4 (continued)

the usual elements of any `pta`, with additional elements to store the results of the Intrastructure of the rows of the two K-tables. In this list, elements of particular interest are:

Step 1: the Interstructure

- `$RV`: The RV coefficients (**Rv**)
- `$RV.eig`: eigenvalues
- `$RV.coo`: scores of the tables

Step 2: the Compromise

- `$tabw`: table weights
- `$tab`: Compromise table (**Z**)
- `$li`: row scores
- `$co`: column scores

Step 3: the Intrastructure

- `$Tli`: projections of the rows of each Z_k table onto the principal axes (stacked vertically)
- `$Tco`: projections of the columns of each Z_k table onto the principal components (stacked vertically)
- `$supIX`: projections of the rows of the first K-table stacked vertically
- `$supIY`: projections of the rows of the second K-table stacked vertically

STATICO is a Partial Triadic Analysis on the sequence of cross product tables, so the Compromise is also a cross product table, with the 13 Ephemeroptera species in rows and the 10 environmental variables in columns, in the `meau` data set. Sites have disappeared from this table, but they can be projected as supplementary elements to help interpret the results of the analysis. The following code shows how computations are performed on the `meau` data set.

```
wit.env <- withinpca(meau$env, meau$design$season,
    scannf = FALSE, scaling = "total")
pca.spe <- dudi.pca(meau$spe, scale = FALSE, scannf = FALSE)
wit.spe <- wca(pca.spe, meau$design$season, scannf = FALSE)
kta.env <- ktab.within(wit.env, colnames = rep(c("S1",
    "S2", "S3", "S4", "S5", "S6"), 4))
kta.spe <- ktab.within(wit.spe, colnames = rep(c("S1",
    "S2", "S3", "S4", "S5", "S6"), 4))
statico.envspe <- statico(kta.env, kta.spe, scannf = FALSE)
```

The `statico.krandtest` function can be used to test the statistical significance of the Coinertia Analyses on the series of pairs of tables. This function produces a `krandtest` object and Fig. 10.4 shows the result of the plot function on this object.

```
plot(statico.krandtest(kta.env, kta.spe))
```

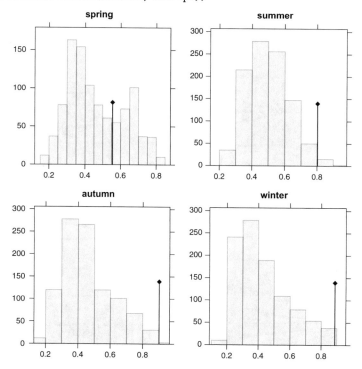

Fig. 10.4 Graphs of the four permutation tests obtained with the `statico.krandtest` function to test the statistical significance of the four Coinertia Analyses.

Figure 10.5 is a compound graph that sums up the first two steps of the STATICO method: Interstructure and Compromise. It is simply obtained with the generic `plot` function.

The Interstructure plot (top-left) shows that autumn and summer are the two most important seasons for defining the Compromise, while winter and spring are slightly less important.

The Compromise plots (top-right and bottom-left) are very similar to the BGCOIA plots (Fig. 10.3). They show that the first axis (horizontal) is also a pollution gradient: clean water on the right, and pollution on the left. The second axis (vertical) is also an upstream-downstream physical gradient: discharge (`Flow`) and temperature (`Temp`) increase downstream (downward on the figure). Nitrates (`Nitr`) also increase along the whole stream instead of having a maximum at site 2 like other pollution variables, and this is why they are located here. The sensitivity of all Ephemeroptera species to pollution and the specificity of some species (`Bpu`, `Hla`, `Eda` upstream and `Bsp`, `Eig`, `Ecd` downstream) are also found again. The `Typological value` plot (bottom-right) shows that autumn has the highest influence in the construction of the Compromise, while spring has the lowest.

```
plot(statico.envspe)
```

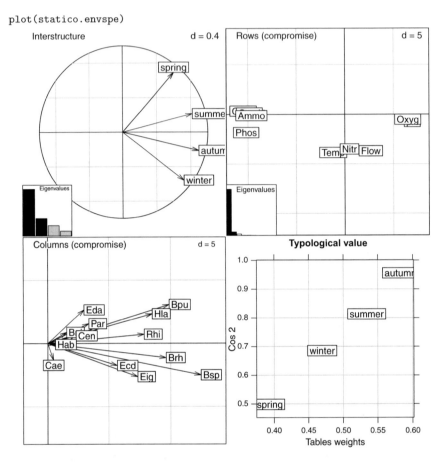

Fig. 10.5 Interstructure and Compromise of STATICO on the meau data set.

Figure 10.6 shows the Intrastructure step for environmental variables (top) and Ephemeroptera species (bottom). It is drawn using the projection of the columns of the two series of tables as supplementary elements in the Compromise analysis (`statico.envspe$Tli` and `statico.envspe$Tco`).

Autumn is clearly the season where the structures are the strongest (arrows are much longer at this date), both for environmental variables and for Ephemeroptera species. Conversely, spring is the season where the structures are the weakest (arrows are all very short). This confirms the interpretations made in Fig. 10.5. However, although the structures may vary in intensity, they are preserved across dates: the first axis is always a pollution gradient, and the second one is always an upstream-downstream opposition.

Figure 10.7 shows the Intrastructure step for the sites. It is drawn using the projection of the rows of the two sequences of tables as supplementary elements in the Compromise analysis (`statico.envspe$supIX` and

```
sa1 <- s.arrow(statico.envspe$Tli, facets = statico.envspe$TL[, 1],
    labels = statico.envspe$TL[, 2], psub.cex = 1.5,
    plabels.col = "red", plabels.boxes.draw = TRUE, plot = FALSE)
sa2 <- s.arrow(statico.envspe$Tco, facets = statico.envspe$TC[, 1],
    labels = statico.envspe$TC[, 2], psub.cex = 1.5,
    plabels.col = "blue", plabels.boxes.draw = TRUE, plot = FALSE)
pos1 <- rbind(c(0, 0, 0.25, 1), c(0.25, 0, 0.5, 1), c(0.5, 0, 0.75, 1),
    c(0.75, 0, 1, 1))
sa1@positions <- sa2@positions <- pos1
ADEgS(list(sa1, sa2), layout = c(2, 1))
```

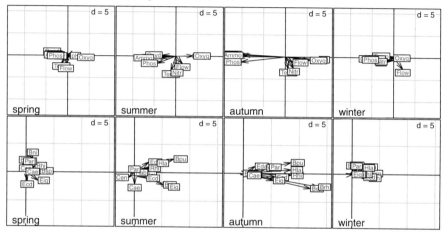

Fig. 10.6 Intrastructure of environmental variables (top) and Ephemeroptera species (bottom) of STATICO on the `meau` data set.

`statico.envspe$supIY`). It is very similar to the graph of sites in Fig. 10.3, but it is split according to seasons instead of sites. The sites of the environmental variables tables are on the first row of graphs while the sites of Ephemeroptera species tables are on the second row. This presentation insists on the comparison between the four seasons, showing mainly the distortions of the upstream-downstream gradient across seasons, as Ephemeroptera species react to pollution increase (maximum reached in autumn) or decrease (minimum in spring).

The differences between sites among the seasons for environmental variables are shown in Fig. 10.7 (top row). In spring, sites are lined up vertically on the upstream-downstream gradient and only site 2 moves slightly to the left. Structures are clearly weaker during this season and the permutation test (Fig. 10.4) is not statistically significant.

In summer, pollution is highest at site 2, and restoration occurs along sites 3, 4 and 5. In autumn, pollution is maximum because stream flow is at its minimum (pollutants concentrations are maximum). In winter, pollution has almost disappeared, because Autrans is a summer mountain resort, but the upstream-downstream gradient is still disturbed.

The position sites for Ephemeroptera species (bottom row) shows the same structures, because the pollution has a negative impact on species abundance

```
st1 <- s.traject(statico.envspe$supIX, facets = statico.envspe$supTI[, 1],
     plabels.cex = 0, psub.cex = 0, plot = FALSE)
sla1 <- s.label(statico.envspe$supIX, facets = statico.envspe$supTI[, 1],
     psub.cex = 1.5, labels = statico.envspe$supTI[, 2],
     plabels.col = "red", plot = FALSE)
st2 <- s.traject(statico.envspe$supIY, facets = statico.envspe$supTI[, 1],
     plabels.cex = 0, psub.cex = 0, plot = FALSE)
sla2 <- s.label(statico.envspe$supIY, facets = statico.envspe$supTI[, 1],
     psub.cex = 1.5, labels = statico.envspe$supTI[, 2],
     plabels.col = "blue", plot = FALSE)
pos1 <- rbind(c(0, 0, 0.25, 1), c(0.25, 0, 0.5, 1),
     c(0.5, 0, 0.75, 1), c(0.75, 0, 1, 1))
st1@positions <- st2@positions <- pos1
sla1@positions <- sla2@positions <- pos1
s1 <- superpose(st1, sla1)
s2 <- superpose(st2, sla2)
ADEgS(list(s1, s2), layout = c(2, 1))
```

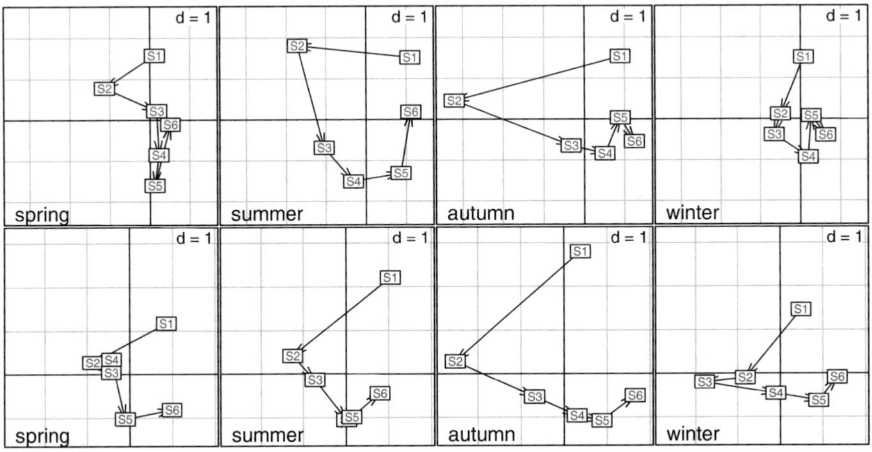

Fig. 10.7 Intrastructure of sites for environmental variables (top) and for Ephemeroptera species (bottom) of STATICO on the `meau` data set.

(horizontal axis) and because of the upstream-downstream preferences of particular species (vertical axis).

10.4   COSTATIS

COSTATIS is also based on K-table methods and on Coinertia. It benefits from the advantages of both STATICO and BGCOIA. Indeed, it has the same optimality properties of K-table analyses as STATICO (i.e., the maximising properties of the Compromise), but it retains the simplicity of BGCOIA.

COSTATIS is simply a Coinertia Analysis of the Compromises of the two K-table analyses. The first step of COSTATIS consists in performing two Partial Triadic

Analyses: one on the environmental variables K-table, and one on the species K-table. The second step is simply a Coinertia Analysis of the Compromises of these two Partial Triadic Analyses. This means that the number of tables does not have to be the same for the two series of tables, but that the number of species, of environmental variables, and of sampling sites must be the same for all the tables.

The Coinertia Analysis of the two Compromises decomposes the total coinertia and maximises the coinertia between species and environmental variable scores. An additional step can be implemented: like in the STATICO method, it is possible to project the rows and columns of all the tables of the two series as supplementary elements into the multidimensional space of this Coinertia Analysis.

Each Compromise represents the "stable structure" of the corresponding series. COSTATIS brings to light the relationships between these two stable structures, and it discards the conflicting variations between the whole sequences. It is therefore very easy to interpret (like a standard Coinertia Analysis), yet it retains the optimality properties of the Compromises of the two Partial Triadic Analyses.

Basic mathematical definitions are recalled in Box 10.5.

In the **ade4** package, the `costatis` function is used to compute a COSTATIS Analysis. All the outputs are grouped in a `dudi` object (subclass `coinertia`), and Box 10.6 recalls the corresponding output elements.

The call to the `costatis` function just passes the two K-tables, using the same syntax as the `statico` function:

```
costatis.envspe <- costatis(kta.env, kta.spe, scannf = FALSE)
```

Box 10.5 COSTATIS Analysis: Basic Mathematical Definitions

Let $X_1, \ldots, X_k, \ldots, X_K$ be K tables of environmental variables with the same n rows (samples) and the same p columns (variables). Let $Y_1, \ldots, Y_k, \ldots, Y_K$ be K tables of species with the same n rows (samples) and the same q columns (species).

COSTATIS consists in two Partial Triadic Analyses (PTA, see Box 9.2) and a Coinertia Analysis (see Box 8.1) of the Compromises of these two PTA.

Step 1.
Two partial Triadic Analyses are performed:

- one on the environmental variables K-table, i.e., (X_k, D_p, D) for $k = 1, K$
- one on the species K-table, i.e., (Y_k, D_q, D) for $k = 1, K$

That leads to the three structures studies and more specifically that of the Compromises. Let $X = \sum_{k=1}^{K} \alpha_k X_k$ be the $(n \times p)$ Compromise of the first PTA (environmental variables) with $\sum_{k=1}^{K} \alpha_k^2 = 1$. Let $Y = \sum_{k=1}^{K} \beta_k Y_k$ be

(continued)

Box 10.5 (continued)

the $(n \times q)$ Compromise of the second PTA (species data) with $\sum_{k=1}^{K} \beta_k^2 = 1$. Let $(\mathbf{X}, \mathbf{D}_p, \mathbf{D})$ and $(\mathbf{Y}, \mathbf{D}_q, \mathbf{D})$ be the two associated triplets.

Step 2.
Coinertia Analysis combines these two analyses in a single one to identify which structures are common to both Compromises. It is therefore defined by the triplet $(\mathbf{Y}^\top \mathbf{DX}, \mathbf{D}_p, \mathbf{D}_q)$. The Coinertia Analysis of these two Compromises decomposes the total coinertia:

$$I_{(\mathbf{Y}^\top \mathbf{DX}, \mathbf{D}_p, \mathbf{D}_q)} = \text{Trace}(\mathbf{Y}^\top \mathbf{DXD}_p \mathbf{X}^\top \mathbf{DYD}_q)$$

and maximises the coinertia between species and environmental variable scores.

An additional step can be implemented, like in the STATICO method: it is possible to project the rows and columns of all the tables of the two sequences as supplementary elements into the multidimensional space of this Coinertia Analysis.

Box 10.6 COSTATIS Analysis: `dudi` Output Elements
In the **ade4** package, the results of a COSTATIS Analysis are stored in an object of class `dudi`, subclass `coinertia`. This object is a list with 20 elements, including the usual elements of any `coinertia`, with additional elements to store the results of the Intrastructure of the rows of the two K-tables. In this list, elements of particular interest are:

- `$tab` covariances between the two Compromises ($\mathbf{Y}^\top \mathbf{DX}$)
- `$c1` coefficients (loadings) for the variables of the Compromise table $\mathbf{X}$
- `$l1` coefficients (loadings) for the variables of the Compromise table $\mathbf{Y}$
- `$1X` scores of rows-sites obtained from the Compromise table $\mathbf{X}$
- `$1Y` scores of rows-sites obtained from the Compromise table $\mathbf{Y}$
- `$supIX`: projections of the rows of the first K-table stacked vertically
- `$supIY`: projections of the rows of the second K-table stacked vertically

---

COSTATIS results are presented in Fig. 10.8. COSTATIS is a Coinertia Analysis, and it is therefore possible to use a permutation test to assess the statistical significance of the relationships between the two tables, just like in a usual Coinertia Analysis. The result of this permutation test (function `costatis.randtest`) gave a p-value of 0.005.

```
sa1 <- s.arrow(costatis.envspe$c1 * 4, xlim = c(-3, 2), ylim = c(-2, 3),
    plot = FALSE)
sc1 <- s.class(costatis.envspe$supIX, meau$design$site, ellipseSize = 0,
    xlim = c(-3, 2), ylim = c(-2, 3), plabels.col = "red",
    plot = FALSE)
s1 <- superpose(sa1, sc1)
sa2 <- s.arrow(costatis.envspe$l1 * 3, xlim = c(-2, 2),
    ylim = c(-2.5, 1.5), plot = FALSE)
sc2 <- s.class(costatis.envspe$supIY, meau$design$site, ellipseSize = 0,
    xlim = c(-2, 2), ylim = c(-2.5, 1.5), plabels.col = "blue",
    plot = FALSE)
s2 <- superpose(sa2, sc2)
ADEgS(list(s1, s2))
```

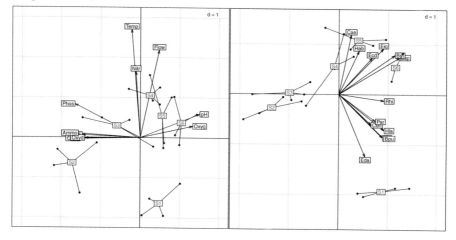

Fig. 10.8 Results of the COSTATIS analysis on the meau data set.

The Coinertia Analysis is done on the Compromises of two *K*-table analyses. Here, we used two Partial Triadic Analyses, but the results of these two analyses are not presented. We show only the plots of the Coinertia Analysis, under the form of two biplots: one for environmental variables (Fig. 10.8, left), and one for Ephemeroptera species (Fig. 10.8, right). These two biplots are at the same scale and in the same space, so they could be superimposed on the same figure. Presenting the results in this way underlines the fact that COSTATIS is looking for the relationships (co-structure) between the stable structures extracted from two series of tables.

The left graph in Fig. 10.8 shows the results for the environmental variables. The same structure as the one detected by STATICO and BGCOIA is observed. The first axis is the pollution gradient (pollution on the left) and the second is the upstream-downstream opposition (downstream is upward). The four dates for each site are projected on this plot and, like in the BGCOIA plot (Fig. 10.3), the four points corresponding to the four sampling dates of each site are grouped to form a star. The gravity centre of these four points is labeled with the number of the site. The four points of site 2 are on the left, as pollution is higher in this site for the four dates (except for site 3 in winter). Pollution decreases downstream along sites 3, 4 and 5, and is the lowest at site 6.

The second biplot is presented at the right of Fig. 10.8. It shows the Ephemeroptera species, with the same opposition between upstream and downstream characteristic species. In the same way as in the figure of environmental variables, the four dates for each site are projected on the plot and the corresponding four points are grouped to form a star. The gravity centre of these four points is labeled with the number of the site. The position of sites corresponds to the abundance of the species in these sites: sites 2 and 3 have the lowest number of Ephemeroptera, so they are far on the left. Site 1 has the highest number of species Eda, and sites 5 and 6 have the highest number of species Bsp, Brh and Eig.

The first axis common to these two biplots (i.e., the first COSTATIS axis) maximises the covariance between the coordinates of the "Compromise variables" and the "Compromise species". The result is that it displays the relationships between the stable structures extracted from the two data sets. On this example, this relationship is the fact that the pollution gradient affects the abundance of Ephemeroptera species. The second axis represents the upstream-downstream opposition, and the relationships between ecological preferences of Ephemeroptera species and physical variables or stream morphology.

10.5   Conclusion

In this chapter, we presented the principles and some examples of use of three methods for analysing a series of pairs of data tables (or a pair of data cubes): BGCOIA, STATICO and COSTATIS. Figure 10.9 shows a comparison of the three approaches.

BGCOIA is a Between-Group Coinertia Analysis. It is therefore simply computed by doing a Coinertia Analysis on the two tables of group means, considering each table as a group (Franquet et al. 1995).

In STATICO, we first use Coinertia Analysis K times to compute the sequence of K cross-covariance tables, and then Partial Triadic Analysis to analyse this new K-table. Symmetrically in COSTATIS, we first use two Partial Triadic Analyses to compute the Compromises of the two K-tables, and then Coinertia Analysis to analyse the relationships between these two Compromises.

The three methods presented here uncover the same features in the example data set. This is a small data set, but with strong structure, and strong structures often are clear with any method. However, the three methods used to analyse even a data set with clear structure can have advantages and drawbacks. The advantages of these methods can be summarised as follows:

- BGCOIA: It is the most straightforward method. It is simple to apply and outputs are easy to interpret. It can be used to favour one point of view (for example, space *vs.* time), by choosing the factor of Between-Class Analysis. It can also be

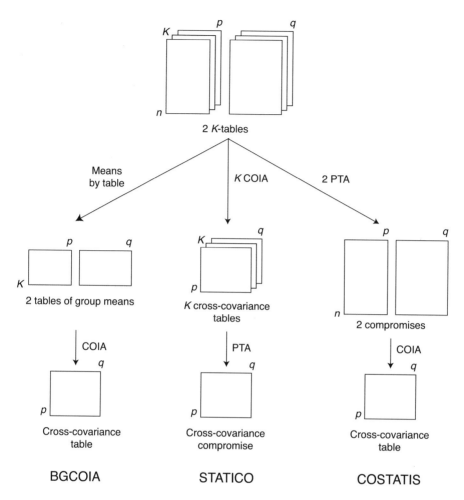

Fig. 10.9 Comparison of the three methods. BGCOIA is a Between-Group Coinertia Analysis, considering each table of the series as a group. STATICO is a Partial Triadic Analysis on the series of cross-product tables obtained by crossing the two tables of a pair at each date. COSTATIS is a Coinertia Analysis of the Compromises computed by the Partial Triadic Analysis of the two K-tables. In BGCOIA, the mean of the variables in each table is computed and arranged in two new tables. A Coinertia Analysis is then done on this couple of new tables. In STATICO, K cross-covariance tables are computed from the two K-tables, resulting in a new K-table. A Partial Triadic Analysis is then done on this new K-table. In COSTATIS, two Partial Triadic Analyses are used to compute the Compromises of the two K-tables. A Coinertia Analysis is then used to analyse the relationships between these two Compromises.

used in conjunction with WGCOIA (Within-Group Coinertia Analysis, Franquet and Chessel 1994) to study an effect (time) after removing the other (space).

- STATICO: The main advantage of this method is the optimality of the Compromise (maximisation of the similarity with all the initial tables). It gives a

Compromise of co-structures, which means that it displays the stable component of species-environment relationship variations. It benefits from the three-step computation scheme of STATIS-like methods (Interstructure, Compromise, Intrastructure), and graphical outputs can be very detailed.

- COSTATIS: This method benefits from the advantages of the two others: optimality of the Partial Triadic Analysis Compromises, ease of use, simplicity of Coinertia Analysis graphical outputs. COSTATIS is the Coinertia Analysis of two Compromises, so it looks for the relationships between two stable structures. This is different from the STATICO point of view (co-structure of two Compromises *vs.* Compromise of a series of co-structures).

Chapter 11
Relating Species Traits to Environment

Abstract This chapter focuses on three-table methods to study the relationships between species traits and environmental variables mediated by species abundances. The RLQ and fourth-corner methods are described.

11.1 Introduction

Methods presented in Chap. 8 are based on the analysis of a pair of tables (species abundances and environmental variables) to understand how environmental gradients influence the composition of species assemblages. This chapter focuses on methods that introduce an additional table containing the measures of several species traits. The aim is to find out if the characteristics of species are related to the environmental conditions of the sites in which they occur. In this context, the RLQ and fourth-corner methods are two efficient alternatives that provide a direct way to analyse trait-environment relationships. RLQ analysis produces a simultaneous ordination of the three tables whereas the fourth-corner method provides bivariate tests. This chapter shows how these two approaches can be handled and combined in a single framework using the **ade4** package.

We consider the `aravo` data set (Choler 2005; Dray et al. 2014), designed to identify relationships between plant functional traits and habitat heterogeneity along a snow melting gradient.

```
library(ade4)
library(adegraphics)
data(aravo)
names(aravo)
```

```
[1] "spe"       "env"       "traits"    "spe.names"
```

It contains the abundances of 82 alpine plant species in 75 sites (`aravo$spe`). Sites are described by 6 environmental variables (`aravo$env`):

- `Aspect`: Relative south aspect (opposite of the sine of aspect with flat coded 0)
- `Slope`: Slope inclination (degree)
- `Form`: Microtopographic landform index. Coded as `factor` with 5 levels (1: convexity, 2: convex slope, 3: right slope, 4: concave slope and 5: concavity)

© Springer Science+Business Media, LLC, part of Springer Nature 2018
J. Thioulouse et al., *Multivariate Analysis of Ecological Data with ade4*,
https://doi.org/10.1007/978-1-4939-8850-1_11

- `PhysD`: Physical disturbance, i.e., percentage of unvegetated soil due to physical processes
- `ZoogD`: Zoogenic disturbance, i.e., quantity of unvegetated soil due to marmot activity. Coded as a `factor` with three levels (`no`, `some` and `high`)
- `Snow`: Mean snowmelt date (Julian day) averaged over 1997–1999

  Species are characterised by eight traits (`aravo$traits`):

- `Height`: Vegetative height (cm)
- `Spread`: Maximum lateral spread of clonal plants (cm)
- `Angle`: Leaf elevation angle estimated at the middle of the lamina
- `Area`: Area of a single leaf
- `Thick`: Maximum thickness of a leaf cross section (avoiding the midrib)
- `SLA`: Specific leaf area
- `N_mass`: Mass-based leaf nitrogen content
- `Seed`: Seed mass

11.2 RLQ Analysis

RLQ analysis (Dolédec et al. 1996) is an extension of Coinertia Analysis (Sect. 8.3) to the case of three tables. It aims to identify the main co-structures between traits and environmental variations mediated by species abundances. It is based on the computation of a crossed array (cross-covariance matrix weighted by the abundances) that measures the relationships between traits and environmental variables. Box 11.1 gives the basic definitions of RLQ analysis in the framework of the duality diagram and Box 11.2 describes the main outputs provided by the `rlq` function.

Box 11.1 RLQ Analysis: Basic Mathematical Definitions

RLQ analyses three tables: $\mathbf{Q}$ ($p \times s$) that describes s traits for p species, $\mathbf{R}$ ($n \times m$) that contains the measurements of m environmental variables in n sites and a third $n \times p$ table $\mathbf{L}$ with the abundances of the p species within n sites. RLQ analysis combines the three separate analyses of $\mathbf{R}$, $\mathbf{L}$ and $\mathbf{Q}$ to identify the main relationships between environmental gradients and traits mediated by species abundances.

Correspondence Analysis is applied to $\mathbf{L}$ (see Sect. 6.2) leading to the triplet $\left(\mathbf{D}_n^{-1}\mathbf{P}_0\mathbf{D}_p^{-1}, \mathbf{D}_p, \mathbf{D}_n\right)$ where $\mathbf{P}_0$ is the doubly centred matrix of relative frequencies and $\mathbf{D}_n$ and $\mathbf{D}_p$ are the associated row and column weights (see Box 6.2 for more details). The separate analyses of $\mathbf{R}$ and $\mathbf{Q}$ should be weighted using CA-derived weights ($\mathbf{D}_n$ and $\mathbf{D}_p$) and lead to the triplets $(\mathbf{R}, \mathbf{D}_m, \mathbf{D}_n)$ and $\left(\mathbf{Q}, \mathbf{D}_s, \mathbf{D}_p\right)$, respectively. According to the type of

---

(continued)

Box 11.1 (continued)

variables, these triplets correspond to different methods: Principal Component Analysis for quantitative variables, Multiple Correspondence Analysis for qualitative variables or Hill and Smith Analysis for a mix of qualitative and quantitative variables (Chap. 5).

RLQ combines the three separate analyses of **R**, **L** and **Q** to investigate their joint co-structures. It corresponds to the statistical triplet $\left(\mathbf{R}^{\mathsf{T}}\mathbf{P_0}\mathbf{Q}, \mathbf{D}_s, \mathbf{D}_m\right)$:

$$
\begin{array}{ccc}
 & \mathbf{D}_s & \\
\mathbb{R}^s & \longrightarrow & \mathbb{R}^{s^*} \\
\mathbf{Q}^{\mathsf{T}}\mathbf{P_0}^{\mathsf{T}}\mathbf{R} \Big\uparrow & & \Big\downarrow \mathbf{R}^{\mathsf{T}}\mathbf{P_0}\mathbf{Q} \\
\mathbb{R}^{m^*} & \longleftarrow & \mathbb{R}^m \\
 & \mathbf{D}_m &
\end{array}
$$

The matrix $\mathbf{R}^{\mathsf{T}}\mathbf{P_0}\mathbf{Q}$ is a crossed array that measures the links between the traits and the environmental variables. It is named the "fourth-corner" by Legendre et al. (1997) and each cell corresponds to a bivariate association that can be tested by the `fourthcorner` or `fourthcorner2` functions.

The Property 3.3 of the duality diagram theory (Box 3.2) shows that RLQ analysis seeks for a principal axis **a** and a principal component **b** maximising:

$$\mathbf{b}^{\mathsf{T}}\mathbf{D}_m\left(\mathbf{R}^{\mathsf{T}}\mathbf{P_0}\mathbf{Q}\right)\mathbf{D}_s\mathbf{a}$$

Vector **b** contains coefficients for the environmental variables and vector **a** contains coefficients for the traits. These loadings are used to compute a score for sites ($\mathbf{x} = \mathbf{R}\mathbf{D}_m\mathbf{b}$) and species ($\mathbf{y} = \mathbf{Q}\mathbf{D}_s\mathbf{a}$) and the previous equation can thus be rewritten as:

$$\mathbf{b}^{\mathsf{T}}\mathbf{D}_m\left(\mathbf{R}^{\mathsf{T}}\mathbf{P_0}\mathbf{Q}\right)\mathbf{D}_s\mathbf{a} = \mathbf{x}^{\mathsf{T}}\mathbf{P_0}\mathbf{y} = \mathrm{cov}_{\mathbf{P}}(\mathbf{x}, \mathbf{y}) = \sqrt{\lambda}$$

RLQ computes a species score **y** (linear combination of traits) and a site score **x** (linear combination of environmental variables). The absolute value of the cross-covariance between these two scores is maximised, and the maximum is equal to the square root of the first RLQ eigenvalue λ.

This cross-covariance can be decomposed as a product of three terms:

$$\mathrm{cov}_{\mathbf{P}}(\mathbf{R}\mathbf{D}_m\mathbf{b}, \mathbf{Q}\mathbf{D}_s\mathbf{a}) = \mathrm{cor}_{\mathbf{P}}(\mathbf{R}\mathbf{D}_m\mathbf{b}, \mathbf{Q}\mathbf{D}_s\mathbf{a}) \cdot \|\mathbf{R}\mathbf{D}_m\mathbf{b}\|_{\mathbf{D}_n} \cdot \|\mathbf{Q}\mathbf{D}_s\mathbf{a}\|_{\mathbf{D}_p}$$

The first term, $\mathrm{cor}_{\mathbf{P}}(\mathbf{R}\mathbf{D}_m\mathbf{b}, \mathbf{Q}\mathbf{D}_s\mathbf{a})$ is optimised by the Correspondence Analysis of table **L**. The second term, $\|\mathbf{R}\mathbf{D}_m\mathbf{b}\|_{\mathbf{D}_n}$ is maximised by the analysis of **R** that aims to identify the main structures in this data set. The last term, $\|\mathbf{Q}\mathbf{D}_s\mathbf{a}\|_{\mathbf{D}_p}$ is maximised by the analysis of **Q**.

Box 11.2 RLQ Analysis: dudi Output Elements
In the **ade4** package, the results of an RLQ analysis are stored in an object of class dudi, subclass rlq. This object is a list with 17 elements, including the usual elements of any dudi. In this list, elements of particular interest are:

- $tab: cross-covariances between original variables ($\mathbf{R}^\top\mathbf{P_0Q}$)
- $eig: eigenvalues ($\mathbf{\Lambda}$)
- $l1: coefficients (loadings) for the environmental variables (**B**)
- $c1: coefficients (loadings) for the traits (**A**)
- $aR: projection of the axes of the analysis of **R** on the RLQ axes
- $aQ: projection of the axes of the analysis of **Q** on the RLQ axes
- $lR: scores of sites ($\mathbf{RD}_m\mathbf{b}$)
- $lQ: scores of species ($\mathbf{QD}_s\mathbf{a}$)
- $mR: normed scores of sites
- $mQ: normed scores of species

The randtest function can be used to check the statistical significance of the link between traits and environment (see Box 11.3).

A preliminary step of RLQ analysis is to perform the three separate analyses of abundances, traits and environmental tables. The method is provided by the rlq function that takes three dudi objects as arguments. Before doing the RLQ analysis, species abundances should be treated by a Correspondence Analysis (dudi.coa). Traits and environmental variables are then analysed with any suitable methods. The only constraint here is that these analyses should use the species and site weights computed by the Correspondence Analysis of the abundance table.

In the case of the aravo data set, the quantitative traits are analysed by a PCA (dudi.pca function) and a Hill and Smith Analysis (dudi.hillsmith function) is applied on the environmental table, as it contains a mix of numeric and categorical variables.

```
coaL.aravo <- dudi.coa(aravo$spe, scannf = FALSE)
pcaR.aravo <- dudi.hillsmith(aravo$env, row.w = coaL.aravo$lw,
        scannf = FALSE)
pcaQ.aravo <- dudi.pca(aravo$traits, row.w = coaL.aravo$cw,
        scannf = FALSE)
rlq.aravo <- rlq(pcaR.aravo,coaL.aravo,pcaQ.aravo,
        scannf = FALSE)
```

The plot function can be used to display the main outputs of the analysis (Fig. 11.1). The barplot of eigenvalues (bottom-right) clearly highlights the importance of the first axis (86.7%) but the second dimension (9.8%) will also be used to interpret the main structures of traits-environment relationships.

RLQ analysis computes coefficients ($c1) for the traits and for the environmental variables ($l1) that are represented on the two graphs at the middle-bottom part of the plot ("R loadings" and "Q loadings"). These loadings are used to compute two sets of scores allowing to position sites by their environmental conditions ($lR,

```
pl1 <- plot(rlq.aravo)
```

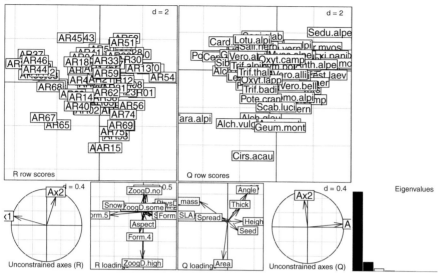

Fig. 11.1 Plot of the outputs of an RLQ analysis. This is a composite plot made of seven graphs (see text for an explanation of the seven graphs).

top-left graph) and species by their traits ($1Q, top-right graph). RLQ analysis maximises the squared cross-covariances, weighted by the abundances, between these two sets of scores.

Note that the outputs of RLQ analysis displayed by the **adegraphics** package are objects and thus can be updated (see Chap. 4). For instance, it is possible to zoom and update the three graphs representing species (Q row scores), environmental variables (R loadings) and traits (Q loadings) to facilitate their interpretation (Fig. 11.2).

The left (negative) part of the first RLQ axis identifies species (*Poa supina* (Poa.supi), *Alchemilla pentaphyllea* (Alch.pent) or *Taraxacum alpinum* (Tara.alpi)) with higher specific leaf area (SLA) and mass-based leaf nitrogen content (N_mass), lower height (Height) and a reduced seed mass (Seed). These species were mostly found in late-melting habitats. The right part of the axis highlights traits attributes (upright and thick leaves) associated with convex landforms, physically disturbed and mostly early-melting sites. Corresponding species are *Sempervivum montanum* (Semp.mont), *Androsace adfinis* (Andr.brig) or *Lloydia serotina* (Lloy.sero). The second RLQ axis outlined zoogenic disturbed sites located in concave slopes. These habitats were characterised by large-leaved species (*Cirsium acaule* (Cirs.acau), *Geum montanum* (Geum.mont) or *Alchemilla vulgaris* (Alch.vulg)).

The two correlation circles on the bottom of Fig. 11.1 show the projection of the first axes of the initial simple analyses (pcaR.aravo and pcaQ.aravo)

```
names(pll)
```

```
[1] "Rrow"       "Qrow"       "Rax"        "Rloadings"
[5] "Qloadings"  "Qax"        "eig"
```

```
col <- rep("transparent", nrow(rlq.aravo$lQ))
col[c(17, 19, 20, 21, 22, 25, 33, 40, 47, 65, 74)] <- "black"
up1 <- update(pll$Qrow, ppoints.cex = 0.5, psub.cex = 1.5,
  plabels = list(col = col, optim = TRUE, box = list(draw = FALSE)),
  plot = FALSE)
up2 <- update(pll$Rloadings, plabels = list(cex = 2), psub.cex = 2,
  plot = FALSE)
up3 <- update(pll$Qloadings, plabels = list(cex = 2), psub.cex = 2,
  plot = FALSE)
ADEgS(list(up1, up2, up3), layout = list(matrix(c(1, 1, 2, 1, 1, 3),
  nrow = 2, ncol = 3, byrow = TRUE)))
```

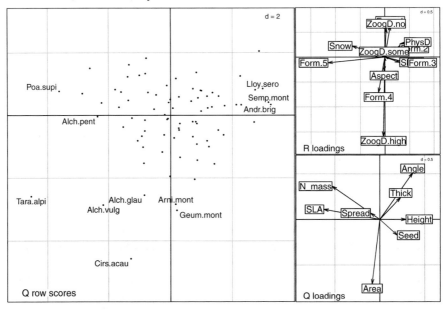

Fig. 11.2 Updated graph showing the species (Q row scores), environmental variables (R loadings) and traits (Q loadings). Only species discussed in the text are labelled.

onto the RLQ axes ($aR and $aQ). These graphs provide a convenient way to look at the relationships between the main structures of each data set (identified by simple analyses) and the co-structures identified by RLQ analysis. For the traits data, the first two axes of the simple PCA are nearly equivalent to the RLQ axes. For environmental data, RLQ has performed an inversion of sign of the first axis and a slight clockwise rotation.

The summary function provides several useful results about the analysis, especially concerning the maximised criteria:

```
summary(rlq.aravo)

RLQ analysis

Class: rlq dudi
Call: rlq(dudiR = pcaR.aravo, dudiL = coaL.aravo,
    dudiQ = pcaQ.aravo, scannf = FALSE)

Total inertia: 1.578

Eigenvalues:
      Ax1       Ax2       Ax3       Ax4       Ax5
1.367618  0.154783  0.045189  0.006948  0.001993

Projected inertia (%):
     Ax1      Ax2      Ax3      Ax4      Ax5
 86.6481   9.8066   2.8630   0.4402   0.1263

Cumulative projected inertia (%):
     Ax1    Ax1:2    Ax1:3    Ax1:4    Ax1:5
   86.65    96.45    99.32    99.76    99.88

(Only 5 dimensions (out of 8) are shown)

Eigenvalues decomposition:
      eig   covar     sdR     sdQ    corr
1  1.3676  1.1695   1.464   1.530  0.5221
2  0.1548  0.3934   1.241   1.152  0.2753

Inertia & coinertia R (pcaR.aravo):
     inertia     max   ratio
1      2.143   2.266  0.9458
12     3.682   4.113  0.8953

Inertia & coinertia Q (pcaR.aravo):
     inertia     max   ratio
1      2.341   2.409  0.9718
12     3.667   3.907  0.9386

Correlation L (coaL.aravo):
     corr     max   ratio
1  0.5221  0.8128  0.6424
2  0.2753  0.6484  0.4246
```

As for any object inheriting from the dudi class, the eigenvalues and percentages of (cumulative) projected inertia are returned (see Sect. 3.4). Information on the eigenvalues and their decomposition is also returned. Eigenvalues in RLQ analysis are squared cross-covariances between linear combinations of species traits ($1Q) and environmental variables ($1R).

The Eigenvalues decomposition table gives the eigenvalues (eig) and their square root (covar). As shown in Box 11.1, the covariance is equal to the product of the correlation between $1R and $1Q (corr), the standard deviation of the environmental score $1R (sdR) and the standard deviation of the species traits score $1Q (sdQ).

The maximal possible values for the standard deviations are produced by the simple analyses of the initial tables (pcaR.aravo, pcaQ.aravo) that identify the main structures of each data set. The two tables, Inertia & coinertia, allow to compare the quantity of variance captured by the RLQ analysis (inertia) to the maximum possible value provided by the simple analysis (max). It is therefore possible to ensure that an important part of the information contained in each table (structures) is preserved in the co-structures.

The last table, `Correlation L`, compares the correlation between the traits-based species scores (`$1Q`) and the environmental site scores (`$1R`) captured by RLQ analysis to the maximum possible value provided by the Correspondence Analysis of the abundance table (`max`). For the `aravo` data set, it is noticeable that the correlation is quite low for the second axis (0.2753). The variance of the environmental scores is well preserved on the first two axes (89.53%). For the traits, the amount of variance preserved (2.341 and 3.667) in nearly equal to the amount obtained in simple Principal Component Analysis (2.409 and 3.907).

The total inertia (i.e., the sum of eigenvalues) is a multivariate measure of the global link between traits and environment. Its significance can be tested by a two-step procedure described in Box 11.3. The link is highly significant:

```
randtest(rlq.aravo, modeltype = 6, nrepet = 999)


class: krandtest lightkrandtest
Monte-Carlo tests
Call: randtest.rlq(xtest = rlq.aravo, nrepet = 999, modeltype = 6)

Number of tests:    2

Adjustment method for multiple comparisons:    none
Permutation number:     999
       Test    Obs Std.Obs    Alter Pvalue
1 Model 2 1.578    27.15 greater  0.001
2 Model 4 1.578    13.24 greater  0.001
```

11.3 Fourth-Corner Analysis

Whereas RLQ analysis provides a global picture of the traits-environment relationships, the fourth-corner (Legendre et al. 1997) allows to test the significance of individual trait-environment associations (i.e., one trait and one environmental variable at a time). Similarly to RLQ analysis, the fourth-corner method computes a matrix containing measures of trait-environment associations (see details in Legendre et al. 1997; Dray and Legendre 2008).

In this array, each cell corresponds to a bivariate association whose statistical significance can be evaluated. Since the fourth-corner method considers variables measured on different statistical units (species and sites), appropriate randomisation techniques should be used to obtain an adequate testing procedure (see Box 11.3). The only valid method consists in combining the outputs of two tests based on different types of permutations.

Fourth-corner is implemented in the `fourthcorner` function and the combined testing procedure can be used if the `modeltype` argument of the `randtest` function is set to 6. As the fourth-corner procedure involves a test for each combination of one single trait and one environmental variable, many tests are performed and p-values could be adjusted to avoid multiple comparison issues using the `p.adjust.method.G` and `p.adjust.method.D` arguments. A very high number of repetitions (`nrepet <- 49999`) is set in order to have enough power in corrected tests. This is time-consuming and could be modified to speed up the different analyses (e.g., `nrepet <- 999`).

Box 11.3 Testing the Significance of Traits-Environment Relationships

Testing the significance of the link between traits (**Q**) and environment (**R**) mediated by the abundance (**L**) is not a trivial issue. As the variables considered are measured on different statistical units (p species and n sites), adapted testing procedures should be considered. Several permutation models have been proposed in the literature to resolve the problem (Model 1–4 in Legendre et al. (1997), Model 5 in Dolédec et al. (1996)):

- Model 1: Permute abundance values for each species independently (i.e., within each column of **L**)
- Model 2: Permute the n sites (i.e., rows of **R** or **L**)
- Model 3: Permute abundance values for each site independently (i.e., within each row of **L**)
- Model 4: Permute the p species (i.e., rows of **Q** or columns of **L**)
- Model 5: Permute the p species and after (or before), permute the n sites (i.e., permute the rows of both tables **R** and **Q**)

It is demonstrated in Dray and Legendre (2008) that all these procedures (Model 1–5) did not truly control the type I error and an alternative based on the combination of two permutation models is proposed. This procedure (Model 6) consists in performing two separate tests using models 2 and 4 and combine the results by keeping the highest p-value (p_{max}) produced by the two permutation tests:

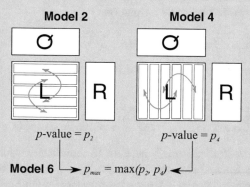

It is demonstrated in ter Braak et al. (2012) that a sequential test with a global significance level α, that controls the type I error in all cases, is simply provided by comparing p_{max} to α.

```
nrepet <- 49999
four.comb.aravo <- fourthcorner(aravo$env, aravo$spe,
```

```
aravo$traits, modeltype = 6, p.adjust.method.G = "none",
    p.adjust.method.D = "none", nrepet = nrepet)
```

Results can be reported using the summary or print methods. The former returns outputs for variables whereas the latter provides detailed results for levels in the case of categorical variables. Outputs can also be plotted. In this example, there are some associations between categorical traits and quantitative environmental variables. These associations can be measured in three different ways (Legendre et al. 1997). The three methods correspond to three possible values of the stat argument in the plot and print functions:

- stat = "D2": the association is measured between the quantitative variable and each category separately. A correlation coefficient is used to indicate the strength of the association between the given category and the small or large values of the quantitative variable.
- stat = "G": the association between the quantitative variable and the whole categorical variable is measured by a global statistic (F).
- stat = "D": the association is estimated between the quantitative variable and each category separately by a measure of the within-group homogeneity. The strength of the association is indicated by the dispersion of the values of the quantitative variable for a given category.

In the rest of the chapter, we focus on the D2 statistic. The correction of p-values by a sequential procedure (Box 11.3, ter Braak et al. 2012) leads to significant associations if the maximal p-value is lower than $\alpha = 0.05$. In this case, there are only 26 significant associations (Fig. 11.3), while there are 51 when $\alpha = \sqrt{0.05}$, i.e., the biased version proposed by Dray and Legendre (2008).

Adjusted p-values for multiple comparisons are obtained with the fdr method using the p.adjust.4thcorner function.

```
four.comb.aravo.adj <- p.adjust.4thcorner(four.comb.aravo,
    p.adjust.method.G = "fdr", p.adjust.method.D = "fdr")
```

Note that adjusted p-values can be obtained directly using the fourthcorner function:

```
fourthcorner(aravo$env, aravo$spe, aravo$traits,
    modeltype = 6, p.adjust.method.G = "fdr",
    p.adjust.method.D = "fdr", nrepet = nrepet)
```

When adjusted p-values are used, there are 18 significant associations (Fig. 11.4). SLA and N_mass showed the same trend (positive correlation with snow (Snow) and landform concavity (Form.5), negative correlation with right slope (Form.3) and physical disturbance (PhysD)). This high number of significant tests is linked to the strong snow-melting gradient (also depicted by RLQ axis 1).

Other significant bivariate tests could be identified, e.g., the associations between plant height (Height) and right slopes (Form.3), and between leaf area (Area) and zoogenic disturbance (ZoogD.high). This last relationship was indeed described by the second RLQ axis.

```
plot(four.comb.aravo, alpha = 0.05, stat = "D2")
```

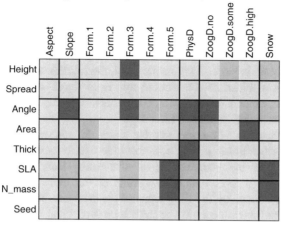

Fig. 11.3 Plot of the outputs of a fourth-corner analysis. Blue cells correspond to negative significant relationships while red cells correspond to positive significant relationships (this can be modified using the argument `col`).

```
plot(four.comb.aravo.adj, alpha = 0.05, stat = "D2")
```

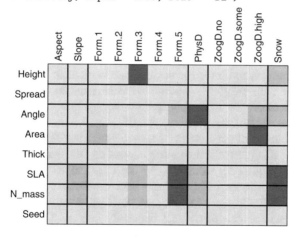

Fig. 11.4 Plot of the outputs of a fourth-corner analysis. *p*-values have been adjusted for multiple comparisons using the false discovery rates. Blue cells correspond to negative significant relationships while red cells correspond to positive significant relationships.

11.4   Combining Both Approaches

RLQ analysis summarises multivariate structures but it does not provide significance tests for the associations. Moreover, the factor maps are difficult to read when the number of variables is large. On the other hand, the fourth-corner analysis only tests the significance of bivariate associations and it does not consider the covariation among traits or among environmental variables. The resulting high number of statistical tests is also difficult to summarise.

To take advantage of both method that share the analysis of a matrix of trait-environment associations, a single framework can be used to summarise and simultaneously test the main ecological structures (Dray et al. 2014). A first approach consists in representing the results of the fourth-corner tests onto the factorial map produced by the RLQ analysis. In that case, RLQ scores are used to position traits and environmental variables on a biplot and significant associations detected by the fourth-corner tests are depicted by lines. This procedure results in a global representation of the significant links as edges of a correlation network. It has the main advantage of summarising the results of the two analyses using a single biplot that facilitates the interpretation of ecological structures.

However, the approach does not solve all the problems described above because the computation of each analysis is performed separately and their outputs are combined *a posteriori*.

Both approaches can be combined if RLQ scores are used to represent traits and environmental variables on a biplot. Then, significant associations revealed by the fourth-corner approach can be represented using segments (blue lines for negative associations, red lines for positive associations, see the `col` argument). Only traits and environmental variables that have at least one significant association are represented. Here, we apply this method using adjusted *p*-values for multiple comparisons and a significance level $\alpha = 0.05$.

The representation of the significant associations identified by the fourth-corner method onto the RLQ factorial map helps interpreting the main patterns of variation and correlation (Fig. 11.5). Compared to the classical RLQ outputs (Fig. 11.1), the interpretation focuses only on traits and environmental variables that are significantly related. Groups of significant positive associations can be identified (e.g., `SLA`, `N_mass` with `Snow` and concavity (`Form.5`), leaf area with high zoogenic disturbance). However, it is much harder to summarise the high number of significant negative associations (blue lines in Fig. 11.5).

Another approach (Dray et al. 2014) is provided by the `fourthcorner.rlq` function and consists in testing directly the links between RLQ axes and traits (`typetest = "Q.axes"`) or environmental variables (`typetest = "R.axes"`).

```
plot(four.comb.aravo.adj, x.rlq = rlq.aravo, alpha = 0.05,
     stat = "D2", type = "biplot")
```

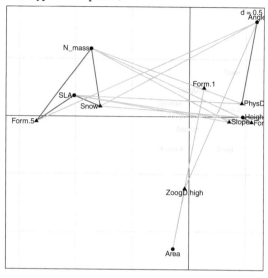

Fig. 11.5 Biplot of the outputs of an RLQ analysis. Relationships are tested by the fourth-corner method and positive significant associations are represented by red lines whereas negative are in blue.

```
testQaxes.comb.aravo <- fourthcorner.rlq(rlq.aravo,
       modeltype = 6, typetest = "Q.axes", nrepet = nrepet,
       p.adjust.method.G = "fdr", p.adjust.method.D = "fdr")
testRaxes.comb.aravo <- fourthcorner.rlq(rlq.aravo,
       modeltype = 6, typetest = "R.axes", nrepet = nrepet,
       p.adjust.method.G = "fdr", p.adjust.method.D = "fdr")
```

The outputs of the different tests can be obtained by the `print` function which allows to specify which statistic should be display:

```
print(testQaxes.comb.aravo, stat = "D")
print(testRaxes.comb.aravo, stat = "D")
```

Results can be represented using a table with colours indicating significance (Fig. 11.6). Significant association with axes can also be reported on the factor map of the RLQ analysis (Fig. 11.7). Testing directly the associations between RLQ axes and traits/environmental variables clearly improves the interpretation of RLQ and fourth-corner results (Figs. 11.6 and 11.7).

The first axis is significantly negatively correlated with snow cover and concavity (late-melting) and positively with physical disturbance and slope (early-melting). Associated traits are higher specific leaf area and nitrogen content for late-melting sites and higher angle and plant height for early melting sites. Choler (2005) hypothesised that high leaf angle in the physically disturbed, early-melting habitats limits nocturnal radiative loss of leaf surfaces and ensures a better structural photoprotection against low-temperature photoinhibition.

```
par(mfrow=c(1,2))
plot(testQaxes.comb.aravo, alpha = 0.05, type = "table", stat = "D2")
plot(testRaxes.comb.aravo, alpha = 0.05, type = "table", stat = "D2")
```

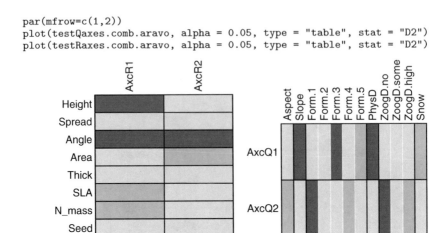

Fig. 11.6 Plot of the outputs of a fourth-corner analysis testing the link between RLQ axes and traits and environmental variables. Blue cells correspond to negative significant relationships while red cells correspond to positive significant relationships.

```
par(mfrow=c(1,2))
plot(testQaxes.comb.aravo, alpha = 0.05, type = "biplot", stat = "D2",
     col = c("black", "blue", "orange", "green"))
plot(testRaxes.comb.aravo, alpha = 0.05, type = "biplot", stat = "D2",
     col = c("black", "blue", "orange", "green"))
```

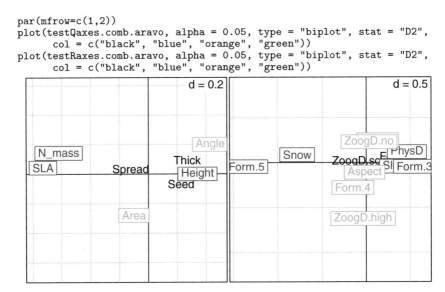

Fig. 11.7 Plot of the outputs of a fourth-corner analysis, with a test of the link between RLQ axes and traits and environmental variables. Significant associations with the first axis are represented in blue, with the second axis in orange, with both axes in green (variables with no significant association are in black).

The second axis opposes convex sites with no zoogenic disturbance and concave slopes where marmots are present. Communities found in these disturbed sites have higher leaf area and lower angle. Zoogenic disturbance and milder habitat conditions in the middle part of the mesotopographical gradient may explain the occurrence of large-leaved, light-demanding rosette forbs such as *Geum montanum* (`Geum.mont`), *Alchemilla glaucescens* (`Alch.glau`) or *Arnica montana* (`Arni.mont`) (Figs. 11.1 and 11.2), a set of species that are more commonly found at lower elevation.

11.5 Extensions

The `fourthcorner2` function computes modified bivariate statistics that sum up to the global statistic provided by the RLQ analysis (Dray and Legendre 2008). Extensions of RLQ and fourth-corner methods have been proposed in the literature to consider spatial and phylogenetic information (e.g., Pavoine et al. 2011) in the analysis of trait-environment relationships. It is also possible to analyse the influence of a partition of sites in several groups (Within- and Between-Class Analyses, Chap. 7) on an object created by the `rlq` function with the `bca.rlq` function (partial RLQ, Wesuls et al. 2012, see `example(bca.rlq)`).

Chapter 12
Analysing Spatial Structures

Abstract In many cases, multivariate data are collected for entities that are geographically located (i.e., georeferenced). This chapter describes several techniques to incorporate the spatial information in multivariate methods using packages **sp**, **spdep** and **adespatial**.

12.1 Introduction

Spatial data are commonly used in Ecology due to the development of technologies for their gathering (e.g., global positioning system, satellite imagery) and management (e.g., geographic information system). Hence, sampled entities (e.g., sites) are described by the measurements of environmental variables and/or species abundances as well as geographical attributes. Since the early work of Goodall (1954), a major concern of Ecology is the identification and explanation of the spatial patterns of ecological structures. Answering these questions leads to the notion of *spatial autocorrelation* and requires multivariate methods that consider explicitly the spatial information. Whereas traditional approaches used polynomial of geographical coordinates (trend-surface analysis) or distances (Mantel-based approaches), this chapter focuses on recent methods that introduce space using a Spatial Weighting Matrix (SWM).

12.2 Managing Spatial Data

The **sp** package provides classes and methods to manage spatial data in **R** (Bivand et al. 2013; Pebesma and Bivand 2005). It allows to deal with raster (grid of cells) and vector (lines, points or polygons) data with or without attributes. This chapter focuses on vector data stored using the `SpatialPoints` and `SpatialPolygons` classes. Usually, spatial data are managed in Geographic Information System (GIS) and the **maptools** package (Bivand and Lewin-Koh 2017) contains functions to import these data directly in **R**. For instance, the

© Springer Science+Business Media, LLC, part of Springer Nature 2018
J. Thioulouse et al., *Multivariate Analysis of Ecological Data with ade4*,
https://doi.org/10.1007/978-1-4939-8850-1_12

readShapeSpatial function offers a convenient way to import a shapefile in **R**.

This chapter will use the mafragh data set (de Bélair and Bencheikh-Lehocine 1987; Pavoine et al. 2011) of the **ade4** package. It contains abundance values of 56 plant species at 97 sites located in the Mafragh plain (Algeria). Species names are recorded in mafragh$spenames, a dataframe with 56 rows and 2 columns: the scientific name in column 1 and a 4-character code in column 2. The geographical coordinates of the sites (mafragh$xy) can be used to build an object of class Spatialpoints (see Fig. 12.1).

In the **adegraphics** package, the s.Spatial function allows to represent these Spatial-inherited objects (Fig. 12.2).

```
library(ade4)
library(adespatial)
library(adegraphics)
library(sp)
data(mafragh)
names(mafragh$flo) <- mafragh$spenames[, 2]
maf.Sp <- mafragh$Spatial.contour
mflo <- mafragh$flo
xy.Sp <- SpatialPoints(mafragh$xy)
plot(xy.Sp, cex = 0.5)
box()
```

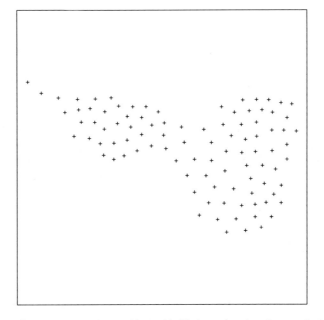

Fig. 12.1 Plot of a SpatialPoints object with 97 sites using the plot method provided by the sp package.

```
s.Spatial(xy.Sp, Sp = maf.Sp, plabels.boxes.draw = FALSE,
        pSp.col = "white")
```

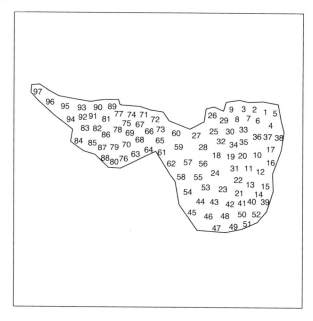

Fig. 12.2 Position of the 97 sampling sites in the Mafragh plain.

A new object belonging to class SpatialPointsDataFrame is created by attaching a dataframe to a SpatialPoints object with the
SpatialPointsDataFrame function. Here, the abundance of the 56 plant
species is attached to the xy.Sp object, producing the xy.SpDF object:

```
xy.SpDF <- SpatialPointsDataFrame(xy.Sp, as.data.frame(mflo))
```

The various classes of **sp** allow to deal with spatial objects that contain
(Spatial*DataFrame) or not (Spatial*) associated data:

```
showClass("Spatial")
```

```
Class "Spatial" [package "sp"]

Slots:

Name:           bbox proj4string
Class:          matrix        CRS

Known Subclasses:
Class "SpatialPoints", directly
Class "SpatialMultiPoints", directly
Class "SpatialGrid", directly
Class "SpatialLines", directly
Class "SpatialPolygons", directly
Class "SpatialPointsDataFrame", by class "SpatialPoints",
        distance 2
Class "SpatialPixels", by class "SpatialPoints", distance 2
Class "SpatialMultiPointsDataFrame", by class
```

```
            "SpatialMultiPoints", distance 2
Class "SpatialGridDataFrame", by class "SpatialGrid", distance 2
Class "SpatialLinesDataFrame", by class "SpatialLines",
        distance 2
Class "SpatialPixelsDataFrame", by class "SpatialPoints",
        distance 3
Class "SpatialPolygonsDataFrame", by class "SpatialPolygons",
        distance 2
```

The s.Spatial function allows to represent these Spatial*DataFrame objects by thematic maps (Fig. 12.3). An alternative to represent spatial data is provided by the other plotting functions of **adegraphics** (for example, s.value, see Sect. 4.4), using the Sp argument.

12.3   From Spatial Data to Spatial Weights

Spatial structures manifest themselves by the relationship (or lack of independence) between values observed at neighbouring sites in space (Dray et al. 2012; Legendre 1993). In many instances, sampling sites that are closer tend to display values that are more similar than sites that are further apart, resulting in positive spatial dependence. In order to detect spatial patterns, a first step is to define spatial neighbouring relationships between sites. These spatial links are stored in a Spatial Weighting Matrix (SWM). In its broader sense, an SWM is usually a square symmetric matrix (sites-by-sites) that contains non-negative values expressing the strengths of the potential exchanges between the spatial units; conventionally, diagonal values are set to zero. In its simplest form, an SWM is a binary matrix, with ones for pairs of sites considered as neighbours and zeros otherwise. The **spdep** package (Bivand and Piras 2015; Bivand et al. 2013) provides tools to create and manipulate spatial weighting matrices.

In the **spdep** package, the user should first create a spatial neighbourhood object (nb class) that will be converted, in a second step, to an SWM (listw object). If sampling sites are polygons (SpatialPolygons), the poly2nb function creates a neighbourhood object by considering that two sites are neighbours if they share a common boundary. For regular grid of points, the cell2nb function allows to define *rook* and *queen* neighbourhoods. If sampling sites are points irregularly spaced, several approaches can be considered. An intuitive way is to define a distance criteria that sees two sites as neighbours if their distance is below a threshold value:

```
library(spdep)
(nb1 <- dnearneigh(xy.Sp, 0, 23))


Neighbour list object:
Number of regions: 97
Number of nonzero links: 316
Percentage nonzero weights: 3.358
Average number of links: 3.258
4 regions with no links:
54 58 96 97
```

```
g1 <- s.Spatial(xy.SpDF[, c("Phco", "Homa", "Mein")],
       scale = FALSE, col = c("black", "palegreen3"), Sp = maf.Sp,
       psub.cex = 2, plot = FALSE)
spobj <- SpatialPolygonsDataFrame(Sr = mafragh$Spatial,
       data = mflo[, c("Phco", "Homa", "Mein")], match.ID = FALSE)
mypal <- colorRampPalette(c("#EDF8FB", "#006D2C"))
g2 <- s.Spatial(spobj, ppalette.quanti = mypal, psub.cex = 2,
       plot = FALSE)
g3 <- s.value(mafragh$xy, mflo[, c("Phco", "Homa", "Mein")],
       symbol = "circle", Sp = maf.Sp, col = c("black",
       "palegreen3"), psub.cex = 2, plot = FALSE)
ADEgS(list(g1, g2, g3), layout = c(3, 1))
```

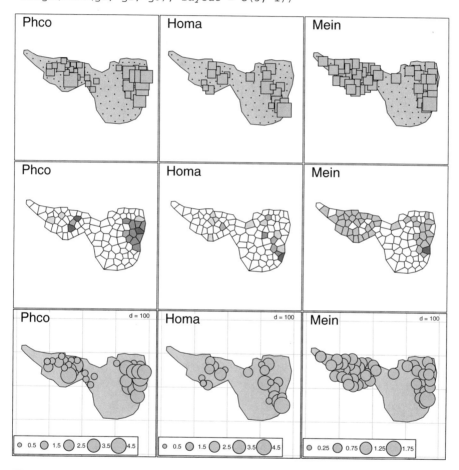

Fig. 12.3 Distribution of the abundance of 3 plant species (*Phalaris coerulescens*, *Hordeum marinum*, and *Medicago intertexta*) in the 97 sites, using the s.Spatial function with a SpatialPoints object (top), with a SpatialPolygons object (middle), and using the s.value function (bottom).

```
g1 <- s.label(mafragh$xy, Sp = maf.Sp, nb = nb1,
       pSp.col = "grey", pnb.edge.col = "red", ppoints.cex = 1.5,
       plabels.cex = 0, plot = FALSE)
g2 <- s.label(mafragh$xy, Sp = maf.Sp, nb = nb2,
       pSp.col = "grey", pnb.edge.col = "red", ppoints.cex = 1.5,
       plabels.cex = 0, plot = FALSE)
ADEgS(list(g1, g2))
```

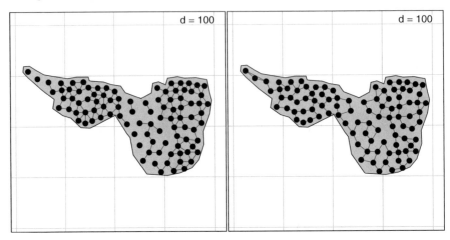

Fig. 12.4 Neighbourhoods obtained using distance (left) and nearest neighbours (right) criteria.

It is also possible to define neighbourhood by a criteria based on nearest neighbours. However, this option can lead to non-symmetric neighbourhood: if site A is the nearest neighbour of site B, it does not mean that site B is the nearest neighbour of site A. The `knearneigh` function creates an object of class knn that can be transformed into an nb object with the `knn2nb` function. The `sym` argument forces the output neighbourhood to be symmetric:

```
(nb2 <- knn2nb(knearneigh(xy.Sp, k = 2), sym = TRUE))
```

```
Neighbour list object:
Number of regions: 97
Number of nonzero links: 260
Percentage nonzero weights: 2.763
Average number of links: 2.68
```

Neighbourhood objects are directly related to the binary matrix representation of graphs where sites correspond to nodes. An edge links two neighbours and is coded by 1 in the associated adjacency matrix (Fig. 12.4).

These definitions of neighbourhood can lead to unconnected subgraphs. The `n.comp.nb` function finds the number of disjoint connected subgraphs:

```
n.comp.nb(nb1)
```

```
$nc
[1] 9

$comp.id
```

```
 [1] 1 1 1 1 1 1 1 1 1 1 1 1 1 1 1 1 1 1 1 1 1 2 2 1 1 3 3
[29] 1 1 1 1 1 1 1 1 1 1 1 1 1 1 2 2 2 1 1 1 1 1 1 2 4 2 2
[57] 2 5 6 6 7 7 7 7 7 7 7 7 7 7 7 7 7 7 7 7 7 7 7 7 7 7 7
[85] 7 7 7 7 7 7 7 7 7 7 8 9
```

More elaborate approaches derived from graph theory are available to depict connectivity (Jaromczyk and Toussaint 1992; Dale and Fortin 2010). For instance, Delaunay triangulation is obtained with the `tri2nb` function that requires the `deldir` package (Turner 2018). Other procedures are also available such as Gabriel graph (see the `gabrielneigh` function) or relative neighbourhood (see the `relativeneigh` function).

The `edit.nb` function provides an interactive tool to add or delete connections from an existing `nb` object. Other utility functions are provided in **spdep** to manipulate neighbourhood objects (see `diffnb`, `intersect.nb`, `union.nb`, `setdiff.nb`, `complement.nb`, `droplinks` and `nblag`).

In a second step, the `nb2listw` function is used to convert the neighbourhood object (class `nb`) into an SWM (object of the `listw` class). As binary spatial links may appear too restrictive to represent complex inter-site relationships, this function allows to explicitly weight the spatial relationships among sampling locations using the `glist` argument. For instance, edges can be weighted by a function of geographical distances using the `nbdists` function. The `style` argument allows to define a global transformation of the SWM such as standardisation by row sum, by total sum, binary coding, etc.

For instance, the row-standardised SWM based on a Gabriel graph with edges weighted by inverse distances is obtained by:

```
xym <- as.matrix(mafragh$xy)
nb3 <- graph2nb(gabrielneigh(xym), sym = TRUE)
invdist <- lapply(nbdists(nb3, xym), function(x) 1/x)
lw3 <- nb2listw(nb3, glist = invdist, style = "W")
names(lw3)
```

```
[1] "style"      "neighbours" "weights"
```

```
lw3$neighbours[[1]]
```

```
[1] 2 4 5 6
```

```
lw3$weights[[1]]
```

```
[1] 0.2563 0.1997 0.2931 0.2509
```

To facilitate the building of spatial neighbourhoods (`nb` object) and associated spatial weighting matrices (`listw` object), the **adespatial** package provides the `listw.candidates` function which is a wrapper to **spdep** functions (Dray et al. 2018). It also provides an interactive graphical interface which can be launched by the call `listw.explore()` assuming that spatial coordinates are still stored in an object of the **R** session (see Fig. 12.5).

When the `listw` object has been specified, it is then possible to compute a spatial autocorrelation index to measure how the values of a variable are more similar when the sampling sites are closer.

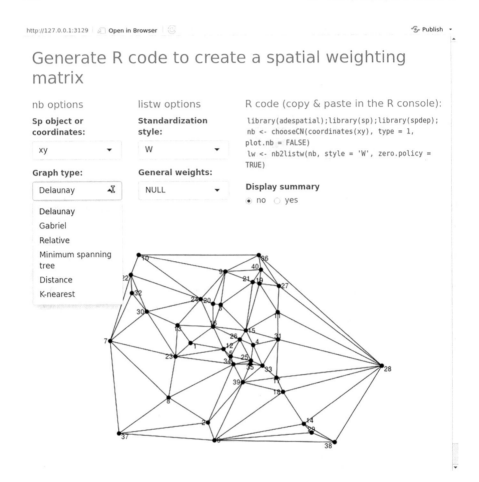

Fig. 12.5 Interactive interface implemented in the `listw.explore` function. It provides code to produce spatial weighting matrices that can be copied and pasted in the console.

12.4   Spatial Autocorrelation

Geary's ratio (Geary 1954) and Moran's coefficient MC (Moran 1948) are standard approaches to measure spatial autocorrelation by quantifying the degree of dependency among observations in a geographical context (see Box 12.1). The `moran.randtest` function (which is a wrapper to the `moran.mc` function of the **spdep** package) allows to compute MC and test its significance by a randomisation procedure:

```
moran.randtest(mflo[, "Boma"], listw = lw3, nrepet = 999)

Monte-Carlo test
Call: moran.randtest(x = mflo[, "Boma"], listw = lw3,
  nrepet = 999)
```

```
Observation: 0.4195

Based on 999 replicates
Simulated p-value: 0.001
Alternative hypothesis: greater

Std.Obs.statistic          Expectation              Variance
       6.629584            -0.011312               0.004222
```

Box 12.1 Moran's Coefficient and Moran Scatterplot

Let us consider the $n \times 1$ vector $\mathbf{x} = (x_1 \cdots x_n)^\top$ containing measurements of a quantitative variable for n spatial units and $\mathbf{W} = [w_{ij}]$ the $n \times n$ spatial weighting matrix. The usual formulation for Moran's coefficient of spatial autocorrelation is:

$$MC(\mathbf{x}) = \frac{n \sum_{(2)} w_{ij}(x_i - \bar{x})(x_j - \bar{x})}{\sum_{(2)} w_{ij} \sum_{i=1}^{n}(x_i - \bar{x})^2} \text{ where } \sum_{(2)} = \sum_{i=1}^{n}\sum_{j=1}^{n} \text{ with } i \neq j$$

MC can be rewritten using matrix notation:

$$MC(\mathbf{x}) = \frac{n}{\mathbf{1}^\top \mathbf{W} \mathbf{1}} \frac{\mathbf{z}^\top \mathbf{W} \mathbf{z}}{\mathbf{z}^\top \mathbf{z}}$$

where $\mathbf{z} = \left(\mathbf{I}_n - \mathbf{1}_n \mathbf{1}_n^\top / n\right) \mathbf{x}$ is the vector of centred values ($z_i = x_i - \bar{x}$) and $\mathbf{1}_n$ is a vector of ones (of length n).

The numerator of MC corresponds to the covariation between contiguous observations. The significance of the observed value of MC can be tested by a Monte-Carlo procedure, in which locations are permuted to obtain a distribution of MC under the null hypothesis of random distribution. An observed value of MC that is greater than that expected at random indicates the clustering of similar values across space (positive spatial autocorrelation), while a significant negative value of MC indicates that neighbouring values are more dissimilar than expected by chance (negative spatial autocorrelation).

If the SWM is row-standardised (i.e., $w_{ij} = \frac{w_{ij}}{\sum_{j=1}^{n} w_{ij}}$), we can define the lag vector $\tilde{\mathbf{z}} = \mathbf{W}\mathbf{z}$ (i.e., $\tilde{z}_i = \sum_{j=1}^{n} w_{ij}x_j$) composed of the weighted (by the spatial weighting matrix) averages of the neighbouring values. MC can then be rewritten as:

$$MC(\mathbf{x}) = \frac{\mathbf{z}^\top \tilde{\mathbf{z}}}{\mathbf{z}^\top \mathbf{z}}$$

(continued)

Box 12.1 (continued)

In this case, MC measures the autocorrelation by giving an indication of the intensity of the linear association between the vector of observed values **z** and the vector of weighted averages of neighbouring values **z̃** (lag vector). MC can then be visualised in the form of a bivariate scatterplot of **z̃** against **z**. A linear regression can be added to this *Moran scatterplot*, with slope equal to MC to represent the degree of spatial autocorrelation and detect the presence of outliers or local pockets of non-stationarity (Anselin 1996).

If the SWM has been row-standardised, it is possible to compute a lag vector that contains the weighted averages of neighbouring values. In this case, MC is equal to the slope of the linear model that explains the variability of the lag vector by the observed values:

```
xlag <- lag.listw(lw3, mflo[, "Mein"])
lm1 <- lm(xlag ~ mflo[, "Mein"])
coefficients(lm1)

   (Intercept) mflo[, "Mein"]
      0.2928           0.3961
```

The relationships between the lag vector and observed values can then be represented on a Moran scatterplot (Fig. 12.6).

12.5   Detecting Spatial Multivariate Structures

When several variables are considered, it is possible to repeat univariate analysis (MC) for each species easily using the `moran.randtest` function of the **adespatial** package:

```
moran.plot(mflo[, "Mein"], listw = lw3)
```

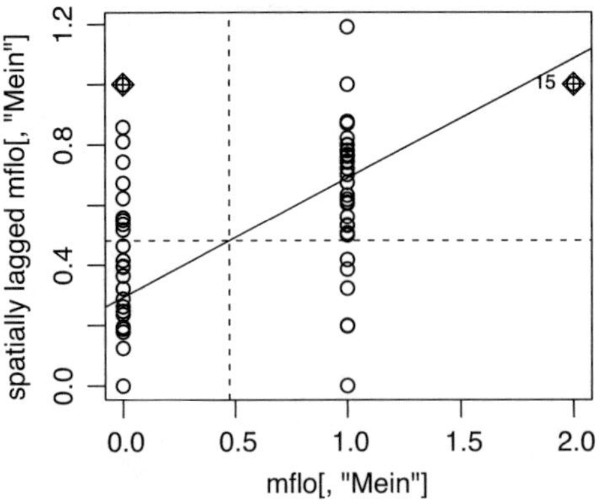

Fig. 12.6 Moran scatterplot of *Medicago intertexta* (`Mein`). The slope of the linear model is equal to MC.

```
(kMC <- moran.randtest(mflo[, c("Boma", "Phco",
      "Homa", "Mein")], listw = lw3))

class: krandtest lightkrandtest
Monte-Carlo tests
Call: moran.randtest(x = mflo[, c("Boma", "Phco", "Homa","Mein")],
      listw = lw3)

Number of tests:    4

Adjustment method for multiple comparisons:    none
Permutation number:    999
   Test     Obs Std.Obs    Alter Pvalue
1 Boma 0.4195   6.350 greater   0.001
2 Phco 0.4887   7.243 greater   0.001
3 Homa 0.2080   3.374 greater   0.004
4 Mein 0.3961   5.778 greater   0.001
```

However, this approach is not optimal as it does not consider properly the multivariate information: each species is treated independently and it is thus not possible to detect similarities between spatial distributions.

The identification of spatial structures requires tools that integrate simultaneously multivariate and spatial aspects. The simplest approach is a two-step procedure where the data are first summarised with a multivariate analysis (PCA, see Sect. 5.2). In a second step, univariate spatial statistics or mapping techniques are applied to PCA scores for each axis separately (Fig. 12.7).

```
pca.spe <- dudi.pca(mflo, scale = FALSE, scannf = FALSE)
mc1 <- moran.mc(pca.spe$li[, 1], lw3, 999)
s.value(mafragh$xy, pca.spe$li[, 1], symbol = "circle",
      Sp = maf.Sp, sub = paste("MC =", round(mc1$statistic, 3)),
      pSp.col = "grey")
```

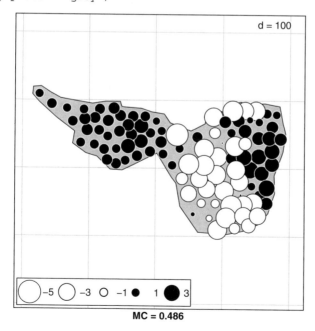

Fig. 12.7 Mapping and MC of the scores on the first PCA axis.

It is very simple to carry out this two-step approach but it has the major disadvantage of being indirect, as it considers the spatial pattern only after summarising the main structures of the multivariate data set. In the next sections, we present several approaches that go one step further by considering the identification of spatial structures and the dimensionality reduction simultaneously.

12.5.1 Moran's Eigenvector Maps (MEMs)

A common practice is to integrate the geographic information by spatial predictors that can be used to evaluate the spatial component of ecological structures. Polynomials of geographic coordinates have been traditionally used but new procedures have been recently proposed as alternatives. Moran's Eigenvector Maps (MEMs) are produced by the diagonalisation of the spatial weighting matrix. These eigenvectors are orthogonal vectors with a unit norm that maximises MC (Box 12.2, Fig. 12.8).

Box 12.2 Moran's Eigenvectors Maps (MEMs)

Let us consider $\mathbf{W} = [w_{ij}]$ the $n \times n$ spatial weighting matrix. If a non-symmetric spatial weighting matrix $\mathbf{W}^*$ has been defined, the results can be generalised using $\mathbf{W} = (\mathbf{W}^* + \mathbf{W}^{*\top})/2$. Moran's eigenvectors maps (MEMs) are the $n - 1$ eigenvectors obtained by the diagonalisation of the doubly-centred SWM:

$$\mathbf{\Omega V} = \mathbf{V\Lambda}$$

where $\mathbf{\Omega} = \mathbf{HWH}$ and $\mathbf{H} = \left(\mathbf{I} - \mathbf{11}^{\top}/n\right)$ is a centring operator.

The upper and lower bounds of MC (de Jong et al. 1984) for a given spatial weighting matrix $\mathbf{W}$ are equal to $\lambda_{\max}(n/\mathbf{1}^{\top}\mathbf{W1})$ and $\lambda_{\min}(n/\mathbf{1}^{\top}\mathbf{W1})$ where $\lambda_{\max}$ and $\lambda_{\min}$ are the extreme eigenvalues of $\mathbf{\Omega}$.

MEMs are stored in matrix $\mathbf{V}$. They are orthogonal vectors with a unit norm that maximise MC (Griffith 1996). MEMs associated with high positive (or negative) eigenvalues have high positive (or negative) autocorrelation. MEMs associated with eigenvalues with small absolute values correspond to low spatial autocorrelation (Dray et al. 2006). Unlike polynomial functions, MEMs have the ability to capture various spatial structures at multiple scales (coarse to fine scales). MEMs have been used for spatial filtering purposes and introduced as spatial predictors in linear models, generalised linear models and multivariate analysis.

MEMs provide a basis of orthonormal vectors that are able to decompose the variance of a variable at multiple scales. They can be used as spatial predictors in

```
(me <- mem(lw3))
```

```
Orthobasis with 97 rows and 96 columns
Only 6 rows and 4 columns are shown
       MEM1    MEM2     MEM3      MEM4
1  0.9859  -2.048  -0.5452  -1.18005
2  0.9438  -1.957  -0.4045  -0.64642
3  0.9090  -1.830  -0.2413  -0.06485
4  1.0213  -1.963  -0.6074  -1.40389
5  0.7473  -1.542  -0.4454  -1.03190
6  1.0157  -2.024  -0.4934  -0.93286
```

```
s.value(mafragh$xy, me[, c(1:3, 94:96)], ppoints.cex = 0.75,
        Sp = maf.Sp, pSp.col = "grey")
```

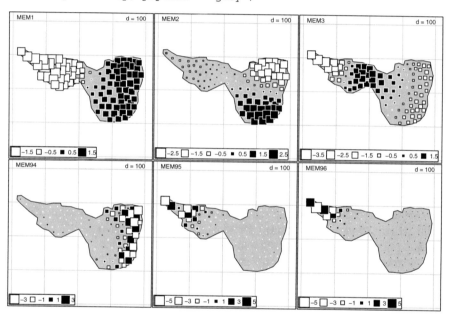

Fig. 12.8 Mapping of the first and last three MEMs. These eigenvectors are orthogonal and maximise MC.

Redundancy Analysis (see Sect. 8.4.1) or variation partitioning methods to identify the main spatial structures of a given data set. However, as the number of MEMs is usually equal to the *number of samples − 1*, a first step of variable selection is required to avoid overfitting. The mem.select function implements different procedures described in Bauman et al. (2018) and will not be detailed further.

Another approach consists in decomposing the total variance of a given variable onto the MEM basis. It is then possible to build a scalogram indicating the part of variance explained by each MEM:

```
scalo <- scalogram(mflo[, "Mein"], me)
sum(scalo$obs)
```

```
[1] 1
```

```
scalo2 <- scalogram(mflo[, "Mein"], me, nblocks = 10)
plot(scalo2)
```

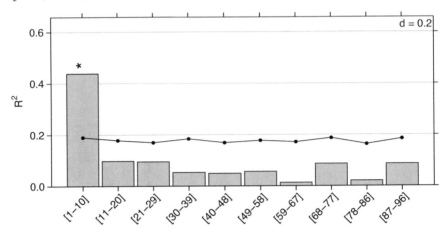

Fig. 12.9 Smoothed scalogram of *Medicago intertexta*. Spatial components are divided in ten groups of successive MEMs (nblocks argument).

Results can be more readable using smoothed scalograms (using the nblocks argument) where spatial components are formed by groups of successive MEMs (Fig. 12.9, Munoz 2009; Dray et al. 2012).

Figure 12.10 shows how the statistically significant spatial components can be related to the spatial distribution of abundances for four species.

It is possible to compute scalograms for all the species of the data table. These scalograms can be stored in a table and analysing this table with a PCA allows to identify the important scales of the data set and the similarities between species based on their spatial distributions (Jombart et al. 2009). This analysis named Multiscale Patterns Analysis (MSPA) is available in the **adespatial** package.

Figure 12.11 shows the biplot of the MSPA of the mafragh data set. The 96 MEMs and the 56 species are plotted, but the spatial maps of 5 important spatial scales (MEM1, MEM2, MEM3, MEM6, MEM96) and 3 associated species (*Borago officinalis* (Boof), *Medicago intertexta* (Mein), and *Halimione portulacoides* (Hapo)) are superimposed over the MSPA factor map. Species are clearly ordered by MSPA according to the similarity of their spatial distribution with MEMs spatial structure.

The number of MEMs can be high, and the results provided by this approach can be difficult to interpret. The nblocks argument of the mspa function allows to create groups of MEMs, which makes easier interpretations.

```
sc1 <- plot(scalogram(mflo[, "Boma"], me, nblocks = 10))
sv1 <- s.value(mafragh$xy, mflo[, "Boma"], Sp = maf.Sp,
        psub = list(text = "Boma", cex = 1.5), plot = FALSE)
sc2 <- plot(scalogram(mflo[, "Mein"], me, nblocks = 10))
sv2 <- s.value(mafragh$xy, mflo[, "Mein"], Sp = maf.Sp,
        psub = list(text = "Mein", cex = 1.5), plot = FALSE)
sc3 <- plot(scalogram(mflo[, "Juma"], me, nblocks = 10))
sv3 <- s.value(mafragh$xy, mflo[, "Juma"], Sp = maf.Sp,
        psub = list(text = "Juma", cex = 1.5), plot = FALSE)
sc4 <- plot(scalogram(mflo[, "Boof"], me, nblocks = 10))
sv4 <- s.value(mafragh$xy, mflo[, "Boof"], Sp = maf.Sp,
        psub = list(text = "Boof", cex = 1.5), plot = FALSE)
ADEgS(list(sc1, sc2, sc3, sc4, sv1, sv2, sv3, sv4),
        layout = c(2, 4))
```

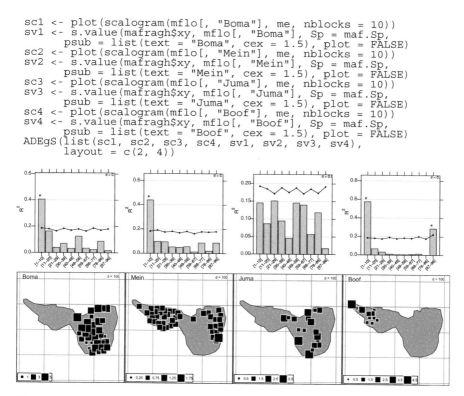

Fig. 12.10 Smoothed scalograms and abundance maps of four species (*Bolboschoenus maritimus, Medicago intertexta, Juncus maritimus* and *Borago officinalis*).

12.5.2 MULTISPATI Analysis

The MEM framework introduced the spatial information into multivariate analysis through the diagonalisation of the spatial weighting matrix. Usually, only a part of the information contained in this matrix is considered because only a subset of MEM are used as regressors in Redundancy Analysis (Sect. 8.4.1). In this last section, we present a multivariate method that considers the Spatial Weighting Matrix in its original form.

MULTISPATI (Multivariate spatial analysis based on Moran's index) aims to identify multivariate spatial structures by studying the link between a table of variables and a table containing their lagged vectors using Coinertia Analysis (8.3). Hence, it extends MC to the multivariate case (Box 12.3).

```
mspa1 <- mspa(pca.spe, me, scannf = FALSE, nf = 2)
oldpar <- adegpar()
adegpar(plegend.drawKey = FALSE, psub.cex = 1.5)
gme <- s.value(mafragh$xy, me[, c(1, 2, 6, 3, 96)], Sp = maf.Sp,
    ppoints.cex = 0.5, plot = FALSE)
gv1 <- s.value(mafragh$xy, mflo[, "Boof"], Sp = maf.Sp,
    ppoints.cex = 0.5, psub.text = "Boof", col = c("black",
    "palegreen2"), plot = FALSE)
gv2 <- s.value(mafragh$xy, mflo[, "Mein"], Sp = maf.Sp,
    ppoints.cex = 0.5, psub.text = "Mein", col = c("black",
    "palegreen2"), plot = FALSE)
gv3 <- s.value(mafragh$xy, mflo[, "Hapo"], Sp = maf.Sp,
    ppoints.cex = 0.5, psub.text = "Hapo", col = c("black",
    "palegreen2"), plot = FALSE)
scl <- scatter(mspa1, posieig = "topright", plot = FALSE)
gil <- insert(gme[[1]], scl, posi = c(0.01, 0.4), plot = FALSE)
gil <- insert(gme[[2]], gil, posi = c(0.43, 0.06), plot = FALSE)
gil <- insert(gme[[3]], gil, posi = c(0.75, 0.01), plot = FALSE)
gil <- insert(gme[[4]], gil, posi = c(0.15, 0.78), plot = FALSE)
gil <- insert(gme[[5]], gil, posi = c(0.50, 0.79), plot = FALSE)
gil <- insert(gv1, gil, posi = c(0.25, 0.54), plot = FALSE)
gil <- insert(gv2, gil, posi = c(0.4, 0.3), plot = FALSE)
gil <- insert(gv3, gil, posi = c(0.78, 0.24))
adegpar(oldpar)
```

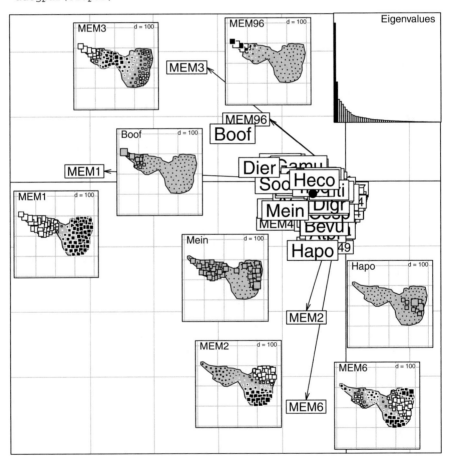

Fig. 12.11 Biplot of MSPA applied to the `mafragh` data set. Plots of important spatial scales (MEM1, MEM2, MEM3, MEM6, MEM96) and associated species (*Borago officinalis*, *Medicago intertexta*, *Halimione portulacoides*) are superimposed over the MSPA factor map.

Box 12.3 MULTISPATI Analysis

MULTISPATI (Multivariate spatial analysis based on Moran's index, Dray et al. 2008) generalised Wartenberg's multivariate spatial correlation method (Wartenberg 1985) by introducing the $n \times n$ row-standardised spatial weighting matrix $\mathbf{W}$ in the analysis of a statistical triplet $(\mathbf{X}, \mathbf{Q}, \mathbf{D})$. Hence, this approach is very general and allows to define spatially constrained versions of various methods (corresponding to different triplets).

By extension of the lag vector (Box 12.1), a lag matrix $\tilde{\mathbf{X}} = \mathbf{WX}$ can be defined. The two tables $\tilde{\mathbf{X}}$ and $\mathbf{X}$ are fully matched, i.e., they have the same columns (variables) and rows (observations). MULTISPATI aims to identify multivariate spatial structures by studying the link between $\tilde{\mathbf{X}}$ and $\mathbf{X}$ using the Coinertia Analysis (Sect. 8.3) of a pair of fully matched tables. It corresponds to the analysis of the statistical triplet $\left(\mathbf{X}, \mathbf{Q}, \frac{1}{2}(\mathbf{W}^\top \mathbf{D} + \mathbf{DW})\right)$. According to Property 3.1 (Box 3.2), MULTISPATI searches for a principal axis $\mathbf{a}$ maximising:

$$Q(\mathbf{a}) = \mathbf{a}^\top \mathbf{Q}^\top \mathbf{X}^\top \frac{1}{2}(\mathbf{W}^\top \mathbf{D}^\top + \mathbf{DW})\mathbf{XQa}$$

$$= \frac{1}{2}(\mathbf{a}^\top \mathbf{Q}^\top \mathbf{X}^\top \mathbf{W}^\top \mathbf{D}^\top \mathbf{XQa} + \mathbf{a}^\top \mathbf{Q}^\top \mathbf{X}^\top \mathbf{DWXQa})$$

$$= \frac{1}{2}\langle \mathbf{XQa}, \mathbf{WXQa}\rangle_\mathbf{D} + \langle \mathbf{WXQa}, \mathbf{XQa}\rangle_\mathbf{D}$$

$$= \mathbf{a}^\top \mathbf{Q}^\top \mathbf{X}^\top \mathbf{DWXQa} = \mathbf{r}^\top \mathbf{DWr} = \mathbf{r}^\top \mathbf{D}\tilde{\mathbf{r}}$$

This analysis maximises the scalar product between a linear combination of original variables ($\mathbf{r} = \mathbf{XQa}$) and a linear combination of lagged variables ($\tilde{\mathbf{r}} = \mathbf{WXQa}$). The maximised quantity can be rewritten as:

$$Q(\mathbf{a}) = \frac{\mathbf{a}^\top \mathbf{Q}^\top \mathbf{X}^\top \mathbf{DWXQa}}{\mathbf{a}^\top \mathbf{Q}^\top \mathbf{X}^\top \mathbf{DXQa}} \mathbf{a}^\top \mathbf{Q}^\top \mathbf{X}^\top \mathbf{DXQa}$$

$$= MC_\mathbf{D}(\mathbf{XQa}) \cdot \|\mathbf{XQa}\|_\mathbf{D}^2 = MC_\mathbf{D}(\mathbf{r}) \cdot \|\mathbf{r}\|_\mathbf{D}^2$$

MULTISPATI finds coefficients ($\mathbf{a}$) to obtain a linear combination of variables ($\mathbf{r} = \mathbf{XQa}$) that maximises a compromise between the classical multivariate analysis ($\|\mathbf{r}\|_\mathbf{D}^2$) and a generalised version of Moran's coefficient ($MC_\mathbf{D}(\mathbf{r})$). The only difference between the classical Moran's coefficient and its generalised version $MC_\mathbf{D}$ is that the second one uses a general matrix of weights $\mathbf{D}$, while the first considers only the usual case of uniform weights ($\mathbf{D} = \frac{1}{n}\mathbf{I}_n$).

In practice, the $\mathbf{Q}$-symmetric matrix $\frac{1}{2}\mathbf{X}^\top(\mathbf{W}^\top \mathbf{D} + \mathbf{DW})\mathbf{Q}$ is diagonalised.

In the **adespatial** package, the `multispati` function is used to compute a MULTISPATI Analysis. This function takes an object of the class `dudi` and a spatial weighting matrix (object of class `listw`) as arguments. It is important to note that this analysis can produce negative eigenvalues, corresponding to negatively autocorrelated spatial structures. Hence, the function asks for the number of positive eigenvalues (`nfposi`) and negative eigenvalues (`nfnega`) corresponding to multivariate structures with positive and negative autocorrelations. Here, we consider only two positive eigenvalues:

```
ms1 <- multispati(pca.spe, lw3, scannf = FALSE, nfposi = 2,
       nfnega = 0)
```

The outputs produced by the analysis are grouped in a `multispati` object and are described in Box 12.4.

Box 12.4 MULTISPATI Analysis: dudi Output Elements
In the **adespatial** package, the results of a MULTISPATI Analysis are stored in an object of class `multispati`. This object is a list with 8 elements. In this list, elements of particular interest are:

- `$eig`: eigenvalues (Λ)
- `$c1`: coefficients (loadings) for the variables ($\mathbf{A}$)
- `$li`: scores of individuals ($\mathbf{R} = \mathbf{XQA}$)
- `$ls`: lagged scores of individuals ($\hat{\mathbf{R}} = \mathbf{WXQA}$)
- `$as`: projection of the axes of the analysis of $\mathbf{X}$ on the MULTISPATI axes

---

Whereas the standard analysis (PCA in this example) identifies the main structures, MULTISPATI seeks for spatial structures. It is therefore important to analyse the differences between the criteria maximised by these two analyses. This comparison is provided by the `summary` function:

```
summary(ms1)

Multivariate Spatial Analysis
Call: multispati(dudi = pca.spe, listw = lw3, scannf = FALSE,
      nfposi = 2, nfnega = 0)

Scores from the initial duality diagram:
      var    cum   ratio   moran
RS1 5.331  5.331  0.2835  0.4863
RS2 1.973  7.304  0.3884  0.4640

Multispati eigenvalues decomposition:
      eig    var    moran
CS1 2.946  4.839  0.6088
CS2 1.217  1.890  0.6437
```

Figure 12.12 includes four graphs. The top graph shows the link between the sites seen by the original data table and seen through the lag vectors. Like in the Coinertia Analysis plot, arrows link the two site coordinates (`ms1$li` and `ms1$ls`). In this case, it corresponds to the score of sites and the lagged score (i.e., average score of the neighbours). The bottom-left graph is the plot of eigenvalues (with positive and negative values), the bottom-right graph is the plot of the PCA (unconstrained) axes projected in the MULTISPATI analysis, and the middle graph shows the species loadings.

`plot(ms1)`

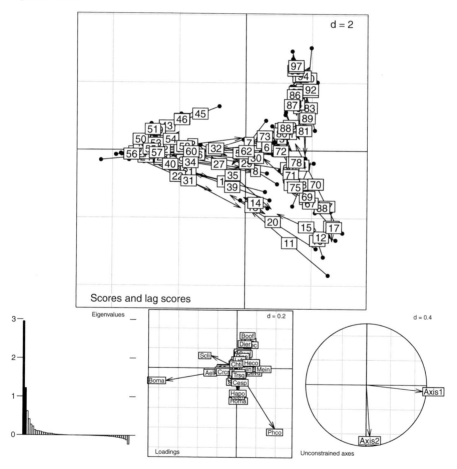

Fig. 12.12 Outputs of MULTISPATI applied to the `mafragh` data set indicating the main spatial structures.

The site score of the analysis (ms1$li) can be mapped to help interpret the outputs (Fig. 12.13). It highlights the main spatial patterns of changes in the composition of floristic communities. For instance, the first axis distinguishes the central part of the study area to the eastern and western parts.

```
s.value(mafragh$xy, ms1$li, Sp = maf.Sp, nb = nb3,
    pSp.col = "grey")
```

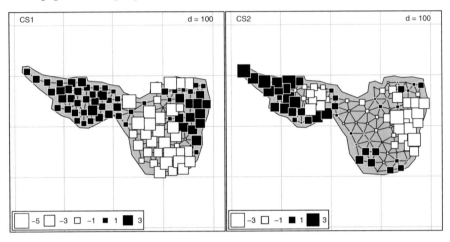

Fig. 12.13 Mapping of MULTISPATI scores corresponding to positive autocorrelated structures.

Figure 12.14 helps interpret species loadings (ms1$c1). It shows the factor map of species with abundance maps for particular species: *Bolboschoenus maritimus* (Boma), *Phalaris coerulescens* (Phco), *Borago officinalis* (Boof) and *Schoenoplectus litoralis* (Scli). These four species have indeed particular spatial distribution, that can be interpreted in relation with environmental factors (see Siberchicot et al. 2017).

Figure 12.15 is the symmetric display of Fig. 12.14 and helps interpret site scores. It shows the MULTISPATI factor map of sites (ms1$li). For particular sites (sites number 11, 60 and 97), it shows the species loadings map with species presence noted with the species label. It is easy to see that these sites present particular species. For instance, *Bolboschoenus maritimus* (Boma) is present in site 60, *Borago officinalis* (Boof) in site 97 and *Phalaris coerulescens* (Phco) in site 11. The site position in the Mafragh plain is given in Fig. 12.2.

```
sa1 <- s.arrow(ms1$c1)
gm1 <- s.value(mafragh$xy, mflo[, c("Scli", "Boma", "Boof",
        "Phco")], Sp = maf.Sp, plegend.drawKey = FALSE,
        ppoints.cex = 0.5, col = c("black", "palegreen3"),
        psub.cex = 1.5, plot = FALSE)
p1 <- list(c(0.1, 0.65), c(0.01, 0.24), c(0.74, 0.7),
        c(0.55, 0.05))
gi2 <- insert(gm1[[1]], sa1, posi = p1[[1]], ratio = 0.25,
        plot = FALSE)
gi2 <- insert(gm1[[2]], gi2, posi = p1[[2]], ratio = 0.25,
        plot = FALSE)
gi2 <- insert(gm1[[3]], gi2, posi = p1[[3]], ratio = 0.25,
        plot = FALSE)
gi2 <- insert(gm1[[4]], gi2, posi = p1[[4]], ratio = 0.25)
```

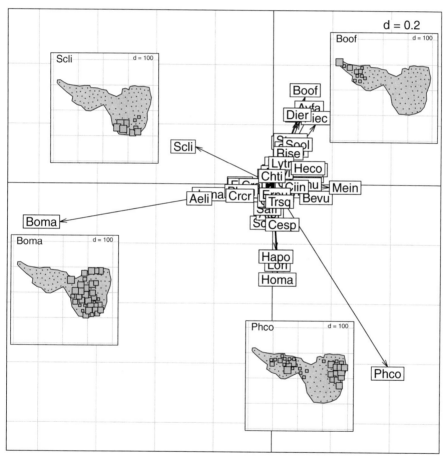

Fig. 12.14 Outputs of MULTISPATI applied to the `mafragh` data set. Loadings for species are represented. Maps of the spatial distributions of *Bolboschoenus maritimus* (`Boma`), *Phalaris coerulescens* (`Phco`), *Borago officinalis* (`Boof`) and *Schoenoplectus litoralis* (`Scli`) are inserted to help the interpretation.

```
sl1 <- s.label(ms1$li)
sl11 <- s.label(ms1$c1, ifelse(mflo[11,] != 0, names(mflo), ""),
        plabels = list(col = "green3", cex = 1.5, optim = TRUE),
        psub = list(text = "site 11", pos = "topleft", cex = 2))
sl60 <- s.label(ms1$c1, ifelse(mflo[60,] != 0, names(mflo), ""),
        plabels = list(col = "green3", cex = 1.5, optim = TRUE),
        psub = list(text = "site 60", pos = "topleft", cex = 2))
sl97 <- s.label(ms1$c1, ifelse(mflo[97,] != 0, names(mflo), ""),
        plabels = list(col = "green3", cex = 1.5, optim = TRUE),
        psub = list(text = "site 97", pos = "topleft", cex = 2))
p1 <- list(c(0.4, 0.72), c(0.01, 0.17), c(0.5, 0.01))
gi3 <- insert(sl97, sl1, posi = p1[[1]], ratio = 0.25,
        plot = FALSE)
gi3 <- insert(sl60, gi3, posi = p1[[2]], ratio = 0.25,
        plot = FALSE)
gi3 <- insert(sl11, gi3, posi = p1[[3]], ratio = 0.25)
```

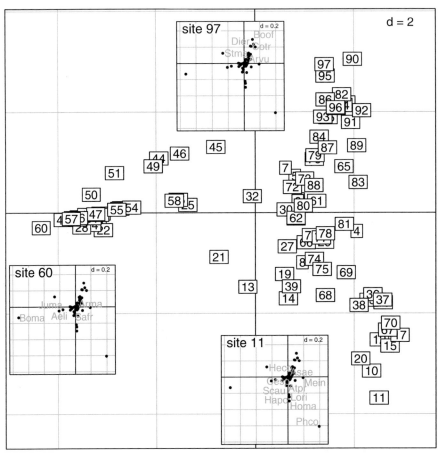

Fig. 12.15 Outputs of MULTISPATI applied to the `mafragh` data set. Representation of site scores. For sites 11, 60 and 97, factorial maps of species are inserted where only species present in these sites are indicated. Geographical map with site numbers is given in Fig. 12.2.

Chapter 13
Analysing Phylogenetic Structures

Abstract This chapter shows how multivariate approaches can be used for investigating phylogenetic structures, focussing on methods for measuring, testing, accounting for and describing a phylogenetic signal.

13.1 Introduction

The constant progress of DNA sequencing technologies combined with powerful phylogenetic reconstruction methods has made phylogenetic trees an increasingly common element of ecological data analysis. The evolutionary relationships underlying a phylogeny often induce non-independence (autocorrelation) in the traits observed in the considered taxa. Simply put, closely related species often tend to look alike and share similar ecological properties. We will refer to such patterns as *phylogenetic structures*. These structures can be a nuisance when modelling biological traits, as they violate the assumption of independence between observations (taxa) made by most likelihood-based approaches as well as tests of association. However, phylogenetic structures can also represent meaningful biological patterns, indicative of interesting evolutionary processes. This dichotomy, at the core of phylogenetic comparative methods (Harvey and Pagel 1991), has motivated a considerable amount of methodological developments over the past decades (Felsenstein 1985; Abouheif 1999; Martins et al. 2002; Blomberg et al. 2003; Revell and Collar 2009).

In this chapter, we introduce methods for the analysis of phylogenetic structures implemented in **adephylo** (Jombart et al. 2010a), a phylogenetic extension of **ade4** for the **R** software. This package provides a range of statistical tools for the exploratory analysis of phylogenetic comparative data and is fully integrated alongside **ade4** and the phylogenetic packages **ape** (Paradis et al. 2004) and **phylobase** (R Hackathon et al. 2017). It includes procedures for data visualisation and handling, computation of phylogenetic proximities and distances, tests and models of phylogenetic signal, and phylogenetic multivariate analyses.

© Springer Science+Business Media, LLC, part of Springer Nature 2018   261
J. Thioulouse et al., *Multivariate Analysis of Ecological Data with ade4*,
https://doi.org/10.1007/978-1-4939-8850-1_13

13.2   Managing Phylogenetic Comparative Data

Phylogenetic comparative data consist of a phylogeny and some biological traits observed for the set of taxa analysed. **adephylo** exploits efficient representations implemented in **ape** for phylogenies (S3 class `phylo`) and in **phylobase** for phylogenies and associated traits (S4 class `phylo4` for trees, and `phylo4d` for trees and traits). Note that the former class `phylog` from **ade4** was less efficient and flexible, and is now deprecated.

In this chapter, the phylogeny and traits associated to its tips are both assumed known. In practice, phylogenies can be obtained in **R** using **ape** for distance-based methods and **phangorn** (Schliep 2011; Schliep et al. 2017) for parsimony and likelihood based methods, or generated by another software and read into **R** using **ape**. Traits are stored as `data.frame` objects, where each row corresponds to a tip of the tree. The essential part in preparing data for analysis in **adephylo** is making sure that the tips of the tree match exactly the rows of the `data.frame`.

The internal structure of `phylo4` and `phylo4d` objects is relatively complex. However, the user does not have to interact directly with the internal content of a tree or a phylogenetic comparative data set. Instead, accessors are used to extract some specific information (see `tdata` function). More information on these objects can be found in a vignette distributed with the **phylobase** package, accessible using the command:

```
vignette("phylobase")
```

after the package has been loaded.

The **phylobase** package implements a very useful formal (S4) class for storing a phylogeny and sets of traits matching the tips, the nodes, or the edges of the tree. This class called `phylo4d` is used throughout **adephylo** to store comparative data. These objects can be obtained either by reading a Nexus file containing tree and traits data, or by *assembling* a tree and data provided for its tips. Nexus files containing both tree and data can be read by **phylobase**'s function `readNexus` (see corresponding help page for more information). Alternatively, a tree and a data frame of traits can be assembled into a `phylo4d` object using the constructor function `phylo4d`. This function takes two arguments: a tree (`phylo` or `phylo4` format) and a `data.frame` containing traits data. We provide in Fig. 13.1 a simple example using a simulated tree (`rtree` function from **ape**); the `table.phylo4d` function is used to display trait values in front of the tree.

The constructor `phylo4d` assumes that the rows of the data frame of traits are in the same order as the tips, whose label is in `$tip.label`. Different ordering can be used as long as the same labelling system is used for the tips of the tree and the rows of the traits `data.frame`, in which case `phylo4d` will reorganise the data adequately. Traits data of a `phylo4d` object can be accessed and modified using the `tdata` function of the **phylobase** package (see `?tdata` for more information). For instance:

```
library(ape)
library(phylobase)
par(mfrow = c(1, 2), mar = c(0.1, 2, 3, 2))
tre <- rtree(10)
plot(tre)
title("simulated tree (phylo object)")
traits <- data.frame(trait1 = c(1, NA, 3:10), trait2 = 10:1)
dat <- phylo4d(tre, traits)
table.phylo4d(dat, center = FALSE, scale = FALSE)
title("tree and traits (phylo4d object)")
```

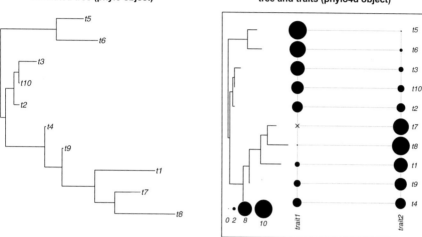

Fig. 13.1 Example of traits matched with a tree using `phylo4d`. The left-hand figure was obtained using the `plot` method for `phylo` objects. The right-hand figure was obtained using `table.phylo4d`. This function plots the tree and displays the traits in front of their tips using symbols of different sizes or colours corresponding to different values. Missing data (NA) are represented by crosses (×).

```
tdata(dat, type = "tip")
```

	trait1	trait2
t8	1	10
t7	NA	9
t1	3	8
t9	4	7
t4	5	6
t2	6	5
t10	7	4
t3	8	3
t6	9	2
t5	10	1

Now that we have seen how to prepare and format the data, we can focus on the analysis of phylogenetic structures. Phylogenetic structures occur when the values of biological traits or ecological features observed in a set of taxa are not independent from their position in the phylogenetic tree. In this chapter, we alternatively refer to this dependence as *phylogenetic autocorrelation* and *phylogenetic signal*. We will say that *positive* phylogenetic autocorrelation occurs when closely related taxa tend to share similar trait values; conversely, we will refer to strong contrasts between sister taxa as *negative* phylogenetic autocorrelation. Several procedures are implemented in **adephylo** to measure and test phylogenetic autocorrelation (see Box 13.1).

13.3 Computing Phylogenetic Proximities

The quantification and analysis of a phylogenetic signal in **adephylo** requires the computation of pairwise phylogenetic proximities between the tips of the tree. These can be obtained using the `proxTips` function, which defines phylogenetic proximities as a function of phylogenetic distances (using argument `f`) so that greater values increasing the contrast between close and distant taxa. Several types of phylogenetic distances are available (see `?distTips`) and can be specified through the `method` argument:

- `patristic`: patristic distance, i.e., sum of branch lengths on the shortest path between two tips
- `nNodes`: number of nodes on the shortest path between two tips
- `Abouheif`: Abouheif's distance (see Box 13.1)
- `sumDD`: sum of the number of direct descendants of all nodes on the shortest path between two tips

The choice of a phylogenetic metric is somehow arbitrary, as different distances reflect different properties of the phylogeny. The patristic distance (`method = "patristic"`) is probably the most biologically intuitive as it corresponds to the amount of evolution separating two taxa. The number of nodes (`method = "nNodes"`) is also fairly intuitive, as it can be used as a proxy for the number of speciation events that separate two taxa. Measures relating to Abouheif's distance (`method = "Abouheif"` or `"sumDD"`) do not have immediate biological interpretations, but seem the most powerful for detecting traits evolving under a Brownian motion model (Pavoine et al. 2008). In practice, it is safer to compare the results obtained using different metrics before drawing conclusions on the data.

Box 13.1 Modelling Phylogenetic Signal Using Proximities

Let $\mathbf{x} \in \mathbb{R}^n$ be the (centred) vector of a quantitative variable measured on the tips of a tree. We note $\mathbf{W} = [w_{ij}]$ a matrix of phylogenetic proximities so that w_{ij} measures the proximity between tips i and j on the tree, with the constraints $\sum_j w_{ij} = 1$, $w_{ij} \geq 0$ for $i, j = 1, \ldots, n$ and $w_{ii} = 0$ for $i = 1, \ldots, n$. Consequently, the i-th row of $\mathbf{W}$ contains weights (terms are positive or null and sum to one) which are greater for taxa (tips) phylogenetically closer to i. The lag vector $\tilde{\mathbf{x}} = \mathbf{W}\mathbf{x}$ contains, for each tip, the mean values of $\mathbf{x}$ observed in the phylogenetic neighbourhood of this tip.

(continued)

Box 13.1 (continued)

$\tilde{\mathbf{x}}$ can be plotted against $\mathbf{x}$ to assess the presence of a phylogenetic signal: a positive (respectively negative) relationship will indicate positive (respectively negative) phylogenetic autocorrelation. The underlying linear model is the basis of autoregressive models (Cheverud and Dow 1985; Cheverud et al. 1985) of the type:

$$\mathbf{x} = \rho\tilde{\mathbf{x}} + \mathbf{Z}\boldsymbol{\beta} + \boldsymbol{\epsilon}$$

where ρ is an autocorrelation coefficient, $\mathbf{Z}$ a matrix of covariates with coefficients $\boldsymbol{\beta}$ and $\boldsymbol{\epsilon}$ is the vector of residuals.

An alternative way of measuring phylogenetic signal is using Moran's index, defined as (Gittleman and Kot 1990):

$$I_{\mathbf{W}}(\mathbf{x}) = \frac{\mathbf{x}^{\top}\mathbf{W}\mathbf{x}}{n\,\mathrm{var}(\mathbf{x})}$$

where $\mathrm{var}(\mathbf{x})$ is the variance of trait $\mathbf{x}$. The expected value of this statistics in the absence of phylogenetic signal is $-1/(n-1)$. Greater (respectively smaller) values are suggestive of positive (respectively negative) phylogenetic autocorrelation. Non-parametric tests of $I_{\mathbf{W}}(\mathbf{x})$ can easily be obtained by randomly permuting the values in $\mathbf{x}$.

Interestingly, Abouheif's test of phylogenetic signal (Abouheif 1999; Pavoine et al. 2008) turns out to be a test of Moran's index with a particular phylogenetic proximity defined as:

$$w_{ij} = \frac{a_{ij}}{\sum_{j, i \neq j} a_{ij}}$$

with

$$a_{ij} = \Big(\prod_{p \in P_{ij}} f(p)\Big)^{-1}$$

where P_{ij} is the set of nodes on the shortest path from tip i to tip j and $f(p)$ is the number of direct descendants from node p.

We illustrate these differences using the data set `maples` of the **ade4** package, which contains a phylogeny and morphological measurements for 17 species of maples (Ackerly and Donoghue 1998). We compute the four different distance matrices, standardise them and merge them with the phylogeny using `phylo4d`:

```
data(maples)
tre <- read.tree(text = maples$tre)
D1 <- as.matrix(distTips(tre, method = "patristic"))
D1 <- D1/max(D1)
D1 <- phylo4d(tre, D1)
D2 <- as.matrix(distTips(tre, method = "nNodes"))
D2 <- D2/max(D2)
D2 <- phylo4d(tre, D2)
D3 <- as.matrix(distTips(tre, method = "Abouheif"))
D3 <- D3/max(D3)
D3 <- phylo4d(tre, D3)
D4 <- as.matrix(distTips(tre, method = "sumDD"))
D4 <- D4/max(D4)
D4 <- phylo4d(tre, D4)
```

The `table.phylo4d` function of the **adephylo** package is then used to plot the distances and the phylogeny (see Fig. 13.2). As it can be seen, the four distances capture different features of the phylogeny.

13.4   Detecting Phylogenetic Structures

When phylogenetic proximities have been defined, they can be used to detect if and how the variation of traits values is related to the phylogenetic structure. Several methods can be envisaged.

13.4.1   Moran's I

The `moran.idx` function of **adephylo** computes Moran's I, an index measuring the phylogenetic autocorrelation in a quantitative trait (see Box 13.1). If the argument `addInfo` is TRUE, the function also returns the null value (`IO`) and the range of variation of I (`Imin` and `Imax`). In this approach, the phylogenetic information is included using a matrix of pairwise phylogenetic proximities between taxa which can be obtained using `proxTips` (see Sect. 13.3).

We illustrate the use of Moran's I using the `ungulates` data set of the **ade4** package, which contains 4 life-history traits for 18 ungulate species along with their phylogeny (Pélabon et al. 1995). Only adult female body weight (`afbw`) and female neonatal body weight (`fnw`) are here analysed.

```
data(ungulates)
tre <- read.tree(text = ungulates$tre)
W <- proxTips(tre, method = "patristic")
afbw <- ungulates$tab$afbw
moran.idx(afbw, W, addInfo = TRUE)
```

```
[1] -0.04101
attr(,"IO")
[1] -0.05882
attr(,"Imin")
[1] -0.1741
attr(,"Imax")
[1] 1.001
```

```
myPal <- colorRampPalette(c("lightgrey", "orange", "red"))
par(mfrow = c(2, 2), mar = c(2, 2, 4, 2), xpd = TRUE)
table.phylo4d(D1, symbol = "colors", cex.symbol = 2,
        col = myPal(100), center = FALSE, scale = FALSE,
        box = FALSE, cex.label = 0.5)
title("Maple data - patristic distance")
table.phylo4d(D2, symbol = "colors", cex.symbol = 2,
        col = myPal(100), center = FALSE, scale = FALSE,
        box = FALSE, cex.label = 0.5)
title("Maple data - 'nNodes' distance")
table.phylo4d(D3, symbol = "colors", cex.symbol = 2,
        col = myPal(100), center = FALSE, scale = FALSE,
        box = FALSE, cex.label = 0.5)
title("Maple data - Abouheif's distance")
table.phylo4d(D4, symbol = "colors", cex.symbol = 2,
        col = myPal(100), center = FALSE, scale = FALSE,
        box = FALSE, cex.label = 0.5)
title("Maple data - 'sumDD' distance")
```

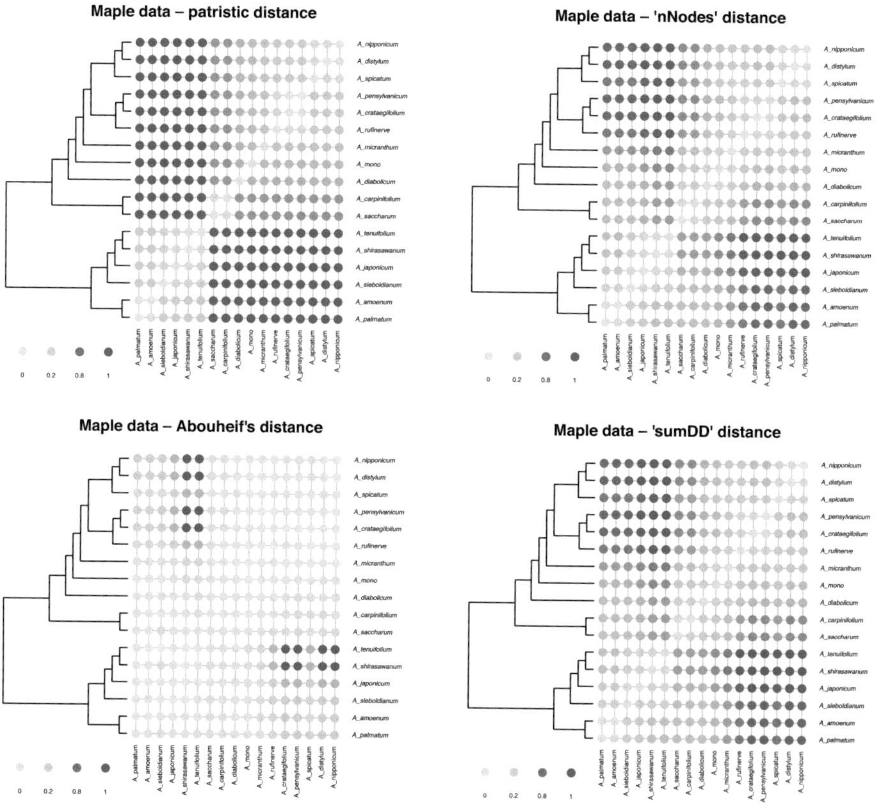

Fig. 13.2 Four distance matrices obtained for the `maples` data set using `distTips`.

```
fnw <- ungulates$tab$fnw
moran.idx(fnw, W, addInfo = TRUE)
```

```
[1] 0.02282
attr(, "I0")
[1] -0.05882
```

```
attr(,"Imin")
[1] -0.1741
attr(,"Imax")
[1] 1.001
```

Moran's index for `afbw` appears to be very close to the null value, suggesting that the trait is not phylogenetically autocorrelated. `fnw` is slightly greater, and may exhibit some phylogenetic pattern. Formal tests are needed to support these intuitions.

It is straightforward to build a non-parametric test based on Moran's I, using `replicate` to permute the values of the variable:

```
Iobs <- moran.idx(afbw, W)
Iperm <- replicate(999, moran.idx(sample(afbw), W))
library(ade4)
Itest <- as.randtest(obs = Iobs, sim = Iperm)
Itest
```

```
Monte-Carlo test
Call: as.randtest(sim = Iperm, obs = Iobs)

Observation: -0.04101

Based on 999 replicates
Simulated p-value: 0.251
Alternative hypothesis: greater

    Std.Obs Expectation    Variance
   0.437735   -0.058230    0.001548
```

Here, `afbw` does not appear to be phylogenetically autocorrelated, as the observed I falls well within the distribution of permuted values.

13.4.2 Abouheif's Test

Abouheif's test of phylogenetic signal has proved to be a powerful version of Moran's I test for the detection of phylogenetic signal (see Box 13.1). It is implemented in **adephylo** by the `abouheif.moran` function, which generalises the testing procedure by proposing different phylogenetic proximity measures in addition to the original one. The simplest way to apply this test to a data set is to use `abouheif.moran` directly on a `phylo4d` object. We illustrate this approach using the `ungulates` data set. `abouheif.moran` runs non-parametric tests of phylogenetic signal on each trait in the `phylo4d` object. It returns a `krandtest` object, which is the standard class in **ade4** for storing multiple Monte Carlo tests.

```
ung <- phylo4d(tre, ungulates$tab)
abouheif.moran(ung)
```

```
class: krandtest lightkrandtest
Monte-Carlo tests
Call: as.krandtest(sim = matrix(res$result, ncol = nvar,
       byrow = TRUE), obs = res$obs, alter = alter,
       names = test.names)
```

```
Number of tests:    4

Adjustment method for multiple comparisons:    none
Permutation number:    999
   Test      Obs Std.Obs    Alter Pvalue
1 afbw 0.1654    1.130 greater   0.134
2  mnw 0.3681    2.725 greater   0.015
3  fnw 0.3843    2.778 greater   0.015
4   ls 0.3002    1.983 greater   0.039
```

In this case, it seems that all variables but afbm are phylogenetically structured.

Note that other proximities than those proposed in abouheif.moran can be used: on has just to pass the appropriate proximity matrix to the function (argument W).

13.5 Describing the Phylogenetic Signal

13.5.1 Orthonormal Bases

Significant phylogenetic signal can reflect a range of biological patterns: from ancient (near-root) divergence of life-history strategies to tight similarities between sister species or local contrasts caused by recent diversifying selection. Beyond the mere testing of phylogenetic signal, there is therefore considerable interest in assessing the nature of phylogenetic patterns. One way to tackle this objective is expressing the trait of interest as a combination of known phylogenetic structures. This approach relies on (1) finding uncorrelated variables which reflect a wide range of phylogenetic structures and (2) regressing the trait of interest onto these variables (see Box 13.2).

Box 13.2 Decomposing Phylogenetic Signal Using Orthonormal Bases

Once the presence of phylogenetic signal has been detected in a trait x ($x \in \mathbb{R}^n$), one may be interested in exploring further this signal and locating where phylogenetic patterns occur in the tree. This can be achieved by decomposing the variation of the trait of interest onto variables ($b_1, \ldots, b_r \in \mathbb{R}^n$) which describe the structure of the tree. For such a decomposition to be practicable, these variables need to be uncorrelated and have the same variance, which means that geometrically, their vectors are *orthonormal*. To decompose fully the variance of x, these variables also need to form a basis B ($B = [b_1, \ldots, b_r]$), so that x can be represented as a linear combination of the columns of $b_1, \ldots, b_r$.

One way to obtain such bases is using Moran's eigenvectors (Dray et al. 2006). Using the same notations as before (Box 13.1), these eigenvectors can be derived from a matrix of phylogenetic proximities by taking the

(continued)

Box 13.2 (continued)

eigenvectors **B** of the symmetric matrix:

$$\mathbf{H}\left(\frac{1}{2}(\mathbf{W}^{\top} + \mathbf{W})\right)\mathbf{H}$$

where **H** is the centring operator defined as $\mathbf{H} = \mathbf{I}_n - \mathbf{1}_n\mathbf{1}^{\top}_n/n$. It can be shown that the $n - 1$ column-vectors of **B** (sorted by decreasing eigenvalue) are orthonormal variables ranging from the largest to the lowest possible phylogenetic autocorrelation (as measured by Moran's I, see Box 13.1, Griffith 1996). Therefore, these variables model different observable phylogenetic structures. Note that there are other ways of obtaining phylogenetic orthonormal bases. For instance, one can use classical orthonormalisation procedures on indicator variables derived from the tree topology to obtain orthonormal vectors reflecting the structure of the tree (Ollier et al. 2005).

Once a phylogenetic orthonormal basis has been obtained, the trait variation can be fully decomposed using multiple regression approach, giving rise to $n - 1$ squared correlation coefficients $(r_1^2, \ldots, r_{n-1}^2)$ between **x** and $(\mathbf{b}_1, \ldots, \mathbf{b}_{n-1})$, where a large r_i^2 indicates that the phylogenetic structure in **x** strongly matches $\mathbf{b}_i$. These values are exploited in the *orthogram* approach (Ollier et al. 2005), which defines four test statistics for detecting phylogenetic signal.

$$\mathrm{R2Max}(\mathbf{x}) = \max(r_1^2, \ldots, r_{n-1}^2)$$

is simply the maximum squared correlation.

$$D\mathrm{max}(\mathbf{x}) = \max_{1 \le m \le n-1}\left(\sum_{i=1}^{m} r_i^2 - \frac{m}{n-1}\right)$$

corresponds to the deviation from a uniform distribution measured by the Kolmogorov–Smirnov statistic.

$$\mathrm{SkR2k}(\mathbf{x}) = \sum_{i=1}^{n-1} i r_i^2$$

measures how close to the tips the phylogenetic structures occur.

$$\mathrm{SCE}(\mathbf{x}) = \sum_{i=2}^{n-1}(r_i^2 - r_{i-1}^2)^2$$

(continued)

> **Box 13.2** (continued)
>
> measures how inequally distributed phylogenetic variation is in the tree: it is close to 0 when phylogenetic patterns are evenly distributed across the phylogeny, and close to 1 when phylogenetic signal affects a single area of the tree.
>
> In the orthogram, these four statistics are tested using non-parametric approaches relying on the permutation of the values within **x**. Associated graphs allow a visual diagnosis of how the phylogenetic signal is structured in the tree.

The first step can be achieved in **adephylo** using Moran's eigenvectors which are implemented by the `me.phylo` function. These vectors are derived from a matrix of pairwise phylogenetic proximities (as returned by `proxTips`). They are scaled to unit variance, are uncorrelated, and allow the full decomposition of any trait, and thus form an orthonormal basis. `me.phylo` returns a `data.frame` with the `orthobasis` class defined in **ade4**; columns of this object are Moran's eigenvectors. We illustrate how orthobases can be obtained using different phylogenetic proximity measures for the `ungulates` data set in Fig. 13.3.

The orthobases obtained in Fig. 13.3 are very similar. We use the first one (based on patristic distances) to decompose the variation of the four traits in the data set. The squared correlations plotted for each trait and each Moran's eigenvector (Fig. 13.4) show that phylogenetic structures are mostly observed at a large phylogenetic scale (close to the root differentiations, Moran's eigenvectors 2 and 3).

13.5.2   Phylogenetic Decomposition with the Orthogram

The phylogenetic decomposition of the variation of a trait onto a phylogenetic orthobasis shown in Fig. 13.4 is more than a graphical tool. As a matter of fact, a series of test statistics can be derived from the r^2 values plotted in this figure (Box 13.2). This approach was originally called *orthogram* by Ollier et al. (2005), and is implemented in the `orthogram` function in **adephylo**. While initially formulated for a specific type of phylogenetic orthobasis, we generalised this approach and the `orthogram` function can now use any phylogenetic orthonormal basis as returned by `me.phylo`.

The orthogram computes four statistics derived from r^2 values of a trait decomposed onto the orthonormal basis, and runs associated non-parametric tests. A graphical display of the results facilitates the biological interpretation. This is illustrated using the female neonatal weight (`fnw`) from the `ungulates` data. We first display the orthonormal basis used in the orthogram (Fig. 13.5), and then obtain the orthogram itself (Fig. 13.6).

```
tre <- read.tree(text = ungulates$tre)
temp <- c("patristic", "nNodes", "Abouheif", "sumDD")
ung.listBases <- lapply(temp, function(e) phylo4d(tre,
      me.phylo(tre, method = e)))
par(mar = rep(0.1, 4), mfrow = c(2, 2))
par(mar = c(1, 1, 4, 1), xpd = TRUE, mfrow = c(2, 2))
for (i in 1:4) {
      table.phylo4d(ung.listBases[[i]], repVar = 1:5,
      cex.symbol = 0.7, how.tip.label = FALSE, show.node = FALSE,
      box = FALSE)
      title(temp[i])
}
```

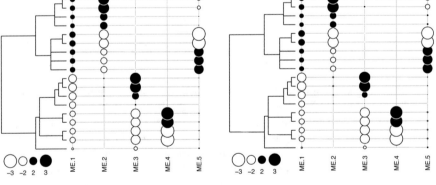

Fig. 13.3 Phylogenetic orthobases formed by Moran's eigenvectors with four different phylogenetic proximity matrices, in the `ungulates` data set.

The orthogram shows that female neonatal weight (`fnw`) exhibits a significant phylogenetic structure at a single, intermediate scale (fourth vector, see Fig. 13.5). This could reflect some important changes in life-history strategies having occurred around node $W10$ (Fig. 13.5).

```
B <- me.phylo(tre)
corTab <- cor(ungulates$tab, B)^2
barplot(corTab, beside = TRUE, col = rainbow(4), las = 3,
        ylab = expression(r^2))
legend("topright", rainbow(4), title = "traits",
        legend = names(ungulates$tab), col = rainbow(4), pch = 15)
```

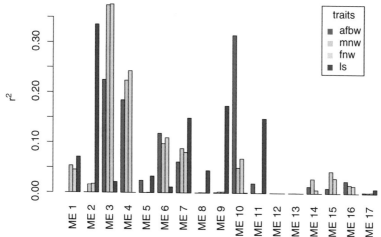

Fig. 13.4 Decomposition of traits variation onto a phylogenetic orthobases derived from patristic distances, in the `ungulates` data set. 'ME' stands for Moran's eigenvectors, numbered from 1 (close-to-the-root structures) to 17 (contrasts between sister species).

13.5.3 Removing Phylogenetic Autocorrelation

Phylogenetic autocorrelation is often seen as a nuisance as it violates the assumption of independence between the observations, required by many statistical approaches including likelihood-based approaches and tests of associations between variables. This is particularly a problem when studying the relationships between several phylogenetically autocorrelated traits.

Moran's eigenvectors can be used to circumvent this issue. Indeed, these vectors can be used in a regression approach to account for phylogenetic signal in the studied traits. The approach is simple: traits are first regressed onto relevant eigenvectors before including relevant covariates in the model. This is illustrated through the study of the link between the average weight at birth (`neonatw`) and the adult female weight (`afbw`) in the `ungulates` data set. We first perform a naive linear regression on the log-transformed (for normality) data, without accounting for the phylogeny:

```
names(ungulates$tab)

[1] "afbw" "mnw"  "fnw"  "ls"

afbw <- log(ungulates$tab[, 1])
neonatw <- log((ungulates$tab[, 2] + ungulates$tab[, 3])/2)
```

```
tre <- read.tree(text = ungulates$tre)
temp <- phylo4d(tre, treePart(tre, result = "orthobasis"))
par(mar = rep(0.1, 4))
table.phylo4d(temp, ratio.tree = 0.3, show.tip = FALSE,
    cex.symbol = 0.6)
```

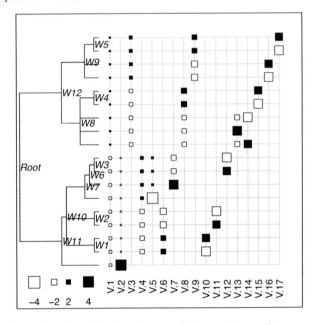

Fig. 13.5 Orthonormal basis used in the orthogram of the ungulates data.

```
lm1 <- lm(neonatw ~ afbw)
anova(lm1)
```

```
Analysis of Variance Table
```

```
Response: neonatw
          Df Sum Sq Mean Sq F value  Pr(>F)
afbw       1  12.16   12.16     159 9.8e-10
Residuals 16   1.22    0.08
```

There seems to be a very strong relationship between the two variables. However, the residuals are clearly not independent:

```
resid1 <- residuals(lm1)
abouheif.moran(phylo4d(tre, resid1))
```

```
class: krandtest lightkrandtest
Monte-Carlo tests
Call: as.krandtest(sim = matrix(res$result, ncol = nvar, byrow
= TRUE), obs = res$obs, alter = alter, names = test.names)
```

```
Number of tests:   1
```

```
Adjustment method for multiple comparisons:    none
Permutation number:     999
   Test    Obs Std.Obs   Alter Pvalue
1    dt 0.4566   3.165 greater  0.003
```

Thus, the tests and estimates of this model (lm1) are probably strongly biased.

```
orthogram(fnw, tre)


class: krandtest lightkrandtest
Monte-Carlo tests
Call: orthogram(x = fnw, tre = tre)
Number of tests:    4
Adjustment method for multiple comparisons:    none
Permutation number:    999
     Test    Obs Std.Obs    Alter Pvalue
1 R2Max 0.4618   2.253  greater  0.032
2 SkR2k 5.5961  -1.879  greater  0.955
3  Dmax 0.4593   2.187  greater  0.030
4   SCE 1.1111   2.599  greater  0.026
```

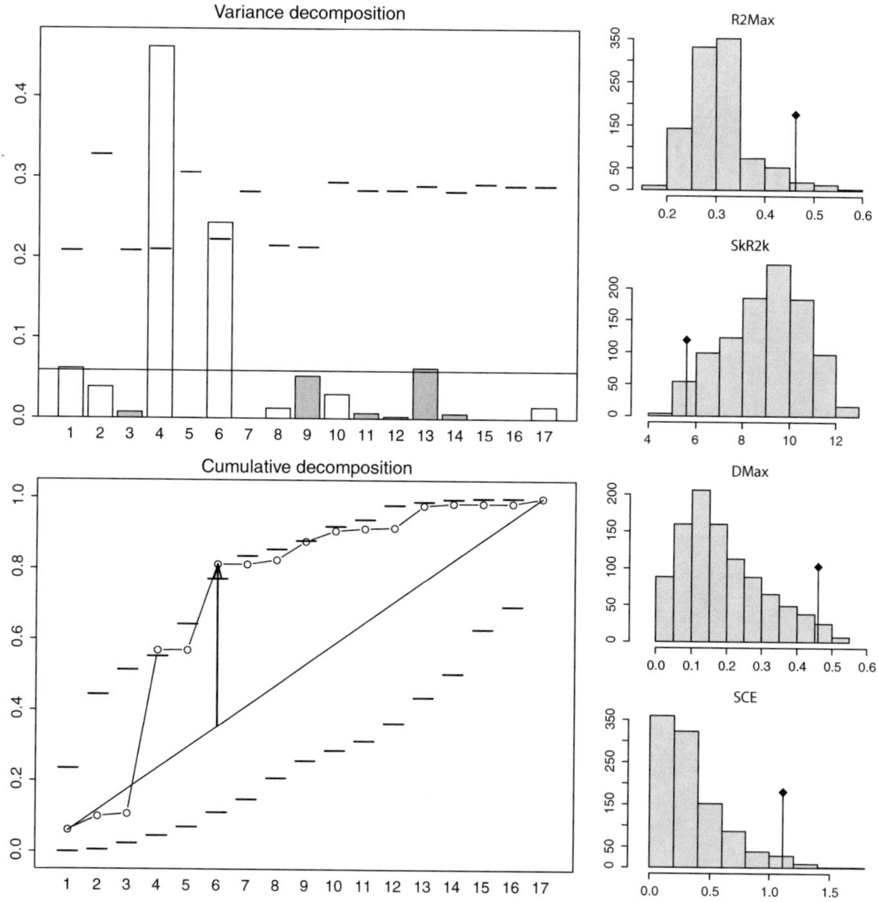

Fig. 13.6 Orthogram of female neonatal weight (fnw, ungulates data set). The two figures on the left indicate the decomposition of the variation (r^2 values) on each vector of the basis, the bottom one corresponding to accumulated values. Bars and dots indicate observed values, while horizontal segments indicate the mean (top) or confidence intervals (bottom) values obtained by permutation (i.e., in the absence of significant phylogenetic signal). The four graphics on the right correspond to the non-parametric tests (see Box 13.2), with histograms indicating permuted values.

We address this issue by regressing the data onto relevant Moran's eigenvectors (here chosen based on the highest correlations with the residuals).

```
B <- me.phylo(tre, method = "patristic")
round(cor(resid1, B)^2, 1)
```

```
      ME 1 ME 2 ME 3 ME 4 ME 5 ME 6 ME 7 ME 8 ME 9 ME 10
[1,]   0.4  0.2  0.1    0    0    0    0  0.1    0    0.1
      ME 11 ME 12 ME 13 ME 14 ME 15 ME 16 ME 17
[1,]   0.1     0     0     0   0.1     0     0
```

```
lm2 <- lm(neonatw ~ B[, 1] + afbw)
anova(lm2, lm1)
```

```
Analysis of Variance Table

Model 1: neonatw ~ B[, 1] + afbw
Model 2: neonatw ~ afbw
  Res.Df   RSS Df Sum of Sq    F Pr(>F)
1     15 0.745
2     16 1.221 -1    -0.476 9.58 0.0074
```

```
summary(lm2)
```

```
Call:
lm(formula = neonatw ~ B[, 1] + afbw)

Residuals:
    Min      1Q  Median      3Q     Max
-0.4825 -0.1140  0.0497  0.1429  0.2771

Coefficients:
            Estimate Std. Error t value Pr(>|t|)
(Intercept)  -1.3193     0.6325   -2.09   0.0545
B[, 1]       -0.1630     0.0527   -3.10   0.0074
afbw          0.8867     0.0560   15.83  9.1e-11

Residual standard error: 0.223 on 15 degrees of freedom
Multiple R-squared:  0.944,       Adjusted R-squared:  0.937
F-statistic:  127 on 2 and 15 DF,  p-value: 3.9e-10
```

The link between the two variables remains statistically very significant (about 94% of the variation in neonatal weight is explained by the phylogeny and the female body mass), but this time the model (lm2) is no longer invalidated by non-independence in the residuals:

```
resid2 <- residuals(lm2)
abouheif.moran(phylo4d(tre, resid2))
```

```
class: krandtest lightkrandtest
Monte-Carlo tests
Call: as.krandtest(sim = matrix(res$result, ncol = nvar,
      byrow = TRUE), obs = res$obs, alter = alter,
      names = test.names)

Number of tests:   1

Adjustment method for multiple comparisons:    none
Permutation number:    999
   Test    Obs Std.Obs  Alter Pvalue
1    dt 0.1607   1.045 greater  0.161
```

13.6 Phylogenetic Principal Component Analysis (pPCA)

Phylogenetic comparative data may often comprise more than a handful of traits, in which case multiple univariate analyses become cumbersome to perform and interpret. More fundamentally, univariate approaches may fail to capture complex relationships between several traits, which may arise when major historical shifts in life-history strategies affect an entire set of traits. To identify such patterns, we can therefore look for combinations of traits exhibiting similar phylogenetic signal.

This is the purpose of the phylogenetic Principal Component Analysis (pPCA, Jombart et al. 2010b) which is an extension of MULTISPATI Analysis (Sect. 12.5.2) where the spatial weights are replaced by phylogenetic proximities. Unlike usual PCA which provides synthetic variables with maximum variance, pPCA explicitly seeks combinations of traits exhibiting both a large variance and an important phylogenetic autocorrelation (as measured by Moran's I, see Box 13.1). The theory of the method is not presented in this chapter as it is strictly equivalent to the description provided in Box 12.3. Therefore, pPCA can provide positive as well as negative eigenvalues, the first corresponding to positive autocorrelation (large, positive I), the latter to negative autocorrelation (large, negative I).

pPCA is implemented in **adephylo** by the `ppca` function. We illustrate this approach using the `maples` data set. Like PCA, pPCA can be applied to any quantitative data. However, missing data need to be replaced, which we do using an *ad hoc* function:

```
any(is.na(maples$tab))
```

```
[1] TRUE
```

```
f1 <- function(x) {
      m <- mean(x, na.rm = TRUE)
      x[is.na(x)] <- m
      return(x)
}
maples$tab <- apply(maples$tab, 2, f1)
any(is.na(maples$tab))
```

```
[1] FALSE
```

Missing data have been replaced, set to the mean of available data, for each trait. We now merge the phylogeny and the traits into a `phylo4d` object:

```
tre <- read.tree(text = maples$tre)
map <- phylo4d(tre, maples$tab)
```

The data are first visualised, but no obvious phylogenetic structure can be observed (Fig. 13.7). It thus makes sense to use pPCA to investigate possibly hidden phylogenetic structures.

By default, the `ppca` function displays a barplot of eigenvalues and asks the user for the number of axes (positively and negatively autocorrelated) to retain. In the case of the `maples` data, only one positive eigenvalue should be retained, and no negative ones (Fig. 13.8).

```
par(mar = rep(1, 4), xpd = TRUE)
table.phylo4d(map, symbol = "color", col = myPal(100),
      cex.symbol = 1.5, cex.label = 0.7, box = FALSE)
```

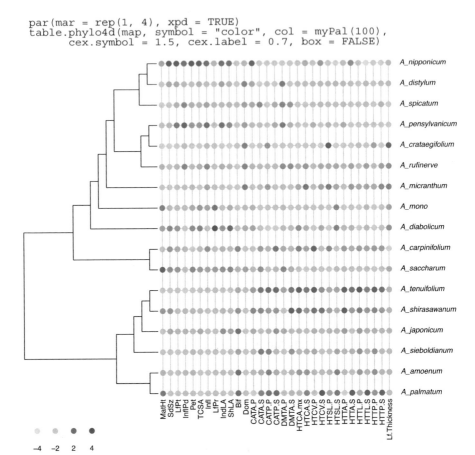

Fig. 13.7 Graphical representation of the `maples` data using `table.phylo4d`. Variables are centred (to mean zero) and scaled (to unit variance) so as to be on comparable scales.

```
ppca1
```

```
#############################################
# phylogenetic Principal Component Analysis #
#############################################
class: ppca
$call: ppca(x = map, scannf = FALSE, nfposi = 1, nfnega = 0)

$nfposi: 1 axes-components saved
$nfnega: 0 axes-components saved
$kept.axes: index of kept axes
Positive eigenvalues: 4.223 0.3593 0.2882 0.1494 0.01034
Negative eigenvalues: -0.9876 -0.6857 -0.4088 -0.3051 -0.1393 ...

  vector length mode     content
1 $eig    16      numeric eigenvalues

  data.frame nrow ncol
1 $c1           31   1
2 $li           17   1
```

```
ppca1 <- ppca(map, scannf = FALSE)
```

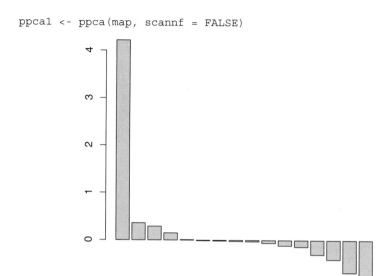

Fig. 13.8 Eigenvalues of the phylogenetic Principal Component Analysis (pPCA) of the `maples` data.

```
3 $ls            17    1
4 $as             2    1
  content
1 principal axes: scaled vectors of traits loadings
2 principal components: coordinates of taxa ('scores')
3 lag vector of principal components
4 pca axes onto ppca axes

$tre: a phylogeny (class phylo4)
$prox: a matrix of phylogenetic proximities

other elements: NULL
```

The `ppca1` object is very similar to usual outputs of the `dudi` functions. A number of procedures allow to summarise and visualise pPCA results (`scatter`, `screeplot`, `summary`, see `?ppca`). The most complete one is `plot` (Fig. 13.9).

Figure 13.9 shows that the `maples` data contains one strong phylogenetic pattern (large positive eigenvalue, outlying in both variance and autocorrelation), corresponding to a strong divergence in life-history traits (see loadings) at the very basis of the tree. The `summary` provides some complementary information on the analysis, detailing the composition of each eigenvalue and comparing them to the results of a usual PCA.

```
summary(ppca1)

### Phylogenetic Principal Component Analysis ###

Call: ppca(x = map, scannf = FALSE, nfposi = 1, nfnega = 0)

== Moran's I statistics ==
     I0    Imin  Imax
 -0.0625 -0.451 1.009
```

```
plot(ppca1)
```

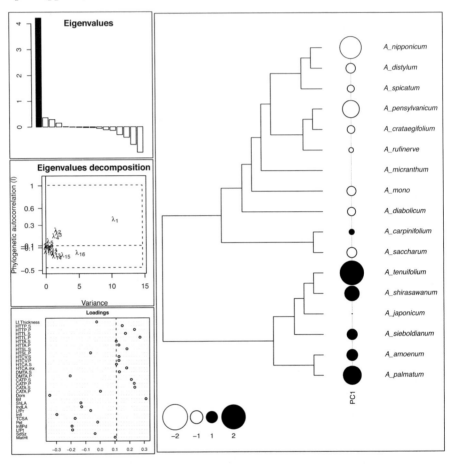

Fig. 13.9 Results of the phylogenetic Principal Component Analysis (pPCA) of the `maples` data. Top-left: eigenvalues of the analysis, middle-left: decomposition of the eigenvalues in terms of variance and autocorrelation (Moran's *I*), as plotted by the `screeplot` function, bottom-left: loadings of the variables for the retained axis, right: first principal component of the analysis, as displayed by the `scatter` function.

```
== PCA scores ==
          var    cum   ratio   moran
Axis 1  13.31  13.31  0.4293  0.2112

== pPCA eigenvalues decomposition ==
          eig    var   moran
Axis 1  4.223  10.52  0.4013
```

In this case, the pPCA is clearly better at identifying phylogenetic structures: the variance of the first component of the analysis is close to that of a PCA (10.52 *vs* 13.31), but its phylogenetic signal is twice as large (0.40 *vs* 0.21).

Chapter 14
Analysing Patterns of Biodiversity

Abstract Patterns of functional or phylogenetic diversity among communities can be described thanks to the Double Principal Coordinate Analysis (DPCoA). This approach depicts differences among communities in low-dimensional plots and explains those differences by their species compositions and the functional or phylogenetic differences among species.

14.1 Introduction

Methods presented in Chap. 6 allow to summarise the structures of ecological communities. These approaches consider only the information gathered by a sites × species table to identify (1) similarities between species distributions and (2) patterns of variation of species composition among sites. This second aspect aims to capture information on species turnover. On the other hand, measurements of species diversity are central tools in Ecology. Whittaker (1972) introduced the important concept of diversity partitioning of total diversity (γ) into within-community (α) and between-community (β) components. Species diversity indices are usually computed as a function of the number of species (species richness) and the number of individuals per species (e.g., Simpson or Shannon indexes). As both ordination methods and diversity measurements try to describe ecological communities, some works have connected these two approaches (ter Braak 1983; Pélissier et al. 2003b). For instance, Pélissier et al. (2003b) showed that Non-Symmetric Correspondence Analysis (function `dudi.nsc`, Kroonenberg and Lombardo 1999) focuses on β diversity measured using Simpson index.

Rao (1982) proposed a new framework to consider dissimilarities between species in the context of diversity partitioning. Whereas standard approaches consider only the number of species and individuals, Rao's diversity coefficient also called quadratic entropy allows to introduce distances among species (e.g., functional distance based on traits, phylogenetic distance) so that α, β and γ

© Springer Science+Business Media, LLC, part of Springer Nature 2018
J. Thioulouse et al., *Multivariate Analysis of Ecological Data with ade4*,
https://doi.org/10.1007/978-1-4939-8850-1_14

diversity measurements take into account species distributions (i.e., number of species and individuals) but also functional or phylogenetic differences among species.

The Double Principal Coordinate Analysis (DPCoA) is an ordination method that allows to introduce differences between species so that diversities are measured by Rao's quadratic entropy.

This approach is illustrated here to characterise the functional diversity of birds along an altitudinal gradient. We used the `tarentaise` data set (Lebreton et al. 1999) of the **ade4** package. It contains a total of 98 bird species seen or listened on 376 points at altitudes varying from 600 m to 3000 m in La Tarentaise, an Alpine Valley in France.

```
library(ade4)
library(adegraphics)
data(tarentaise)
names(tarentaise)
```

```
[1] "ecol"     "frnames"  "alti"     "envir"    "traits"   "latnames"
```

14.2   Ordination of the Faunistic Table

We can define here a bird community as the set of bird species observed at one given point (site). The `tarentaise$ecol` object contains the occurrences of the 98 bird species for the 376 communities:

```
fau <- tarentaise$ecol
dim(fau)
```

```
[1] 376   98
```

As described in Chap. 6, this table can be summarised by an ordination method. We can apply a Non-Symmetric Correspondence Analysis, using the `dudi.nsc` function:

```
nsc1 <- dudi.nsc(fau, scannf = FALSE, nf = 2)
```

This ordination method considers only abundance data, so similarities among sites are only due to changes in species composition. To interpret the results, we used the altitude of sampling points as a supplementary variable: it is not used in the computation but it helps interpreting the results. Altitude has been coded as a categorical variable with 14 classes:

```
alti <- tarentaise$envir$alti
nlevels(alti)
```

```
[1] 14
```

Figure 14.1 represents the factorial map of sites grouped by level of altitude. It demonstrates that variations in species composition are strongly linked to the altitudinal gradient.

```
s.class(nsc1$li, alti, col = terrain.colors(14),
        pbackground.col = "darkgrey", plabels.boxes.col = "black")
```

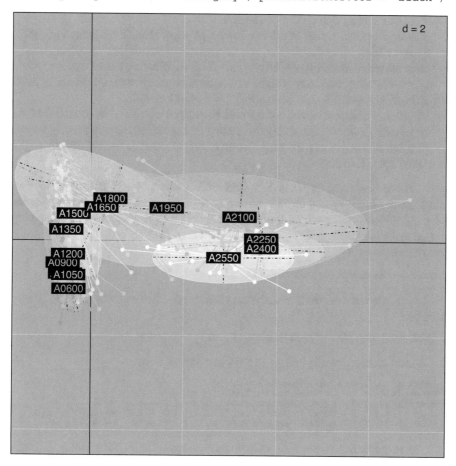

Fig. 14.1 Ordination of sites by non-symmetric correspondence analysis. Sites are grouped by altitude levels.

14.3   From Trait Data to Dissimilarities

Species were characterised by six biological traits (`tarentaise$traits`):

- **Diet habits** are described by a fuzzy variable (see Sect. 5.5) with five attributes denoted as follows: `di.inv` = invertebrates; `di.ver` = vertebrates; `di.car` = carcass, waste; `di.see` = permanent plant resources (e.g., seeds, resiniferous needles; Ericaceae leaves); `di.fru` = fruits and berries.
- **Foranging substrates** are described by a fuzzy variable with four attributes denoted as follows: `fo.air` = aerial; `fo.fol` = in the foliage; `fo.tru` = on trunks and branches; `fo.gro` = on the ground.

- **Nest substrates** are described by a fuzzy variable with four attributes denoted as follows: ne.foi = in the foliage; ne.tru = on/in truncks; ne.roc = on rock faces or cavities; ne.gro = on the ground.
- **Size** is an ordinal variable with five levels:]0, 15g];]15g, 25g];]25g, 80g];]80g, 250g]; >250.
- **Reproductive investment** is an ordinal variable defined by the ratio of the weight of the clutch to the body weight of the female parent with six levels: ≤30%;]30%,40%];]40%,50%];]50%,60%];]60%,80%]; >80%.
- **Migratory status** is an ordinal variable calculated with the time of arrival of the species on La Tarentaise Valley (in number of days since January first): ≤50days (this interval contains sedentary species only);]50, 70] days;]70, 90] days;]90, 110] days;]110, 200] days.

Methods presented in Chap. 5 to summarise one table do not allow to treat simultaneously fuzzy and ordinal variables. An alternative is provided by Pavoine et al. (2009) to handle mixed trait data sets. This approach consists in computing functional distances among species. First, a data frame that includes the first three fuzzy traits is built:

```
tabF <- tarentaise$traits[1:13]
```

The number of categories in each fuzzy trait is specified using the prep.fuzzy function:

```
tabF <- prep.fuzzy(tabF, c(5, 4, 4))
```

A second data frame is built with the three ordinal traits:

```
tabO <- as.data.frame(matrix(0, 98, 3))
names(tabO) <- c("Size", "ReIn", "Migr")
for (i in 1:5) tabO[tarentaise$traits[, i + 13] == 1, 1] <- i
for (i in 1:6) tabO[tarentaise$traits[, i + 18] == 1, 2] <- i
for (i in 1:5) tabO[tarentaise$traits[, i + 24] == 1, 3] <- i
```

The two data frames are then transformed in a ktab object (see Sect. 9.2.2) with the ktab.list.df function:

```
w <- ktab.list.df(list(tabF, tabO))
```

A global functional distance matrix among species (object dis) is computed with the dist.ktab function:

```
dis <- dist.ktab(w, type = c("F", "O"))
```

Principal Coordinate Analysis (see Sect. 6.5) can be performed to summarise the main differences among species based on their functional traits:

```
pco1 <- dudi.pco(dis, scannf = FALSE, nf = 2)
```

The link between the ordinations of species based on their functional traits (pco1$li) and their distributions among the sampling points (nsc1$li) can be evaluated *a posteriori* by computing correlations between scores:

```
cor(pco1$li, nsc1$co)
```

```
       Comp1      Comp2
A1  0.1167  -0.08549
A2  0.2325  -0.16083
```

The link is very low: this indirect method is not optimal because composition and trait data sets are analysed separately. The Double Principal Coordinate Analysis provides a relevant alternative that considers both data sets simultaneously.

14.4 Double Principal Coordinate Analysis (DPCoA)

DPCoA (Pavoine et al. 2004) generalises the Principal Coordinate Analysis (PCoA, see Chap. 6) when two embedded types of objects are studied. Here, species can be considered as embedded in communities. The objective of DPCoA is to describe differences in the composition of communities knowing some sort of differences among these species. Differences among species might be defined according to functional traits, taxonomy or phylogeny. DPCoA then defines differences among communities based on the abundance of each species present in the communities and the (functional, taxonomic or phylogenetic) differences among the species.

DPCoA is defined by the two steps described in Box 14.1. The first step represents species and communities so that the differences among species are optimally represented. This is achieved by performing a Principal Coordinate Analysis to represent functional differences (as described in Sect. 14.3) and then by positioning communities by weighted averaging (see Box 6.1).

The second step aims to optimally represent the functional differences among communities. It corresponds to a Principal Component Analysis of community compositions that turns out to be a PCoA of distances among communities. Hence, DPCoA connects a PCoA of the species with a PCoA of the communities.

DPCoA defines a new space where species and communities are positioned and where the positions of the communities depend on the positions of the species they contain. Species positions are based on biological characteristics, for instance functional traits, or phylogenetic positions. When species are positioned based on functional traits for instance, DPCoA optimally represents the *functional* differences among communities.

Box 14.1 DPCoA: Basic Mathematical Definitions

Here we consider a general definition of the DPCoA where communities are compared using their species composition and some functional or phylogenetic distances among species.

Let $\mathbf{Y} = [y_{ij}]$ be an $n \times s$ abundance table with communities as rows and species as columns. As in Correspondence Analysis (see Box 6.2), the table of frequencies $\mathbf{P} = [y_{ij}/y_{..}]$ (where $y_{..}$ is the grand total of $\mathbf{Y}$) and

---

(continued)

Box 14.1 (continued)

the two vectors $\mathbf{n} = \mathbf{P1}_s = (p_{1\bullet} \cdots p_{n\bullet})^{\top}$ and $\mathbf{s} = \mathbf{P}^{\top}\mathbf{1}_n = (p_{\bullet 1} \cdots p_{\bullet s})^{\top}$ of communities and species weights are computed. The diagonal matrices of weights are:

$$\mathbf{D}_n = \mathrm{diag}(\mathbf{n}) \text{ and } \mathbf{D}_s = \mathrm{diag}(\mathbf{s})$$

To perform DPCoA, the following two steps are required.

Step 1: Principal Coordinate Analysis (PCoA) of the distances among species

Let $\mathbf{\Delta} = [\delta_{kl}]$ and $\mathbf{\Phi} = [-\frac{1}{2}\delta_{kl}^2]$ be the $s \times s$ matrices where δ_{kl} is a distance between species k and l with Euclidean properties. The matrix $\mathbf{\Omega}$ is the doubly centred (by rows and columns) version of $\mathbf{\Phi}$. Using matrix notation, we have $\mathbf{\Omega} = \mathbf{H}\mathbf{\Phi}\mathbf{H}^{\top}$ where $\mathbf{H} = (\mathbf{I}_n - \mathbf{1}_n\mathbf{1}_n^{\top}\mathbf{D}_n)$ is the centring operator. PCoA consists in the following diagonalisation (see Box 6.4):

$$\mathbf{\Omega} = \mathbf{X}\mathbf{X}^{\top}$$

The $s \times k$ matrix $\mathbf{X}$ contains the coordinates of species based on the functional distances. These coordinates are computed for the k dimensions that allow a perfect estimation of the distances. Each community can then be positioned by weighted averaging (see Box 6.1) and their coordinates are given by:

$$\mathbf{Z} = \mathbf{D}_n^{-1}\mathbf{P}\mathbf{X}$$

Note that, by construction, the cloud of communities is centred (i.e., $\mathbf{Z}^{\top}\mathbf{D}_n\mathbf{1}_n = \mathbf{0}_n$).

Step 2: Weighted Principal Component Analysis (PCA) of the coordinates of the communities

The table of communities coordinates $\mathbf{Z}$ is then summarised by a PCA. In this analysis, communities are weighted by their relative proportion using $\mathbf{D}_n$. Hence, DPCoA corresponds to the analysis of the triplet $(\mathbf{Z}, \mathbf{I}_k, \mathbf{D}_n)$. The total inertia of this analysis is equal to the β component of functional diversity (see Box 14.3, Pavoine et al. 2004).

The principal axes ($\mathbf{A}$) maximises the quantity $\|\mathbf{Z}\mathbf{a}\|_{\mathbf{D}_n}^2 = \|\mathbf{D}_n^{-1}\mathbf{P}\mathbf{X}\mathbf{a}\|_{\mathbf{D}_n}^2$. The analysis seeks coefficients ($\mathbf{a}$) for the principal axes obtained in Step 1 to get a score for species ($\mathbf{X}\mathbf{a}$). Communities are then positioned by weighted averaging ($\mathbf{D}_n^{-1}\mathbf{P}\mathbf{X}\mathbf{a}$). Hence, the eigenvalues of this analysis maximise the variance between communities, i.e., the functional β diversity.

In the **ade4** package, the dpcoa function can be used to compute a DPCoA. All the outputs are grouped in a dpcoa object and Box 14.2 recalls the corresponding elements.

The function dpcoa takes two arguments: a sites × species table containing abundance (or presence-absence) data (df) and an object of class dist containing dissimilarities between species (dis). By default, dis is NULL so that species are equidistant. In this case, DPCoA is equivalent to the Non-Symmetric Correspondence Analysis (see Sect. 14.2):

```
dpcoa1 <- dpcoa(fau, scannf = FALSE, nf = 2)
head(nsc1$eig / dpcoa1$eig)
```

```
[1]  98  98  98  98  98  98
```

```
head(nsc1$li / dpcoa1$li)
```

```
  Axis1 Axis2
1 -9.899 9.899
2 -9.899 9.899
3 -9.899 9.899
4 -9.899 9.899
5 -9.899 9.899
6 -9.899 9.899
```

Box 14.2 DPCoA: dudi Output Elements

In the **ade4** package, the results of a DPCoA are stored in an object of class dpcoa. This object is a list with 14 elements. In this list, elements of particular interest are:

- $dw: weights of the species (diagonal of $\mathbf{D}_s$)
- $lw: weights of the communities (diagonal of $\mathbf{D}_n$)
- $eig: eigenvalues ($\Lambda$)
- $dls: coordinates of the species (data frame $\mathbf{XA}$)
- $li: coordinates of the communities (data frame $\mathbf{ZA}$)
- $c1: loadings for the principal coordinates of the species ($\mathbf{A}$)

The coordinates of the species ($dls) and those of the communities ($li) can be superimposed to draw a biplot.

When the dis argument is specified, it is important to ensure that species are in the same order in the abundance table (df) and in the functional distance matrix (dis):

```
fau <- fau[, attributes(dis)$Labels]
```

Then, the DPCoA and associated graphs can be performed (Fig. 14.2):

```
dpcoa2 <- dpcoa(fau, dis, scannf = FALSE, nf = 2,
        RaoDecomp = FALSE)
```

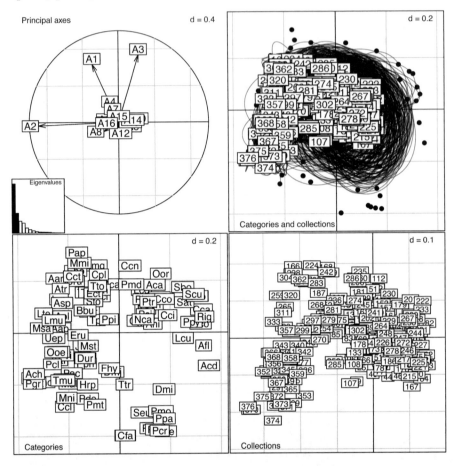

Fig. 14.2 Main plots for DPCoA. The top-left panel contains the projection of the principal axes of the species on the principal axes of the communities. It also contains the eigenvalue barplot. The top-right panel is a biplot that contains the species and the communities. Each community is characterised by its label indicating its position and by an ellipse that indicates the locations of the species the community contains. The bottom-left panel indicates the positions of species and the bottom-right panel the positions of communities. Latin names for species can be found in `tarentaise$latnames`.

Figure 14.3 shows that communities are distributed on the first axis along an elevation gradient. According to species coordinates, species traits are different in different parts of this elevation gradient (Fig. 14.4). Communities of the highest elevations contain bird with the largest body size and the lowest reproductive investment. The most altitudinal parts (>2250 m) are dominated by sedentary, specialised species that can cope with the stressful environment including, for instance, *Cinclus cinclus* (White-throated Dipper) and *Montifringilla nivalis* (White-winged

```
s.class(dpcoa2$li, alti, col = terrain.colors(14),
        pbackground.col = "darkgrey", plabels.boxes.col = "black")
```

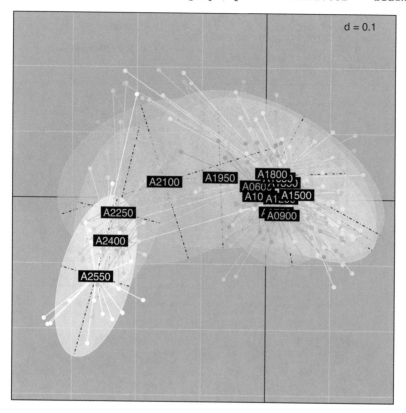

Fig. 14.3 Ordination of communities by DPCoA. Communities are grouped by altitude levels.

Snowfinch). Regarding diet habits, the rapace species are in high elevation, all other diet categories are represented throughout the elevation gradient (Fig. 14.4, top-right panel). Foraging substrate and nest position can be simply explained by the rarefaction of the forest strata at high elevation. At low elevation, a high proportion of species forages in the foliage whereas at higher elevation most species forage on the ground or during flights (Fig. 14.4, bottom-left panel). Similarly, at low elevation, a high proportion of species have their nests in the foliage whereas at higher elevation most species have their nests on the ground, on rock faces or in cavities, which corresponds to modifications in the habitat (Fig. 14.4, bottom-right panel).

The second axis highlights the fact that species at the highest altitudes are sedentary (Fig. 14.4, top-left panel, variable `Migr`). These species better exploit truncks for foraging and nesting and also rocks for nesting (Fig. 14.4, bottom panels).

```
g1 <- s.corcircle(cor(tabO, dpcoa2$dls, method = "spearman"),
      plot = FALSE)
g2 <- s.distri(dpcoa2$dls, tabF[, 1:5], plabels.cex = 1,
      col = TRUE, plot = FALSE)
g3 <- s.distri(dpcoa2$dls, tabF[, 6:9], plabels.cex = 1,
      col = TRUE, plot = FALSE)
g4 <- s.distri(dpcoa2$dls, tabF[, 10:13], plabels.cex = 1,
      col = TRUE, plot = FALSE)
ADEgS(list(g1, g2, g3, g4))
```

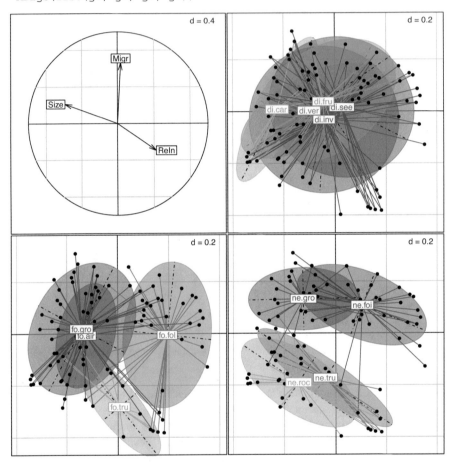

Fig. 14.4 Top-left: Spearman correlation between the three ordinal traits (ReIn = reproduction investment; Size = adult body size and Migr = migratory status) and species' coordinates on the first principal axis (horizontal axis) and the second principal axis (vertical axis) of DPCoA (the correlation circle gives the scale: the radius of the circle equals one); top-right: species's positions on the first two principal axes grouped by type of diet; bottom-left: species grouped by foraging substrate; bottom-right: species grouped by nest position. In the top-right and bottom panels, on the first two principal axes of the communities, points indicate species and labels indicate the attributes of the factor (either diet type, foraging substrate or nest position depending on the panel). Labels are positioned at the barycentre of the species concerned by each attribute (i.e., trait value). A barycentre is weighted by the affinity level species have for each attribute. Segments connect attributes with the concerned species. An ellipse indicates the dispersion of the points of the species that share the same attribute.

14.5 DPCoA and Diversity

DPCoA provides an ordination of communities that considers dissimilarities between species so that diversities are measured by Rao's quadratic entropy. DPCoA analyses the component β as described in Box 14.3.

Box 14.3 DPCoA and Diversity

We used the same notations as in Box 14.1. If we consider the distances among species provided by $-\boldsymbol{\Phi} = \left[\frac{\delta_{kl}^2}{2}\right]$, the diversity of the community i, measured by Rao's quadratic entropy, is equal to:

$$H(\mathbf{p}_i) = \sum_{k=1}^{s} \sum_{l=1}^{s} p_{ik} p_{il} \frac{\delta_{kl}^2}{2}$$

where $\mathbf{p}_i = [p_{ij}/p_{i\bullet}]$ is a vector that contains the relative frequencies of species in community i.

The α diversity is the average diversity within all communities:

$$\alpha = \sum_{i=1}^{n} p_{i\bullet} H(\mathbf{p}_i)$$

The γ diversity is measured over all mixed communities:

$$\gamma = H\left(\sum_{i=1}^{n} p_{i\bullet}\mathbf{p}_i\right) = \sum_{k=1}^{s} \sum_{l=1}^{s} \left(\sum_{i=1}^{n} p_{ik}\right)\left(\sum_{i=1}^{n} p_{il}\right) \frac{\delta_{kl}^2}{2}$$

The component β measures the average differences in the compositions of the communities. It can be simply measured as the difference between γ and α:

$$\beta = \gamma - \alpha$$

It can also be expressed by considering the $n \times n$ matrix $\boldsymbol{\Psi} = [\psi_{ij}]$ of distances among communities. If $\boldsymbol{\Psi}$ is defined as follows:

$$\psi_{ij} = \left(2H\left(\frac{\mathbf{p}_i + \mathbf{p}_j}{2}\right) - H(\mathbf{p}_i) - H(\mathbf{p}_j)\right)$$

then

(continued)

Box 14.3 (continued)

$$\beta = H(\mathbf{n}) = \sum_{i=1}^{n} \sum_{j=1}^{n} p_{i\bullet} p_{\bullet j} \psi_{ij}$$

In DPCoA, the Euclidean distance between the community i and the community j is equal to $\sqrt{2\psi_{ij}}$ (Pavoine et al. 2004). The total variance of the coordinates of communities in DPCoA (i.e., total inertia) is thus equal to the β component of diversity.

The α, β and γ components of functional diversity can be obtained with the apqe function:

```
apqe(as.data.frame(t(fau)), dis)
```

```
$call
apqe(samples = as.data.frame(t(fau)), dis = dis)

$results
                   diversity
Between samples     0.02254
Within samples      0.14861
Total               0.17114
```

In the $results table above, the Between samples row, the Within samples row and the Total row correspond, respectively, to components β, α and γ.

The sum of all eigenvalues in DPCoA is equal to component β, i.e., the component of functional diversity among communities that measures the functional differences in the compositions of the communities:

```
sum(dpcoa2$eig)
```

```
[1] 0.02254
```

The diversity within each community can be obtained with function divc while the distances among communities are provided by the disc function:

```
div.com <- divc(as.data.frame(t(fau)), dis)
dis.com <- disc(as.data.frame(t(fau)), dis)
```

Figure 14.5 shows that the α component of functional diversity decreases strongly with the altitudinal gradient as species become more specialised at higher altitude.

For smaller data sets, a graphical representation of the matrix of distances among collections can be obtained with the table.image function.

The randtest.dpcoa function allows to test whether the differences in the community compositions are higher than expected in the case of random distribution. The default null model considers a random permutation of the columns of fau

```
plot(alti, div.com[, 1], ylab = "Alpha functional diversity",
     col = terrain.colors(14), las = 2)
```

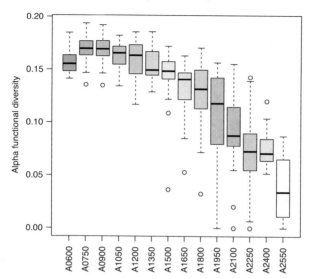

Fig. 14.5 Boxplot of the functional diversity within each bird community in the region La Tarentaise here displayed as a function of the altitude classes (in increasing order).

Table 14.1 Functional structure tested by the `randtest.dpcoa` function. `alter` is one of the parameters used by this function to define the alternative hypothesis.

alter	Structure	Meaning
"greater"	Functional clustering	Coexisting species are similar
"less"	Functional over-dispersion	Coexisting species are different
"two-sided"	Functional non-randomness	Species coexistence depends on traits

(i.e., species) but keeps the `dis` object unchanged. The null hypothesis of this test states that the distribution of species across the communities is independent of their functional traits. Other null models are available (see `?randtest.dpcoa`).

Three alternative hypotheses can be considered (Table 14.1). By default, the `randtest.dpcoa` function uses `alter = "greater"` assuming that coexisting species have similar traits. The statistic of the test is the ratio β/γ as defined in Box 14.1 (Pavoine and Dolédec 2005).

```
randtest(dpcoa2, nrep = 999)

Monte-Carlo test
Call: randtest.dpcoa(xtest = dpcoa2, nrep = 999)

Observation: 0.1317

Based on 999 replicates
Simulated p-value: 0.001
Alternative hypothesis: greater

     Std.Obs Expectation      Variance
   4.773e+00   8.822e-02     8.288e-05
```

Here the test is statistically significant indicating functional clustering, i.e., coexisting species have similar traits.

14.6 Conclusions

DPCoA describes the differences among communities based on known biological differences among their species. In this chapter, we analysed functional diversity but phylogenetic diversity can be analysed exactly in the same way by replacing functional distances among species with phylogenetic distances.

DPCoA is very general and can be applied to other issues. For instance, using the transpose of table `fau` and environmental distances among sites, we could compare the environmental niches of the bird species in La Tarentaise Valley instead of the functional diversity of the sites. In this context, DPCoA can be viewed as a generalisation of Canonical Correspondence Analysis (see Sect. 8.4.2, ter Braak 1986), as demonstrated by Pavoine et al. (2004). If the focus is on the populations of a single species, instead of communities of several species, then DPCoA can be used to analyse the genetic structures of populations and metapopulations (Pavoine and Bailly 2007). Individuals of several populations can then be compared based on genetic distances, such as nucleotide differences between haplotypes (e.g., Turroni et al. 2009). DPCoA has been applied in different contexts such as phylogenetic diversity in ectoparasite assemblages (Krasnov et al. 2012), functional diversity in urban plant assemblages (Valet et al. 2010), song diversity in bird communities (Cardoso and Price 2010) or human intestinal microbial flora (Eckburg et al. 2005). An extension of DPCoA is provided by Dray et al. (2015) to consider external information measured on communities.

Appendix A
A Euclidean Viewpoint on Statistics

This appendix gives the main algebraic and geometric principles used in the descriptive statistic methods presented in this book.

A.1 Inner and Dot Products

Let us consider two vectors $\mathbf{x}$ and $\mathbf{y}$ of $\mathbb{R}^n$. The inner product is a function that associates a real number to the pair of vectors $\mathbf{x}$ and $\mathbf{y}$:

$$\langle \, | \, \rangle : \mathbb{R}^n \times \mathbb{R}^n \to \mathbb{R}$$

with the following properties:

- **Symmetric:** $\langle \mathbf{x}|\mathbf{y}\rangle = \langle \mathbf{y}|\mathbf{x}\rangle,\ \forall \mathbf{x}, \mathbf{y} \in \mathbb{R}^n$
- **Bilinear:**

  - $\langle \mathbf{x}|\mathbf{y} + \mathbf{z}\rangle = \langle \mathbf{x}|\mathbf{y}\rangle + \langle \mathbf{x}|\mathbf{z}\rangle,\ \forall \mathbf{x}, \mathbf{y}, \mathbf{z} \in \mathbb{R}^n$
  - $\langle \mathbf{x}|\alpha\mathbf{y}\rangle = \alpha \langle \mathbf{x}|\mathbf{y}\rangle,\ \forall \mathbf{x}, \mathbf{y} \in \mathbb{R}^n$ and $\forall \alpha \in \mathbb{R}$

- **Positive definite:** $\langle \mathbf{x}|\mathbf{x}\rangle \geq 0,\ \forall \mathbf{x} \in \mathbb{R}^n$
- **Non-degenerate:** $\langle \mathbf{x}|\mathbf{x}\rangle = 0 \Rightarrow \mathbf{x} = \mathbf{0},\ \forall \mathbf{x} \in \mathbb{R}^n$

In $\mathbb{R}^n$, the dot product is the inner product defined in the standard basis by:

$$\langle \mathbf{x}|\mathbf{y}\rangle = \sum_{i=1}^{n} x_i\, y_i = \mathbf{y}^\top \mathbf{x}$$

If $\mathbf{A}$ is an $n \times n$ symmetric positive definite matrix, then the bilinear form $\mathbf{y}^\top \mathbf{A} \mathbf{x}$ satisfies the four properties and defines thus an inner product denoted:

© Springer Science+Business Media, LLC, part of Springer Nature 2018
J. Thioulouse et al., *Multivariate Analysis of Ecological Data with ade4*,
https://doi.org/10.1007/978-1-4939-8850-1

$$\langle \mathbf{x}|\mathbf{y}\rangle_{\mathbf{A}} = \sum_{i=1}^{n}\sum_{j=1}^{n} a_{ij}x_j y_i$$

In $\mathbb{R}^n$, the usual dot product defined in the standard basis is obtained by setting $\mathbf{A}$ to the identity matrix $\mathbf{I}_n$. More generally, given a basis $\{\mathbf{v}_1, \ldots, \mathbf{v}_n\}$ of $\mathbb{R}^n$, the matrix $\mathbf{A}$ defined by $a_{ij} = \langle \mathbf{v}_i|\mathbf{v}_j\rangle_{\mathbf{A}}$ is the unique matrix representing the dot product $\langle \mathbf{x}|\mathbf{y}\rangle_{\mathbf{A}}$. Indeed, we have $\mathbf{x} = \sum_{i=1}^{n} x_i\mathbf{v}_i$ and $\mathbf{y} = \sum_{i=1}^{n} y_i\mathbf{v}_i$, $\forall \mathbf{x}, \mathbf{y} \in \mathbb{R}^n$, and:

$$\langle \mathbf{x}|\mathbf{y}\rangle_{\mathbf{A}} = \left\langle \sum_{i=1}^{n} x_i\mathbf{v}_i \middle| \sum_{j=1}^{n} y_j\mathbf{v}_j \right\rangle_{\mathbf{A}} = \sum_{i=1}^{n'}\sum_{j=1}^{n} x_i \langle \mathbf{v}_i|\mathbf{v}_j\rangle_{\mathbf{A}} y_j$$

$$= \sum_{i=1}^{n}\sum_{j=1}^{n} x_i a_{ij} y_j = \mathbf{y}^{\top}\mathbf{A}\mathbf{x}$$

A.2   Length, Projection, Angle and Distance

The norm (or length) of a vector $\mathbf{x}$ is defined by:

$$\|\mathbf{x}\|_{\mathbf{A}} = \sqrt{\langle \mathbf{x}|\mathbf{x}\rangle_{\mathbf{A}}}$$

Note that $\|\alpha\mathbf{x}\|_{\mathbf{A}} = |\alpha|\, \|\mathbf{x}\|_{\mathbf{A}}$.

The distance between two vectors $\mathbf{x}$ and $\mathbf{y}$ is the norm of their difference:

$$d_{\mathbf{A}}(\mathbf{x}, \mathbf{y}) = \|\mathbf{x} - \mathbf{y}\|_{\mathbf{A}}$$

The projection of $\mathbf{y}$ on the nonzero vector $\mathbf{x}$ is a vector $\mathbf{z}$ parallel to $\mathbf{x}$ so that $\mathbf{y} - \mathbf{z}$ is orthogonal to $\mathbf{x}$. It is given by:

$$\mathbf{z} = \frac{\langle \mathbf{x}|\mathbf{y}\rangle_{\mathbf{A}}}{\langle \mathbf{x}|\mathbf{x}\rangle_{\mathbf{A}}}\mathbf{x}$$

It follows that

$$\cos(\theta_{\mathbf{xy}}) = \frac{\|\mathbf{z}\|_{\mathbf{A}}}{\|\mathbf{y}\|_{\mathbf{A}}} = \frac{\langle \mathbf{x}|\mathbf{y}\rangle_{\mathbf{A}}}{\|\mathbf{x}\|_{\mathbf{A}}\,\|\mathbf{y}\|_{\mathbf{A}}}$$

$$0 \le \theta_{\mathbf{xy}} \le \pi$$

and thus

$$\langle \mathbf{x}|\mathbf{y}\rangle_{\mathbf{A}} = \|\mathbf{x}\|_{\mathbf{A}}\,\|\mathbf{y}\|_{\mathbf{A}}\,\cos(\theta_{\mathbf{xy}})$$

Hence, two vectors $\mathbf{x}$ and $\mathbf{y}$ are orthogonal if $\langle \mathbf{x}|\mathbf{y}\rangle_{\mathbf{A}} = 0$. Moreover, we have

$$\left|\langle \mathbf{x}|\mathbf{y}\rangle_{\mathbf{A}}\right| \le \|\mathbf{x}\|_{\mathbf{A}}\,\|\mathbf{y}\|_{\mathbf{A}} \quad \text{(Cauchy-Schwartz inequality)}$$

and

$$\|\mathbf{x} + \mathbf{y}\|_{\mathbf{A}} \le \|\mathbf{x}\|_{\mathbf{A}} + \|\mathbf{y}\|_{\mathbf{A}} \quad \text{(triangular inequality)}$$

A.3 Mean and Variance

The observed values of a quantitative variable for n individuals are stored in $\mathbf{x} = (x_1, \cdots, x_n)^{\mathsf{T}}$, a vector of $\mathbb{R}^n$. The mean of $\mathbf{x}$ is equal to

$$\mathrm{m}(\mathbf{x}) = \frac{1}{n}\sum_{i=1}^{n} x_i$$

and its variance is

$$\mathrm{v}(\mathbf{x}) = \frac{1}{n}\sum_{i=1}^{n} (x_i - \mathrm{m}(\mathbf{x}))^2$$

Let us consider the uniform inner product of $\mathbb{R}^n$ associated to the diagonal matrix $\frac{1}{n}\mathbf{I}_n$. In a geometric viewpoint, the standard mean is computed by an inner product and corresponds to a Euclidean projection (Fig. A.1):

$$\mathrm{m}(\mathbf{x}) = \langle \mathbf{x}|\mathbf{1}_n\rangle_{\frac{1}{n}\mathbf{I}_n}$$

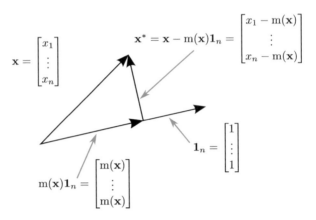

Fig. A.1 Centring a variable seen as an orthogonal projection.

The variance is equal to the squared norm of the centred vector $\mathbf{x}^*$

$$v(\mathbf{x}) = \left\| \mathbf{x} - m(\mathbf{x})\mathbf{1}_n \right\|^2_{\frac{1}{n}\mathbf{I}_n} = \left\| \mathbf{x}^* \right\|^2_{\frac{1}{n}\mathbf{I}_n}$$

A.4   Weighted Mean and Varianc

A weighting function can be defined to give some individuals more influence on the result than other individuals. Weights for the n individuals are stored in a vector $\mathbf{w}$ of $\mathbb{R}^n$. They are positive and their sum is equal to 1:

$$\mathbf{w} = (w_1 \cdots w_n)^\top \text{ with } \sum_{i=1}^{n} w_i = 1 \text{ and } w_i > 0$$

Using $\mathbf{w}$, the weighted mean of $\mathbf{x}$ is

$$m_\mathbf{w}(\mathbf{x}) = \sum_{i=1}^{n} w_i x_i$$

and the weighted variance equals

$$v_\mathbf{w}(\mathbf{x}) = \sum_{i=1}^{n} w_i \left(x_i - m_\mathbf{w}(x) \right)^2$$

Considering the diagonal matrix $\mathbf{D_w} = \text{diag}(\mathbf{w})$ as the inner product of $\mathbb{R}^n$, the weighted mean and variance are given by:

$$m_{\mathbf{w}}(\mathbf{x}) = \langle \mathbf{x} | \mathbf{1}_n \rangle_{\mathbf{D_w}}$$

and

$$v_{\mathbf{w}}(\mathbf{x}) = \| \mathbf{x} - m_{\mathbf{w}}(\mathbf{x}) \mathbf{1}_n \|_{\mathbf{D_w}}^2$$

The standard mean and variance $(m(\mathbf{x}), v(\mathbf{x}))$ correspond to the particular cases of weighted statistics $(m_{\mathbf{w}}(\mathbf{x}), v_{\mathbf{w}}(\mathbf{x}))$ when uniform weights $w_i = \frac{1}{n}$ are chosen. From a geometric viewpoint, computing standard or weighted statistics corresponds to the same operation (i.e., a projection) but using different inner products.

A.5   Covariance and Correlation

The values of two quantitative variables are stored in the vectors $\mathbf{x}$ and $\mathbf{y}$. This information can be considered either as n points (individuals) in $\mathbb{R}^2$ or as 2 points (variables) of $\mathbb{R}^n$. In the first case, data centring corresponds to moving the origin of the system of axes (Fig. A.2a). In the second case, it corresponds to two orthogonal projections on the vector $\mathbf{1}_n$ (Fig. A.2b).

The vectors $\mathbf{x}^*$ and $\mathbf{y}^*$ contain centred data. The standard covariance is equal to

$$\text{cov}(\mathbf{x}, \mathbf{y}) = \text{cor}(\mathbf{x}, \mathbf{y})\sqrt{v(\mathbf{x})}\sqrt{v(\mathbf{y})}$$

$$= \frac{1}{n}\sum_{i=1}^{n}(x_i - m(\mathbf{x}))(y_i - m(\mathbf{y})) = \frac{1}{n}\sum_{i=1}^{n}x_i^* y_i^*$$

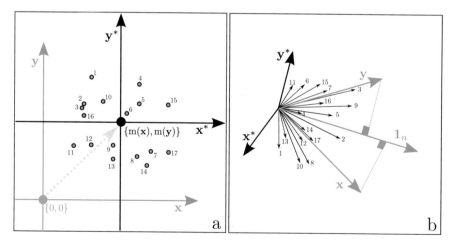

Fig. A.2 Two geometric viewpoints on centring (example with 2 variables and 17 individuals). It corresponds to (**a**) move the origin in $\mathbb{R}^2$ and to (**b**) two orthogonal projections in $\mathbb{R}^{17}$.

It can be rewritten as:

$$\text{cov}(\mathbf{x}, \mathbf{y}) = \langle \mathbf{x}^* | \mathbf{y}^* \rangle_{\frac{1}{n}\mathbf{I}_n}$$

$$= \|\mathbf{x}\|_{\frac{1}{n}\mathbf{I}_n} \|\mathbf{y}\|_{\frac{1}{n}\mathbf{I}_n} \cos(\theta_{\mathbf{xy}})$$

As $\|\mathbf{x}\|_{\frac{1}{n}\mathbf{I}_n} = \sqrt{v(\mathbf{x})}$ and $\|\mathbf{y}\|_{\frac{1}{n}\mathbf{I}_n} = \sqrt{v(\mathbf{y})}$, it follows that:

$$\text{cor}(\mathbf{x}, \mathbf{y}) = \cos(\theta_{\mathbf{xy}})$$

Hence, the covariance is equal to the dot product between the two vectors whereas the correlation is the cosine of the angle formed by the two vectors. Note that weighted covariance and correlation could be obtained by using the appropriate inner product $\mathbf{D_w}$.

A.6   Linear Regression

The linear model that aims to explain the variation of $\mathbf{y}$ by the dependent variable $\mathbf{x}$ can be written as:

$$\mathbf{y} = \beta\mathbf{x} + \alpha\mathbf{1}_n + \boldsymbol{\epsilon}$$

Estimates of α and β are chosen to minimise the sum of squared residuals $\sum_{i=1}^{n} \epsilon_i^2 = \sum_{i=1}^{n} (y_i - \alpha - \beta x_i)^2$ (Fig. A.3a). The least squares estimates of parameters are given by:

$$\hat{\alpha} = m(\mathbf{y}) - \hat{\beta}m(\mathbf{x}) \text{ and } \hat{\beta} = \frac{\text{cov}(\mathbf{x}, \mathbf{y})}{v(\mathbf{x})}$$

Considering the centred variables $\mathbf{x}^*$ and $\mathbf{y}^*$, the estimate of the slope can be rewritten as:

$$\hat{\beta} = \frac{\langle \mathbf{x}^* | \mathbf{y}^* \rangle_{\frac{1}{n}\mathbf{I}_n}}{\|\mathbf{x}^*\|^2_{\frac{1}{n}\mathbf{I}_n}}$$

Thus, the vector of predicted values $\hat{\mathbf{y}}$ can be decomposed as follows:

$$\hat{\mathbf{y}} = \hat{\beta}\mathbf{x} + (m(\mathbf{y}) - \hat{\beta}m(\mathbf{x}))\mathbf{1}_n$$

$$= \hat{\beta}(\mathbf{x}^* + m(\mathbf{x})\mathbf{1}_n) + (m(\mathbf{y}) - \hat{\beta}m(\mathbf{x}))\mathbf{1}_n$$

$$= \hat{\beta}\mathbf{x}^* + m(\mathbf{y})\mathbf{1}_n$$

$$= \frac{\langle \mathbf{x}^* | \mathbf{y}^* \rangle_{\frac{1}{n}\mathbf{I}_n}}{\|\mathbf{x}^*\|^2_{\frac{1}{n}\mathbf{I}_n}} \mathbf{x}^* + \langle \mathbf{y} | \mathbf{1}_n \rangle_{\frac{1}{n}\mathbf{I}_n} \mathbf{1}_n$$

The previous equation shows that the vector of predicted values $\mathbf{y}$ can be computed as the sum of two vectors (Fig. A.3b). The first vector corresponds to the projection of the centred variable $\mathbf{y}^*$ on $\mathbf{x}^*$. The second vector corresponds to the projection of $\mathbf{y}$ on $\mathbf{1}_n$.

As $\mathbf{x} = \mathbf{x}^* + m(\mathbf{x})\mathbf{1}_n$, the three vectors $\mathbf{x}$, $\mathbf{x}^*$ and $\mathbf{1}_n$ are linearly dependent and thus lie in the same plane. It follows that vector of fitted values $\hat{\mathbf{y}}$ corresponds to the orthogonal projection of $\mathbf{y}$ on the plane spanned by the vectors $\mathbf{x}$ and $\mathbf{1}_n$. Applying the Pythagorean theorem to the triangle formed by the vectors $\mathbf{y}$, $\hat{\mathbf{y}}$ and $\epsilon = \mathbf{y} - \hat{\mathbf{y}}$, we obtained the well-known decomposition of variance (Fig. A.4):

$$\|\mathbf{y}\|^2_{\frac{1}{n}\mathbf{I}_n} = \underbrace{\|\hat{\mathbf{y}}\|^2_{\frac{1}{n}\mathbf{I}_n}}_{\text{explained variance}} + \underbrace{\|\mathbf{y} - \hat{\mathbf{y}}\|^2_{\frac{1}{n}\mathbf{I}_n}}_{\text{residual variance}}$$

The coefficient of determination, $R^2_{\mathbf{y}|\mathbf{x}}$ measures the proportion of variance of the dependent variable $\mathbf{y}$ explained by the explanatory variable $\mathbf{x}$. Geometrically, it is the cosine of the angle formed by the vectors $\hat{\mathbf{y}}$ and $\mathbf{y}$ (Fig. A.4):

$$R^2_{\mathbf{y}|\mathbf{x}} = \frac{\|\hat{\mathbf{y}}\|^2_{\frac{1}{n}\mathbf{I}_n}}{\|\mathbf{y}\|^2_{\frac{1}{n}\mathbf{I}_n}} = \cos(\theta_{\hat{\mathbf{y}}\mathbf{y}})$$

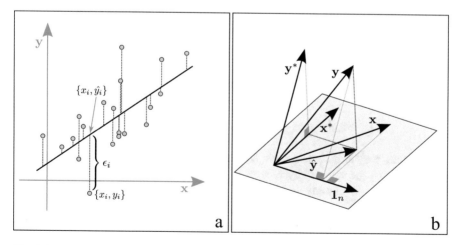

Fig. A.3 Two geometric viewpoints on linear regression with intercept (example with one explanatory variable and 20 individuals). In $\mathbb{R}^2$ (**a**), the usual representation shows that the regression line minimises the residual sum of squares. In $\mathbb{R}^{20}$ (**b**), fitted values are obtained by orthogonal projection of $\mathbf{y}$ on the plane spanned by vectors $\mathbf{x}$ and $\mathbf{1}_n$.

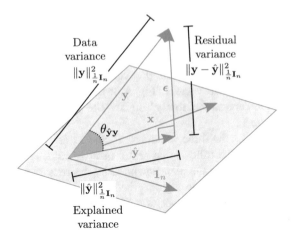

Fig. A.4 Geometric decomposition of the variance using the Pythagorean theorem.

A.7   Categorical Variables

A categorical variable is a variable that can take one of a finite number of possible values, each individual being assigned to a particular group (category, level or class). If we consider a categorical variable with m categories measured for n individuals, the information can be coded as a vector $\mathbf{q}$ of integers. An $n \times m$ table $\mathbf{X} = [\mathbf{x}_1 | \ldots | \mathbf{x}_m]$ of dummy variables can be built. For the k-th category, the dummy variable $\mathbf{x}_k$ is equal to 1 if the individual belongs to this category and 0 otherwise:

	Category		$\mathbf{q}$		$\mathbf{x}_1$	$\mathbf{x}_2$	$\mathbf{x}_3$	$\cdots$	$\mathbf{x}_m$
1	blue		1		1	0	0	$\cdots$	0
2	red		2		0	1	0	$\cdots$	0
3	blue		1		1	0	0	$\cdots$	0
4	green		3		0	0	1	$\cdots$	0
$\vdots$	$\vdots$	$\rightarrow$	$\vdots$	$\rightarrow$	$\vdots$	$\vdots$	$\vdots$	$\vdots$	$\vdots$
n	black		m		0	0	0	$\cdots$	1

Whereas a quantitative variable corresponds to a vector, a categorical variable defines a subspace spanned by vectors $\mathbf{x}_1, \ldots, \mathbf{x}_m$. If we consider a diagonal matrix of weights $\mathbf{D_w}$, the dummy variables are orthogonal by definition (i.e., $\langle \mathbf{x}_i | \mathbf{x}_j \rangle_{\mathbf{D_w}}$ for $i \neq j$). The weight w_k^+ associated to the k-th category is equal to the sum of the weights of the individuals belonging to this category. It is equal to the squared norm of the associated dummy variable, $w_k^+ = \|\mathbf{x}_k\|_{\mathbf{D_w}}^2$.

Let us consider a quantitative variable $\mathbf{y}$. The projection of $\mathbf{y}$ on the k-th dummy variable is equal to:

$$\mathcal{P}_{\mathbf{x}_k}(\mathbf{y}) = \frac{\langle \mathbf{y} | \mathbf{x}_k \rangle_{\mathbf{D_w}}}{\|\mathbf{x}_k\|_{\mathbf{D_w}}^2} \mathbf{x}_k = \frac{\displaystyle\sum_{i/q_i=k} w_i y_i}{w_k^+} \mathbf{x}_k = m_{\mathbf{w}_{/k}}(\mathbf{y}) \mathbf{x}_k$$

The value $m_{w_{/k}}(\mathbf{y})$ is the conditional mean of $\mathbf{y}$ given k (i.e., the weighted mean of the variable $\mathbf{y}$ computed only on the individuals belonging to the k-th category). Hence, the vector $\mathcal{P}_{\mathbf{x}_k}(\mathbf{y})$ takes the value $m_{w_{/k}}(\mathbf{y})$ for the individuals of the k-th category and 0 otherwise.

It follows that the projection of the centred variable $\mathbf{y}^* = \mathbf{y} - m_{\mathbf{w}}(\mathbf{y})\mathbf{1}_n$ on $\mathbf{x}_k$ is simply given by:

$$\mathcal{P}_{\mathbf{x}_k}(\mathbf{y}^*) = (m_{w_{/k}}(\mathbf{y}) - m_{\mathbf{w}}(\mathbf{y}))\mathbf{x}_k$$

As the dummy variables are orthogonal, the projection on the subspace spanned by the vectors $\mathbf{x}_1, \ldots, \mathbf{x}_m$ is simply the sum of the individual projections on each vector $\mathbf{x}_k$:

$$\mathcal{P}_{\mathbf{X}}(\mathbf{y}^*) = \sum_{k=1}^{m} \mathcal{P}_{\mathbf{x}_k}(\mathbf{y}^*)$$

After some substitutions, the squared norm of this projection can be rewritten as:

$$\left\| \mathcal{P}_{\mathbf{X}}(\mathbf{y}^*) \right\|_{\mathbf{D}_{\mathbf{w}}}^2 = \sum_{k=1}^{m} w_k^+ (m_{w_{/k}}(\mathbf{y}) - m_{\mathbf{w}}(\mathbf{y}))^2 = b(\mathbf{y})$$

The quantity $b(\mathbf{y})$ is the between-group variance that measures the differences among categories. Using the Pythagorean theorem, the within-group variance is defined by

$$w(\mathbf{y}) = \left\| \mathbf{y}^* - \mathcal{P}_{\mathbf{X}}(\mathbf{y}^*) \right\|_{\mathbf{D}_{\mathbf{w}}}^2$$

and we obtain the standard ANOVA decomposition of variance:

$$\left\| \mathbf{y}^* \right\|_{\mathbf{D}_{\mathbf{w}}}^2 = \underbrace{\left\| \mathcal{P}_{\mathbf{X}}(\mathbf{y}^*) \right\|_{\mathbf{D}_{\mathbf{w}}}^2}_{\text{between-group variance}} + \underbrace{\left\| \mathbf{y}^* - \mathcal{P}_{\mathbf{X}}(\mathbf{y}^*) \right\|_{\mathbf{D}_{\mathbf{w}}}^2}_{\text{within-group variance}}$$

The correlation ratio $\eta^2(\mathbf{q}, \mathbf{y}) = \frac{b(\mathbf{y})}{v_{\mathbf{w}}(\mathbf{y})}$ measures the proportion associated to the between-group variance. It varies between 0 and 1. Geometrically, it is the cosine of the angle formed by the vectors $\mathcal{P}_{\mathbf{X}}(\mathbf{y}^*)$ and $\mathbf{y}^*$.

A.8   Weighted Multiple Regression

Multiple regression aims to explain the variation of a response variable $\mathbf{y}$ by several dependent variables $\mathbf{x}_1, \ldots, \mathbf{x}_p$ stored in column in an $n \times p$ table $\mathbf{X}$

$(\mathbf{X} = [\mathbf{x}_1|\dots|\mathbf{x}_p] = [x_{ij}])$. For a given weighting matrix $\mathbf{D_w}$, the aim of multiple regression is to predict the observation y_i by a linear model:

$$\hat{y}_i = \beta_1 x_{i1} + \cdots + \beta_p x_{ip} + \alpha = y_i - \epsilon_i$$

The weighted least-squares estimation leads to minimise the residual sum of squares:

$$RSS = \sum_{i=1}^{n} w_i(\hat{y}_i - y_i)^2 = \|\mathbf{y} - \hat{\mathbf{y}}\|_{\mathbf{D_w}}^2$$

The minimisation of the RSS is provided by the orthogonal projection of $\mathbf{y}$ on the subspace spanned by the vectors $\mathbf{x}_1, \dots, \mathbf{x}_p, \mathbf{1}_n$. The vector $\mathbf{1}_n$ is added to consider the intercept in the model so that

$$\hat{\mathbf{y}} = \beta_1 \mathbf{x}_1 + \cdots + \beta_p \mathbf{x}_p + \alpha \mathbf{1}_n$$

The vector of predicted values $\hat{\mathbf{y}}$ exists and is unique. The uniqueness of the coefficients $\beta_1, \cdots, \beta_p, \alpha$ is ensured only if the vectors $\mathbf{x}_1, \dots, \mathbf{x}_p, \mathbf{1}_n$ are independent (i.e., no multicollinearity). This independence is obtained if and only if the centred vectors $\mathbf{x}_1^*, \dots, \mathbf{x}_p^*$ are independent, with $\mathbf{x}_i^* = \mathbf{x}_i - m_\mathbf{w}(\mathbf{x}_i)\mathbf{1}_n$. If the centred vectors are independent, the covariance matrix $\mathbf{X}^{*\top}\mathbf{D_w}\mathbf{X}^*$ is invertible (with $\mathbf{X}^* = [\mathbf{x}_1^*|\dots|\mathbf{x}_p^*]$). In this case, we have:

$$\hat{\mathbf{y}} = \mathcal{P}_{\mathbf{X}^*}(\mathbf{y}) + \mathcal{P}_{\mathbf{1}_n}(\mathbf{y})$$

$$= \mathcal{P}_{\mathbf{X}^*}(\mathbf{y}^*) + \mathcal{P}_{\mathbf{1}_n}(\mathbf{y}^*) + \mathcal{P}_{\mathbf{X}^*}(m_\mathbf{w}(\mathbf{y})\mathbf{1}_n) + \mathcal{P}_{\mathbf{1}_n}(m_\mathbf{w}(\mathbf{y})\mathbf{1}_n)$$

By definition, the centred vectors $\mathbf{x}_1^*, \dots, \mathbf{x}_p^*, \mathbf{y}^*$ are orthogonal to $\mathbf{1}_n$ so that the previous equation simplifies to

$$\hat{\mathbf{y}} = \mathcal{P}_{\mathbf{X}^*}(\mathbf{y}^*) + \mathcal{P}_{\mathbf{1}_n}(m_\mathbf{w}(\mathbf{y})\mathbf{1}_n)$$

In the standard basis, the projection operator $\mathcal{P}_{\mathbf{X}^*}(.)$ is simply equal to $\mathbf{X}^*(\mathbf{X}^{*\top}\mathbf{D_w}\mathbf{X}^*)^{-1}\mathbf{X}^*\mathbf{D_w}$ and the previous equation can be rewritten as:

$$\hat{\mathbf{y}} = \mathbf{X}^*(\mathbf{X}^{*\top}\mathbf{D_w}\mathbf{X}^*)^{-1}\mathbf{X}^*\mathbf{D_w}\mathbf{y}^* + m_\mathbf{w}(\mathbf{y})\mathbf{1}_n$$

The estimates of the parameters are then obtained by

$$\begin{bmatrix} \hat{\beta}_1 \\ \vdots \\ \hat{\beta}_p \end{bmatrix} = (\mathbf{X}^{*\top}\mathbf{D_w}\mathbf{X}^*)^{-1}\mathbf{X}^*\mathbf{D_w}\mathbf{y}^*$$

and

$$\hat{\alpha} = m_\mathbf{w}(\mathbf{y}) - \hat{\beta}_1 m_\mathbf{w}(\mathbf{x}_1^*) - \cdots - \hat{\beta}_p m_\mathbf{w}(\mathbf{x}_p^*)$$

As in simple regression, the part of variance explained by the model is equal to the ratio of two squared norms (and thus the cosine of the angle formed by these two vectors):

$$R_{\mathbf{y}|\mathbf{X}}^2 = \frac{\|\hat{\mathbf{y}}\|_{\mathbf{D_w}}^2}{\|\mathbf{y}\|_{\mathbf{D_w}}^2}$$

Appendix B
Graphical User Interface

Abstract This chapter is a short presentation of **ade4TkGUI**, a Tcl/Tk Graphical User Interface (GUI) package for some basic functions of **ade4**. The **ade4TkGUI** package tries to mix the advantages of a GUI (ease of use, no need to learn numerous commands) with the possibility to use **R** expressions in the dialog boxes, to generate understandable **R** commands, and to manage a session .Rhistory file.

B.1   Introduction

This chapter is based on the paper by Thioulouse and Dray (2007), but only the most interesting features of **ade4TkGUI** are detailed here. The **ade4** package is a part of a previous software that was written in C. This software was mainly used by ecologists, and it had a rich and very useful GUI, written in HyperTalk and based successively on HyperCard, WinPlus and MetaCard (see Chapter 1, Thioulouse et al. 1997).

Switching to **R** and to the command line interface of **ade4** was a hard task for many users, and we decided to make it easier by providing them with a GUI. The first aim of **ade4TkGUI** was to give the users of "Classical ADE-4" an easy access to the main functions of **ade4**. As most users would also be new to **R**, we wanted it to be easy to install, and using **Tcl/Tk** was a guarantee of easiness and multi-platform compatibility.

Only one-table and two-table methods are currently available in **ade4TkGUI** and graphical functions are limited to the basic classes. *K*-table methods are not included.

We decided to use the **Tcl/Tk** language to implement **ade4TkGUI** because the **tcltk** package is available in **R**, and included by default in the base distribution. Many other GUI development systems are available, but they do not offer the same level of availability and platform independence as **tcltk**.

© Springer Science+Business Media, LLC, part of Springer Nature 2018
J. Thioulouse et al., *Multivariate Analysis of Ecological Data with ade4*,
https://doi.org/10.1007/978-1-4939-8850-1

B.2   Overview of the ade4TkGUI Package

It is not possible to give here a detailed description of all the functions of **ade4TkGUI**, and only the main characteristics will be presented. The core of the package is the `ade4TkGUI()` function, which opens the main GUI window (Fig. B.1).

In the main GUI window, buttons are grouped in 6 rows, according to their function: Data sets, One table analyses, One table analyses with groups, Two tables analyses, Graphic functions, and Advanced graphics. To avoid cluttering this window, only a limited subset of functions is displayed. Less frequently used functions are available through the menus of the menu bar, located at the top of the window. Right-clicking the buttons opens the **ade4** help window for the corresponding function. The question-head button opens the help window of **ade4TkGUI**.

The `ade4TkGUI()` function takes two boolean arguments, `show` and `history`. The first one determines whether the **R** commands generated by the GUI

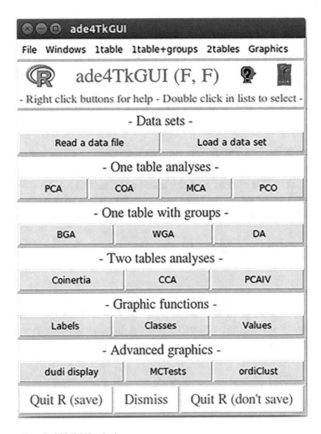

Fig. B.1 The main **ade4TkGUI** window.

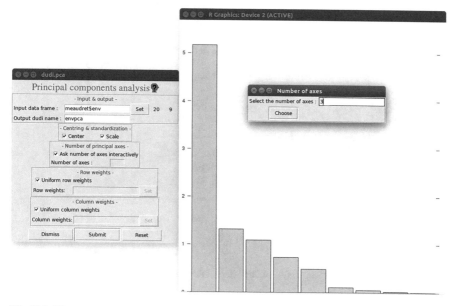

Fig. B.2 The `dudi.pca` function GUI window (left), the eigenvalues barchart (right) and the selection of the number of axes by the user (top-right).

should be printed in the console. When users interact with the GUI, they modify the status of **tcltk** widgets, and when they click on the "`Submit`" button, an **R** command is generated from the status of these widgets. This command is executed and can optionally be displayed in the console. If the `history` argument is set to TRUE, the commands generated by the GUI are also stored in the `.Rhistory` file, where they can easily be retrieved by users. The state of the two parameters is recalled in the main window heading "`ade4TkGUI(T,T)`".

The "`Read a data file`" button opens a dialog window that can be used to set the parameters of the `read.table` command to read a data text file. The "`Load a data set`" just displays the list of **ade4** data sets. This list can be used to choose a particular data set and to load it in memory using the `data` command.

When the "`PCA`" button is clicked, a new window appears (Fig. B.2): this is the GUI window of the `dudi.pca` function.

In this new window, the "`Set`" button can be used to choose the PCA input data frame through a listbox showing the list of data frames in the user global environment. After the "`Input data frame`" text field has been filled by the user, the number of rows and columns (20, 9) are displayed next to it. The output of the `dudi.pca` function is an object of class `dudi` and the user can type the name of this object in the "`Output dudi name`" field. If this field is left empty, the name "`Untitled1`" is used automatically.

The remaining widgets can be used to set particular options for the PCA: centring and standardisation, number of principal axes used to compute row and column coordinates, and row and column weights.

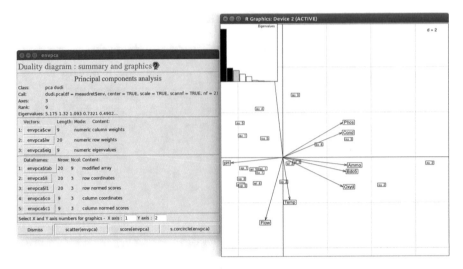

Fig. B.3 The dudi object display window (left) and the biplot obtained by clicking on the "scatter" button (right).

Most of the windows created by **ade4TkGUI** are non-blocking, which means that the user can do other things in the GUI or in the **R** console before taking the action required by this window. This was designed to make the interface more flexible and easier to use.

Clicking the "Submit" button starts the PCA computations. When they are completed, the barplot of eigenvalues is displayed (right of Fig. B.2) and, if this option was chosen in the previous dialog window, the user is asked to select the number of axes on which the row and column scores should be computed.

After scores are computed, the dudi window is displayed (Fig. B.3, left). This window shows a summary of the analysis, and displays the elements of the dudi object under the form of buttons. All these buttons can be used to draw graphs of the corresponding elements. For example, the row and column coordinates buttons draw the classical factor maps. In the lower part of the window, the user can choose which axes are used to draw these graphs.

The last row of buttons gives access to special graphs, according to the particular properties of the dudi that is displayed. For example, in the case of a normed PCA, the "s.corcircle" button allows to draw a correlation circle. The "scatter" button draws a biplot, with a small barchart for eigenvalues (Fig. B.3, right). These additional buttons are adapted to the type of dudi that is displayed, and they allow to draw graphs that illustrate particular properties of this dudi.

An example of GUI for one of the graphical functions of **adegraphics** is given in Fig. B.4. This is the s.class function, which allows to draw factor maps with groups of individuals. The user can choose the data frame containing the row scores (here they come from the "envpca" dudi), and the factor that should be used

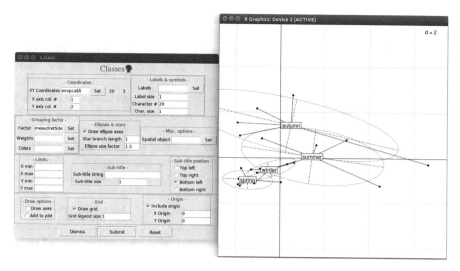

Fig. B.4 The s.class GUI window (left) and the corresponding graph (right).

to draw the groups on the factor map. Many other options can be set to enrich the graphs.

B.3   Conclusion

The main advantage of a GUI is the ease of use for beginners, occasional users, or teachers and students. It makes easier learning how to use a software by making the learning curve smoother, or to get back to work after a long period. This is particularly important in the case of **ade4** in ecological data analysis, because ecologists are mostly occasional users of **R**.

An important feature in **ade4** is the dudi, a complex **R** object containing all the information relating to a duality diagram. The dudi GUI window (Fig. B.3) was designed to display all the components of a dudi, and to draw automatically default graphs for each of these components. Therefore, it offers a centralised and synthetic view of an analysis, and it allows to see rapidly and interactively many graphs. In command line mode, the user must know all the components of a dudi, and remember which one is needed to draw a particular graph; this is particularly difficult for occasional users.

The **ade4TkGUI** package also facilitates the use of **ade4** by pre-selecting the type of objects that are proposed to users when they must do a selection. For example, in the dudi.pca dialog window (Fig. B.2), when the user clicks on the "Set" button to select a data frame, the dialog box contains only data frames present in the global environment (or in lists present in the global environment). In the same window, if the user wants to set non-uniform row weights, the "Set" button for row weights displays only vectors of length equal to the number of rows of the data frame. More generally, lists are filtered to propose only objects with properties consistent with the aim of the action. In the same way, in the dudi window, the buttons and their functions are coherent with the type of dudi and with the mathematical properties of its components.

Obviously, a GUI is not well adapted to scripting, and even to simple repetitive tasks. It is also not good for batch, online or remote use, and it is not easy to integrate into Sweave or R Markdown documents and vignettes. This is probably the main drawback of GUIs: they are made for *personal* and *instant* use, while the command line interface (CLI) allows many operations like scripting, re-doing the same analysis later, sharing pieces of code among colleagues, and batch use for time-consuming computations.

GUIs and CLIs should not be opposed, but considered as complementary. GUIs make the learning curve smoother for beginners, and can be used in education to introduce students to CLI mode. CLI mode is more powerful, it allows to build more complex analyses, particularly when using several packages jointly. When possible, the joint use of both CLI and GUI is attractive, as the user gets the benefits of the two approaches. Joint use can be very intimate: for example, it is possible to use **R** expressions in the GUI dialogs, and the GUI can return **R** expressions that can be copied and pasted in the console. In the case of **ade4TkGUI**, the strings typed by the user in the text fields of the GUI are parsed, and it is therefore possible to use **R** expressions, for example, to specify a subset of a data frame in a PCA.

When ade4TkGUI is called with argument "show = TRUE", **R** commands built by the GUI are echoed to the console. It is then possible to copy/paste these commands and execute them when needed in the console. This is also an effective way for beginners to learn how to use elaborate **R** function calls. Occasional users can thus analyse these command lines and possibly adapt them to their needs, with the additional benefit of gradually learning the **R** language.

In addition to this **Tcl/Tk** GUI, we are developing a new Shiny application to use the main ade4 functionalities through a Web application. Shiny is an **R** package that makes very easy building interactive Web Apps in **R**. The main advantage is that users do not have to install **R** and multiple packages: they only need a web browser. As an example, a first piece of this "in progress" work is deployed on the *shinyapps.io* web site. It can be used to perform a PCA at this URL: https://ade4. shinyapps.io/ShinyPCA. We plan to develop this approach in the near future and hope to be able to propose a complete Shiny GUI to the ade4 package.

Appendix C
Index of Boxes

C.1 Chapter 3: The `dudi` Class

C.2 Chapter 4: Multivariate Analysis Graphs

C.3 Chapter 5: Description of Environmental Variables Structures

C.4 Chapter 6: Description of Species Structures

© Springer Science+Business Media, LLC, part of Springer Nature 2018
J. Thioulouse et al., *Multivariate Analysis of Ecological Data with ade4*,
https://doi.org/10.1007/978-1-4939-8850-1

C.5   Chapter 7: Taking into Account Groups of Sites

C.6   Chapter 8: Description of Species-Environment Relationships

C.7   Chapter 9: Analysing Changes in Structures

C.8   Chapter 10: Analysing Changes in Co-structures

C.9   Chapter 11: Relating Species Traits to Environment

C.10   Chapter 12: Analysing Spatial Structures

C.11   Chapter 13: Analysing Phylogenetic Structures

C.12   Chapter 14: Analysing Patterns of Biodiversity

References

Abdi H, Williams LJ, Valentin D, Bennani-Dosse M (2012) STATIS and DISTATIS: optimum multitable principal component analysis and three way metric multidimensional scaling. Wiley Interdiscip Rev Comput Stat 4:124–167

Abouheif E (1999) A method for testing the assumption of phylogenetic independence in comparative data. Evol Ecol Res 1:895–909

Ackerly DD, Donoghue MJ (1998) Leaf size, sapling allometry, and corner's rules: phylogeny and correlated evolution in maples (acer). Am Nat 152(6):767–791

Anselin L (1996) The Moran scatterplot as an ESDA tool to assess local instability in spatial association. In: Fischer MM, Scholten HJ, Unwin D (eds) Spatial analytical perspectives on GIS. Taylor and Francis, London, pp 111–125

Auda Y (1983) Rôle des méthodes graphiques en analyse des données: application au dépouille-ment des enquêtes écologiques. Thèse de 3ème cycle, Université Lyon 1

Austin MP (2002) Spatial prediction of species distribution: an interface between ecological theory and statistical modelling. Ecol Model 157:101–118

Austin M, Noy-Meir I (1971) The problem of non-linearity in ordination: experiments with two-gradient models. J Ecol 59:763–773

Bady P, Dolédec S, Dumont B, Fruget JF (2004) Multiple co-inertia analysis: a tool for assessing synchrony in the temporal variability of aquatic communities. C R Biol 327:29–36

Bauman D, Drouet T, Dray S, Vleminckx J (2018) Disentangling good from bad practices in the selection of spatial or phylogenetic eigenvectors. Ecography. https://doi.org/10.1111/ecog.03380

Beals EW (1973) Ordination: mathematical elegance and ecological naivete. J Ecol 61:23–35

de Bélair G, Bencheikh-Lehocine M (1987) Composition et déterminisme de la végétation d'une plaine côtière marécageuse: La Mafragh (Annaba, Algérie). Bull d'Ecologie 18(4):393–407

Benzécri JP (1969) Statistical analysis as a tool to make patterns emerge from data. In: Watanabe S (ed) Methodologies of pattern recognition. Academic, New York, pp 35–60

Bertin J (1967) Les diagrammes, les réseaux, les cartes. Mouton & Gautier-Villars, Paris

Bertrand F, Maumy M (2010) Using partial triadic analysis for depicting the temporal evolution of spatial structures: assessing phytoplankton structure and succession in a water reservoir. Case Stud Bus Ind Gov Stat 4:23–43

Bivand R, Lewin-Koh N (2017) maptools: tools for reading and handling spatial objects. https://CRAN.R-project.org/package=maptools, R package version 0.9-2

Bivand R, Piras G (2015) Comparing implementations of estimation methods for spatial econo-metrics. J Stat Softw 63(18):1–36

© Springer Science+Business Media, LLC, part of Springer Nature 2018
J. Thioulouse et al., *Multivariate Analysis of Ecological Data with ade4*,
https://doi.org/10.1007/978-1-4939-8850-1

Bivand RS, Pebesma E, Gomez-Rubio V (2013) Applied spatial data analysis with R, 2nd edn. Springer, New York

Blomberg SP, Garland T, Ives AR (2003) Testing for phylogenetic signal in comparative data: behavioral traits are more labile. Evolution 57(4):717–745

Blondel J, Farré H (1988) The convergent trajectories of bird communities along ecological successions in European forests. Oecologia 75:83–93

Borcard D, Gillet F, Legendre P (2011) Numerical Ecology with R. Springer, New York

Bougeard S, Dray S (2018) Supervised multiblock analysis in R with the ade4 package. J Stat Soft 86(1):1–17. http://doi.org/10.18637/jss.v086.i01

Bouroche JM (1975) Analyse des données ternaires: la double analyse en composantes principales. PhD thesis, Thèse de troisième cycle, Université Paris VI

ter Braak CJF (1983) Principal components biplots and alpha and beta diversity. Ecology 64(3):454–462

ter Braak C (1986) Canonical correspondence analysis: a new eigenvector technique for multivariate direct gradient analysis. Ecology 67:1167–1179

ter Braak CJF (1985) Correspondence analysis of incidence and abundance data: properties in terms of a unimodal reponse model. Biometrics 41:859–873

ter Braak CJF (1987) The analysis of vegetation-environment relationships by canonical correspondence analysis. Vegetatio 69:69–77

ter Braak CJF, Looman CWN (1986) Weighted averaging, logistic regression and the Gaussian response model. Vegetatio 65:3–11

ter Braak CJF, Verdonschot PFM (1995) Canonical correspondence analysis and related multivariate methods in aquatic ecology. Aquat Sci 57:255–289

ter Braak C, Cormont A, Dray S (2012) Improved testing of species traits-environment relationships in the fourth corner problem. Ecology 93:1525–1526

Cardoso GC, Price TD (2010) Community convergence in bird song. Evol Ecol 24:447–461

Chessel, D. (1992) Echanges interdisciplinaires en analyse des données écologiques. Mémoire d'Habilitation à Diriger des Recherches. 107 pages, Université Lyon 1, 69622 Villeurbanne Cedex, France.

Chessel D, Hanafi M (1996) Analyse de la co-inertie de K nuages de points. Rev Stat Appl 44:35–60

Chessel D, Dufour AB, Thioulouse J (2004) The ade4 package - I: one-table methods. R News 4:5–10

Cheverud JM, Dow MM (1985) An autocorrelation analysis of genetic variation due to lineal fission in social groups of Rhesus macaques. Am J Phys Anthropol 67:113–121

Cheverud JM, Dow MM, Leutenegger W (1985) The quantitative assessment of phylogenetic constaints in comparative analyses: sexual dimorphism in body weights among primates. Evolution 39:1335–1351

Choler P (2005) Consistent shifts in Alpine plant traits along a mesotopographical gradient. Arct Antarct Alp Res 37(4):444–453

Culhane A, Perriere G, Considine E, Cotter T, Higgins D (2002) Between-group analysis of microarray data. Bioinformatics 18:1600–1608

Curtis JT, McIntosh RP (1951) An upland forest continuum in the prairie-forest border region of Wisconsin. Ecology 32(3):476–496

Dale M, Fortin MJ (2010) From graphs to spatial graphs. Ann Rev Ecol Evol Syst 41(1):21–38

Dolédec S, Chessel D (1987) Rythmes saisonniers et composantes stationnelles en milieu aquatique. I- Description d'un plan d'observations complet par projection de variables. Acta Oecol Oecol Generalis 8:403–426

Dolédec S, Chessel D (1994) Co-inertia analysis: an alternative method for studying species-environment relationships. Freshw Biol 31:277–294

Dolédec S, Chessel D, ter Braak CJF, Champely S (1996) Matching species traits to environmental variables: a new three-table ordination method. Environ Ecol Stat 3:143–166

Dormann CF, Elith J, Bacher S, Buchmann C, Carl G, Carré G, Marquéz JRG, Gruber B, Lafourcade B, Leitão PJ, Münkemüller T, McClean C, Osborne PE, Reineking B, Schröder B, Skidmore AK, Zurell D, Lautenbach S (2013) Collinearity: a review of methods to deal with it and a simulation study evaluating their performance. Ecography 36:27–46

Dragulescu AA, Arendt C (2018) xlsx: read, write, format Excel 2007 and Excel 97/2000/XP/2003 files. https://CRAN.R-project.org/package=xlsx, R package version 0.6.1

Dray S (2008) On the number of principal components: a test of dimensionality based on measurements of similarity between matrices. Comput Stat Data Anal 52:2228–2237

Dray S, Dufour A (2007) The ade4 package: implementing the duality diagram for ecologists. J Stat Softw 22(4):1–20

Dray S, Jombart T (2011) Revisiting Guerry's data: introducing spatial constraints in multivariate analysis. Ann Appl Stat 5:2278–2299

Dray S, Josse J (2015) Principal component analysis with missing values: a comparative survey of methods. Plant Ecol 216:657–667

Dray S, Legendre P (2008) Testing the species traits-environment relationships: the fourth-corner problem revisited. Ecology 89:3400–3412

Dray S, Chessel D, Thioulouse J (2003) Co-inertia analysis and the linking of ecological data tables. Ecology 84:3078–3089

Dray S, Legendre P, Peres-Neto PR (2006) Spatial modeling: a comprehensive framework for principal coordinate analysis of neighbor matrices (PCNM). Ecol Model 196:483–493

Dray S, Dufour A, Chessel D (2007) The ade4 package–II: two-table and K-table methods. R News 7:47–52

Dray S, Saïd S, Débias F (2008) Spatial ordination of vegetation data using a generalization of Wartenberg's multivariate spatial correlation. J Veg Sci 19:45–56

Dray S, Pélissier R, Couteron P, Fortin MJ, Legendre P, Peres-Neto PR, Bellier E, Bivand R, Blanchet FG, De Caceres M, Dufour AB, Heegaard E, Jombart T, Munoz F, Oksanen J, Thioulouse J, Wagner HH (2012) Community ecology in the age of multivariate multiscale spatial analysis. Ecol Monogr 82(3):257–275

Dray S, Choler P, Dolédec S, Peres-Neto PR, Thuiller W, Pavoine S, ter Braak CJ (2014) Combining the fourth-corner and the RLQ methods for assessing trait responses to environmental variation. Ecology 95(1):14–21

Dray S, Pavoine S, Aguirre de Carcer D (2015) Considering external information to improve the phylogenetic comparison of microbial communities: a new approach based on constrained Double Principal Coordinates Analysis (cDPCoA). Mol Ecol Resour 15:242–249

Dray S, Blanchet G, Borcard D, Clappe S, Guenard G, Jombart T, Larocque G, Legendre P, Madi N, Wagner HH (2018) adespatial: multivariate multiscale spatial analysis. https://CRAN.R-project.org/package=adespatial, R package version 0.2-0

Eckburg PB, Bik EM, Bernstein CN, Purdom E, Dethlefsen L, Sargent M, Gill SR, Nelson KE, Relman DA (2005) Diversity of the human intestinal microbial flora. Science 308:1635–1638

Escofier B, Pagès J (1994) Multiple Factor Analysis (AFMULT package). Comput Stat Data Anal 18:121–140

Escofier Y (1973) Le traitement des variables vectorielles. Biometrics 29:750–760

Escofier Y (1987) The duality diagram: a means of better practical applications. In: Legendre P, Legendre L (eds) Development in numerical ecology. NATO advanced Institute, Serie G. Springer, Berlin, pp 139–156

Felsenstein J (1985) Phylogenies and the comparative method. Am Nat 125:1–15

Foucart T (1978) Sur les suites de tableaux de contingence indexées par le temps. Statistique et Analyse des données 3:67–85

Franquet E, Chessel D (1994) Approche statistique des composantes spatiales et temporelles de la relation faune-milieu. Comptes Rendus de l'Académie des sciences Série 3 317:202–206

Franquet E, Dolédec S, Chessel D (1995) Using multivariate analyses for separating spatial and temporal effects within species-environment relationships. Hydrobiologia 300:425–431

Friday L (1987) The diversity of macroinvertebrate and macrophyte communities in ponds. Freshw
    Biol 18:87–104
Friendly M, Dray S (2014) Guerry: maps, data and methods related to Guerry (1833) "Moral
    statistics of France". http://CRAN.R-project.org/package=Guerry, R package version 1.6-1
Gabriel K (1971) The biplot graphical display of matrices with application to principal component
    analysis. Biometrika 58:453–467
Geary RC (1954) The contiguity ratio and statistical mapping. Inc Stat 5(3):115–145
Gimaret-Carpentier C, Dray S, Pascal JP (2003) Broad-scale biodiversity pattern of the endemic
    tree flora of the Western Ghats (India) using canonical correlation analysis of herbarium
    records. Ecography 26:429–444
Gittleman JL, Kot M (1990) Adaptation: statistics and a null model for estimating phylogenetic
    effects. Syst Zool 39:227–241
Gleason HA (1926) The individualistic concept of the plant association. Bull Torrey Bot Club
    53(1):7–26
Goodall DW (1954) Objective methods for the classification of vegetation. III. An essay on the use
    of factor analysis. Aust J Bot 2:304–324
Gower JC (1966) Some distance properties of latent root and vector methods used in multivariate
    analysis. Biometrika 53:325–338
Gower JC (1984) Distance matrices and their euclidean approximation. In: Diday E, Jambu M,
    Lebart L, Pagès J, Tomassone R (eds) Data analysis and informatics III. Elsevier, Amsterdam,
    pp 3–21
Gower J, Legendre P (1986) Metric and euclidean properties of dissimilarity coefficients. J Classif
    3:5–48
Green RH (1971) A multivariate statistical approach to the Hutchinsonian niche: bivalve molluscs
    of Central Canada. Ecology 52:543–556
Green RH (1974) Multivariate niche analysis with temporally varying environmental factors.
    Ecology 55:73–83
Greenacre M (1984) Theory and applications of correspondence analysis. Academic, London
Griffith DA (1996) Spatial autocorrelation and eigenfunctions of the geographic weights matrix
    accompanying geo-referenced data. Can Geogr 40(4):351–367
Harvey PH, Pagel M (1991) The comparative method in evolutionary biology. Oxford University
    Press, Oxford
Hill M (1973) Reciprocal averaging: an eigenvector method of ordination. J Ecol 61:237–249
Hill MO (1974) Correspondence Analysis: a neglected multivariate method. J R Stat Soc Ser C
    (Appl Stat) 23:340–354
Hill M, Smith A (1976) Principal component analysis of taxonomic data with multi-state discrete
    characters. Taxon 25:249–255
Holmes S (2006) Multivariate analysis: the french way. In: Nolan D, Speed T (eds) Festschrift for
    David Freedman. IMS, Beachwood, OH, pp 1–14
Hotelling H (1933) Analysis of a complex of statistical variables into principal components. J Educ
    Psychol 24:417–441
Hotelling H (1936) Relations between two sets of variates. Biometrika 28:321–377
Jaffrenou P (1978) Sur l'analyse des familles finies de variables vectorielles. Bases algébriques et
    application à la description statistique. PhD thesis, Thèse de troisième cycle, Université Lyon 1
Jaromczyk JW, Toussaint GT (1992) Relative neighborhood graphs and their relatives. Proc IEEE
    80(9):1502–1517
Jarraud S, Mougel C, Thioulouse J, Lina G, Meugnier H, Forey F, Nesme X, Etienne J, Vandenesch
    F (2002) Relationships between staphylococcus aureus genetic background, virulence factors,
    agr type (alleles), and human disease type. Infect Immun 70:631–641
Jolliffe I (2002) Principal component analysis, 2nd edn. Springer, New York
Jombart T, Dray S, Dufour AB (2009) Finding essential scales of spatial variation in ecological
    data: a multivariate approach. Ecography 32:161–168
Jombart T, Balloux F, Dray S (2010a) adephylo: new tools for investigating the phylogenetic signal
    in biological traits. Bioinformatics 26:1907–1909

Jombart T, Pavoine S, Dufour AB, Pontier D (2010b) Putting phylogeny into the analysis of biological traits: a methodological approach. J Theor Biol 264:693–701

de Jong P, Sprenger C, van Veen F (1984) On extreme values of Moran's I and Geary's c. Geogr Anal 16(1):17–24

Krasnov BR, Mouillot D, Khokhlova IS, Shenbrot G, Poulin R (2012) Compositional and phylogenetic dissimilarity of host communities drives dissimilarity of ectoparasite assemblages: geographical variation and scale-dependence. Parasitology 139:338–347

Kroonenberg PM (1983) Three-mode principal component analysis: theory and applications. DWO Press, Leiden

Kroonenberg PM (1989) The analysis of multiple tables in factorial ecology. III. Three-mode Principal Component Analysis: "Analyse triadique complète". Acta Oecol Oecol Generalis 10:245–256

Kroonenberg PM, Lombardo R (1999) Nonsymmetric correspondence analysis: a tool for analysing contingency tables with a dependence structure. Multivar Behav Res 34(3):367–396

Lafosse R, Hanafi M (1997) Concordance d'un tableau avec K tableaux: définition de K + 1 uples synthétiques. Revue de Statistique Appliquée 45:111–126

Lavit C (1988) Analyse conjointe de tableaux quantitatifs. Masson, Paris,

Lavit C, Escoufier Y, Sabatier R, Traissac P (1994) The ACT (STATIS method). Comput Stat Data Anal 18:97–119

Lebart L, Morineau A, Warwick K (1984) Multivariate descriptive statistical analysis. Wiley, New York

Lebreton JD, Chessel D, Prodon R, Yoccoz NG (1988a) L'analyse des relations espèces-milieu par l'analyse canonique des correspondances. I. Variables de milieu quantitatives. Acta Oecol Oecol Generalis 9(1):53–67

Lebreton JD, Chessel D, Richardot-Coulet M, Yoccoz NG (1988b) L'analyse des relations espèces-milieu par l'analyse canonique des correspondances. II. Variables de milieu qualitatives. Acta Oecol Oecol Generalis 9(2):137–151

Lebreton P, Lebrun P, Martinot J, Miquet A, Tournier H (1999) Approche écologique de l'avifaune de la vanoise. Travaux scientifiques du Parc national de la Vanoise 21:7–304

Legendre P (1993) Spatial autocorrelation: trouble or new paradigm? Ecology 74(6):1659–1673

Legendre P, Anderson M (1999) Distance-based redundancy analysis: testing multi-species responses in multi-factorial ecological experiments. Ecol Monogr 69:1–24

Legendre P, Legendre L (1998) Numerical ecology. Elsevier, Amsterdam

Legendre P, Galzin R, Harmelin-Vivien ML (1997) Relating behavior to habitat: solutions to the fourth-corner problem. Ecology 78(2):547–562

LeRoux B, Rouanet H (2004) Geometric data analysis. Academic, Dordrecht

Martins EP, Diniz-Filho JAF, Housworth EA (2002) Adaptive constraints and the phylogenetic comparative method: a computer simulation test. Evolution 56(1):1–13

McIntosh RP (1978) Matrix and plexus techniques. In: Whittaker RH (ed) Ordination of plant communities. Springer, Netherlands, pp 151–184

Mendes S, Gómez JF, Pereira MJ, Azeiteiro UM, Galindo-Villardón MP (2010) The efficiency of the Partial Triadic Analysis method: an ecological application. Biometr Lett 47:83–106

Miller JK (1975) The sampling distribution and a test for the significance of the bimultivariate redundancy statistic: a Monte Carlo study. Multivar Behav Res 10(2):233–244

Miller JK, Farr SD (1971) Bimultivariate redundancy: a comprehensive measure of interbattery relationship. Multivar Behav Res 6(3):313–324

Moran PAP (1948) The interpretation of statistical maps. J R Stat Soc Ser B-Methodol 10:243–251

Munoz F (2009) Distance-based eigenvector maps (DBEM) to analyse metapopulation structure with irregular sampling. Ecol Model 220(20):2683–2689

Neuwirth E (2014) RColorBrewer: ColorBrewer palettes. https://CRAN.R-project.org/package= RColorBrewer, R package version 1.1-2

Nishisato S (1980) Analysis of categorical data: dual scaling and its applications. University of Toronto Press, Toronto

Obadia J (1978) L'analyse en composantes explicatives. Revue de Statistique Appliquée 26(4): 5–28

Oksanen J (1987) Problems of joint display of species and site scores in correspondence analysis. Vegetatio 72:51–57

Oksanen J, Minchin PR (2002) Continuum theory revisited: what shape are species responses along ecological gradients? Ecol Model 157:119–129

Ollier S, Couteron P, Chessel D (2005) Orthonormal transform to detect and characterize phylogenetic signal. Biometrics 62:471–477

Paradis E, Claude J, Strimmer K (2004) APE: analyses of phylogenetics and evolution in R language. Bioinformatics 20:289–290

Pavoine S, Bailly X (2007) New analysis for consistency among markers in the study of genetic diversity: development and application to the description of bacterial diversity. BMC Evol Biol 7:156

Pavoine S, Dolédec S (2005) The apportionment of quadratic entropy: a useful alternative for partitioning diversity in ecological data. Environ Ecol Stat 12:125–138

Pavoine S, Dufour AB, Chessel D (2004) From dissimilarities among species to dissimilarities among communities: a double principal coordinate analysis. J Theor Biol 228:523–537

Pavoine S, Blondel J, Baguette M, Chessel D (2007) A new technique for ordering asymmetrical three-dimensional data sets in ecology. Ecology 88:512–523

Pavoine S, Ollier S, Pontier D, Chessel D (2008) Testing for phylogenetic signal in life history variable: Abouheif's test revisited. Theor Popul Biol 73:79–91

Pavoine S, Vallet J, Dufour AB, Gachet S, Daniel H (2009) On the challenge of treating various types of variables: application for improving the measurement of functional diversity. Oikos 118(3):391–402

Pavoine S, Vela E, Gachet S, de Bélair G, Bonsall MB (2011) Linking patterns in phylogeny, traits, abiotic variables and space: a novel approach to linking environmental filtering and plant community assembly. J Ecol 99(1):165–175

Pearson K (1901) On lines and planes of closest fit to systems of points in space. Philos Mag 2:559–572

Pebesma EJ, Bivand RS (2005) Classes and methods for spatial data in R. R News 5(2):9–13

Pegaz-Maucet D (1980) Impact d'une perturbation d'origine organique sur la dérive des macro-invertébrés benthiques d'un cours d'eau. Comparaison avec le benthos. PhD thesis, Thèse de troisième cycle, Université Lyon 1

Pélabon C, Gaillard JM, Loison A, Portier C (1995) Is sex-biased maternal care limited by total maternal expenditure in polygynous ungulates? Behav Ecol Sociobiol 37(5):311–319

Pélissier R, Couteron P, Dray S, Sabatier D (2003a) Consistency between ordination techniques and diversity measurements: two alternative strategies for species occurrence data. Ecology 84:242–251

Pélissier R, Couteron P, Dray S, Sabatier D (2003b) Consistency between ordination techniques and diversity measurements: two strategies for species occurrence data. Ecology 84(1):242–251

Peres-Neto PR, Legendre P, Dray S, Borcard D (2006) Variation partitioning of species data matrices: estimation and comparison of fractions. Ecology 87:2614–2625

R Hackathon et al (2017) phylobase: base package for phylogenetic structures and comparative data. https://CRAN.R-project.org/package=phylobase, R package version 0.8.4

Rao CR (1964) The use and interpretation of Principal Component Analysis in applied research. Sankhya: Indian J Stat Ser A 26:329–358

Rao CR (1982) Diversity and dissimilarity coefficients: a unified approach. Theor Popul Biol 21:24–43

Revell LJ, Collar DC (2009) Phylogenetic analysis of the evolutionary correlation using likelihood. Evolution 63(4):1090–1100

Rolland A, Bertrand F, Maumy M, Jacquet S (2009) Assessing phytoplankton structure and spatio-temporal dynamics in a freshwater ecosystem using a powerful multiway statistical analysis. Water Res 43:3155–3168

Sarkar D (2008) Lattice: multivariate data visualization with R. Springer, New York

Schliep KP (2011) phangorn: phylogenetic analysis in R. Bioinformatics 27(4):592–593

Schliep, Klaus, Potts, J A, Morrison, A D, Grimm, W G (2017) Intertwining phylogenetic trees and networks. Meth Ecol Evol 8(10):1212–1220

Schutten GJ, hong Chan C, Leeper TJ (2016) readODS: read and write ODS files. https://CRAN. R-project.org/package=readODS, R package version 1.6.4

Siberchicot A, Julien-Laferrière A, Dufour AB, Thioulouse J, Dray S (2017) adegraphics: an S4 lattice-based package for the representation of multivariate data. R J 9(2):198–212

Simier M, Blanc L, Pellegrin F, Nandris D (1999) Approche simultanée de k couples de tableaux: applications à l'étude des relations pathologie végétale-environnement. Revue de Statistique Appliquée 47:31–46

Slimani N, Guilbert E, El Ayni F, Jrad A, Boumaiza M, Thioulouse J (2017) The use of STATICO and COSTATIS, two exploratory three-ways analysis methods. An application to the ecology of aquatic Heteroptera in the Medjerda watershed (Tunisia). Environ Ecol Stat 24:269–295

Swan J (1970) An examination of some ordination problems by use of simulated vegetational data. Ecology 51:89–102

Tenenhaus M, Young FW (1985) An analysis and synthesis of multiple correspondence analysis, optimal scaling, dual scaling, homogeneity analysis and other methods for quantifying categorical multivariate data. Psychometrika 50(1):91–119

Tennekes M (2017) treemap: treemap visualization. https://CRAN.R-project.org/package= treemap, R package version 2.4-2

Thioulouse J (1989) Statistical analysis and graphical display of multivariate data on the Macintosh. Comput Appl Biosci 5(4):287–292

Thioulouse J (1990) Macmul and Graphmu: two Macintosh programs for the display and analysis of multivariate data. Comput Geosci 16(8):1235–1240

Thioulouse J (1996) Outils logiciels, méthodes statistiques et implications biologiques: une approche de la biométrie. Mémoire d'habilitation à diriger des recherches, Université Lyon 1

Thioulouse J (2011) Simultaneous analysis of a sequence of paired ecological tables: a comparison of several methods. Ann Appl Stat 5:2300–2325

Thioulouse J, Chessel D (1987) Les analyses multitableaux en écologie factorielle. I: de la typologie d'état à la typologie de fonctionnement par l'analyse triadique. Acta Oecol Oecol Generalis 8:463–480

Thioulouse J, Chessel D (1992) A method for reciprocal scaling of species tolerance and sample diversity. Ecology 73(2):670–680

Thioulouse J, Dray S (2007) Interactive multivariate data analysis in R with the ade4 and ade4TkGUI packages. J Stat Softw 22(5):1–14

Thioulouse J, Chessel D, Dolédec S, Olivier J (1997) ADE-4: a multivariate analysis and graphical display software. Stat Comput 7(1):75–83

Thioulouse J, Simier M, Chessel D (2004) Simultaneous analysis of a sequence of paired ecological tables. Ecology 85:272–283

Tucker LR (1966) Some mathematical notes on three-mode factor analysis. Psychometrika 31:279–311

Turner R (2018) deldir: Delaunay triangulation and Dirichlet (Voronoi) tessellation. https://CRAN. R-project.org/package=deldir, R package version 0.1-15

Turroni F, Foroni E, Pizzetti P, Giubellini V, Ribbera A, Merusi P, Cagnasso P, Bizzarri B, de'Angelis GL, Shanahan F, Sinderen Dv, Ventura M (2009) Exploring the diversity of the bifidobacterial population in the human intestinal tract. Appl Environ Microbiol 75:1534–1545

Valet J, Daniel H, Beaujouan V, Rozé F, Pavoine S (2010) Using biological traits to assess how urbanization filters plant species of small woodlands. Appl Veg Sci 13:412–424

Verneaux J (1973) Cours d'eau de Franche-Comté (Massif du Jura). Recherches écologiques sur le réseau hydrographique du Doubs. Essai de biotypologie. Thèse de Doctorat d'Etat, Besançon

Wartenberg D (1985) Multivariate spatial correlation: a method for exploratory geographical analysis. Geogr Anal 17(4):263–283

Wesuls D, Oldeland J, Dray S (2012) Disentangling plant trait responses to livestock grazing from spatio-temporal variation: the partial RLQ approach. J Veg Sci 23:98–113

Whittaker R (1956) Vegetation of the great smoky mountains. Ecol Monogr 26(1):1–80

Whittaker RH (1972) Evolution and measurement of species diversity. Taxon 21:213–251

Wickham H, Hester J, Chang W (2018) devtools: tools to make developing R packages easier. https://CRAN.R-project.org/package=devtools, R package version 1.13.5

van den Wollenberg AL (1977) Redundancy analysis, an alternative for canonical analysis. Psychometrika 42(2):207–219

Index

Printed in the United States
By Bookmasters